UCLA Symposia on Molecular and Cellular Biology, New Series

Series Editor, C. Fred Fox

Please contact the publisher for information about previous titles in this series.

Growth Regulation
of Cancer

Growth Regulation of Cancer

Proceedings of an Ortho-UCLA Symposium
on Growth Regulation of Cancer,
Held at Park City, Utah,
January 17–23, 1987

Editor

Marc E. Lippman

National Cancer Institute
National Institutes of Health
Bethesda, Maryland

Alan R. Liss, Inc. • New York

Address all Inquiries to the Publisher
Alan R. Liss, Inc., 41 East 11th Street, New York, NY 10003

Library of Congress Cataloging-in-Publication Data

Ortho-UCLA Symposium on Growth Regulation of Cancer
   (1987 : Park City, Utah)
   Growth regulation of cancer.

   (UCLA symposia on molecular and cellular biology   ;
new ser., v. 74)
   Includes bibliographies and index.
   1. Cancer cells—Growth—Regulation—Congresses.
2. Growth promoting substances—Congresses.
3. Oncogenes—Congresses. 4. Cell transformation—
Congresses. I. Lippman, Marc E., 1945–
II. Ortho Pharmaceutical Corporation. III. University
of California, Los Angeles. IV. Title. V. Series.
[DLNM: 1. Cell Transformation, Neoplastic—congresses
2. Epidermal Growth Factor-Urogastrone—physiology—
congresses. 3. Fibroblast Growth Factor—physiology—
congresses. 4. Growth Substances—physiology—
congresses. 5. Neoplasms—physiopathology—congresses.
6. Oncogenes—congresses. 7. Receptors, Endogenous
Substances—congresses. W3 U17N new ser. v.74 /
QZ 202 077g 1987]
RC269.078 1987   616.99′4071   88-1217
ISBN 0-8451-2673-3

Pages 1–144 of this volume are reprinted from the Journal of Cellular Biochemistry, Volumes 35 and 36. The Journal is the only appropriate literature citation for the articles printed on these pages. The page numbers in the table of contents, contributors list, and index of this volume correspond to the page numbers at the foot of these pages.

The table of contents does not necessarily follow the pattern of the plenary sessions. Instead, it reflects the thrust of the meeting as it evolved from the combination of plenary sessions, poster sessions, and workshops, culminating in the final collection of invited papers, submitted papers, and workshop summaries. The order in which articles appear in this volume does not follow the order of citation in the table of contents. Many of the articles in this volume were published in the Journal of Cellular Biochemistry, and they are reprinted here. These articles appear in the order in which they were accepted for publication and then published in the Journal. They are followed by papers which were submitted solely for publication in the proceedings.

Contents

VI. STEROIDS AND REGULATION OF CANCER

Contributors

S.A. Aaronson, Laboratory of Cellular and Molecular Biology, National Cancer Institute, Bethesda, MD 20892 **[189]**

Adriana Albini, Laboratory for Developmental Biology and Anomalies, National Institute of Dental Research, National Institutes of Health, Bethesda, MD 20892 **[137]**

Abbas ar-Rushdi, The Wistar Institute of Anatomy and Biology, Philadelphia, PA 19104 **[31]**

J. Ashraf, Department of Human Biological Chemistry and Genetics, The University of Texas Medical Branch, Galveston, TX 77550 **[221]**

J.R. Barber, Molecular Biology and Virology Laboratory, The Salk Institute, San Diego, CA 92138 **[175]**

Susan Bates, Medical Breast Cancer Section, Medicine Branch, National Cancer Institute, Bethesda, MD 20892 **[1]**

James F. Battey, NCI-Navy Medical Oncology Branch, National Cancer Institute, Bethesda, MD 20814 **[85]**

Susan L. Berent, Wadley Institutes of Molecular Medicine, Dallas, TX 75235 **[121]**

Paul J. Bertics, Department of Physiological Chemistry, University of Wisconsin-Madison, Madison, WI 53706 **[157]**

Joseph B. Bolen, Laboratory of Tumor Virus Biology, National Cancer Institute, Bethesda, MD 20892 **[39]**

Arthur P. Bollon, Wadley Institutes of Molecular Medicine, Dallas, TX 75235 **[121]**

Diane Bronzert, Medical Breast Cancer Section, Medicine Branch, National Cancer Institute, Bethesda, MD 20892 **[1]**

Françoise Capony, Unité d'Endocrinologie Cellulaire et Moléculaire, INSERM and University of Montpellier, Montpellier, France **[17]**

Cliff D. Carpenter, Department of Medicine, Division of Endocrinology and Metabolism, University of California-San Diego, La Jolla, CA 92093 **[157]**

Vincent Cavaillès, Unité d'Endocrinologie Cellulaire et Moléculaire, INSERM and University of Montpellier, Montpellier, France **[17]**

Monique Chambon, Unité d'Endocrinologie Cellulaire et Moléculaire, INSERM and University of Montpellier, Montpellier, France **[17]**

William S. Chen, Department of Medicine, Division of Endocrinology and Metabolism, University of California-San Diego, La Jolla, CA 92093 **[157]**

Shaun R. Coughlin, Department of Medicine, Cardiovascular Research Institute, and Howard Hughes Medical Institute, University of California, San Francisco, CA 94143 **[151]**

Carlo M. Croce, The Wistar Institute of Anatomy and Biology, Philadelphia, PA 19104 **[31]**

Frank Cuttitta, NCI-Navy Medical Oncology Branch, National Cancer Institute, and Department of Medicine, Uniformed Services University of the Health Sciences, National Navy Medical Center, Bethesda, MD 20814 **[85]**

The number in brackets is the opening page number of the contributor's article.

Krzysztof Darlak, Department of Chemistry, University of Louisville, Louisville, KY 40292 **[109]**

Virginia DeSeau, Laboratory of Tumor Virus Biology, National Cancer Institute, Bethesda, MD 20892 **[39]**

Robert B. Dickson, Medical Breast Cancer Section, Medicine Branch, National Cancer Institute, Bethesda, MD 20892 **[1]**

P.P. Di Fiore, Laboratory of Cellular and Molecular Biology, National Cancer Institute, Bethesda, MD 20892 **[189]**

Jaime A. Escobedo, Department of Medicine, Cardiovascular Research Institute, and Howard Hughes Medical Institute, University of California, San Francisco, CA 94143 **[151]**

Isaiah J. Fidler, Department of Cell Biology, The University of Texas, M.D. Anderson Hospital and Tumor Institute, Houston, TX 77030 **[205]**

Arlette J. Franchi, Centre de Biochimie, CNRS, Université de Nice, Parc Valrose, 06034 Nice, France **[97]**

Glen Franklin, Department of Biochemistry, University of Louisville, Louisville, KY 40292 **[109]**

Gilles Freiss, Unité d'Endocrinologie Cellulaire et Moléculaire, INSERM and University of Montpellier, Montpellier, France **[17]**

Robert R. Friis, Ludwig Institute for Cancer Research, Inselspital, CH-3010 Bern, Switzerland **[213]**

B. Gametchu, Department of Human Biological Chemistry and Genetics, The University of Texas Medical Branch, Galveston, TX 77550 **[221]**

Marcel Garcia, Unité d'Endocrinologie Cellulaire et Moléculaire, INSERM and University of Montpellier, Montpellier, France **[17]**

Edward P. Gelmann, Medical Breast Cancer Section, Medicine Branch, National Cancer Institute, Bethesda, MD 20892 **[1]**

Gordon N. Gill, Department of Medicine, Division of Endocrinology and Metabolism, University of California-San Diego, La Jolla, CA 92093 **[157]**

Bernd Groner, Ludwig Institute for Cancer Research, Inselspital, CH-3010 Bern, Switzerland **[213]**

J.M. Harmon, Department of Pharmacology, Uniformed Services University of the Health Sciences, Bethesda, MD 20814 **[221]**

Meenhard Herlyn, The Wistar Institute of Anatomy and Biology, Philadelphia, PA 19104 **[65]**

Joseph M. Hill, Wadley Institutes of Molecular Medicine, Dallas, TX 75235 **[121]**

Norwood O. Hill, Wadley Institutes of Molecular Medicine, Dallas, TX 75235 **[121]**

Laura Hubler, Department of Physiological Chemistry, University of Wisconsin-Madison, Madison, WI 53706 **[157]**

Karen Huff, Medical Breast Cancer Section, Medicine Branch, National Cancer Institute, Bethesda, MD 20892 **[1]**

Anthony C. Huggett, Laboratory of Experimental Carcinogenesis, Division of Cancer Etiology, National Cancer Institute, Bethesda, MD 20892 **[55]**

Mark A. Israel, Molecular Genetics Section, Pediatric Branch, National Cancer Institute, National Institutes of Health, Bethesda, MD 20892 **[201]**

Rolf Jaggi, Ludwig Institute for Cancer Research, Inselspital, CH-3010 Bern, Switzerland **[213]**

Feng Lan Jia, Wadley Institutes of Molecular Medicine, Dallas, TX 75235 **[121]**

Anwar Joher, Wadley Institutes of Molecular Medicine, Dallas, TX 75235 **[121]**

Attan Kasid, Medical Breast Cancer Section, Medicine Branch, National Cancer Institute, Bethesda, MD 20892 **[1]**

Mark T. Keating, Department of Medicine, Cardiovascular Research Institute, and Howard Hughes Medical Institute, University of California, San Francisco, CA 94143 **[151]**

Amanullah Khan, Wadley Institutes of Molecular Medicine, Dallas, TX 75235 **[121]**

W.R. Kidwell, Laboratory of Tumor Immunology and Biology, National Cancer Institute, Bethesda, MD 20892 **[145]**

C.R. King, Laboratory of Cellular and Molecular Biology, National Cancer Institute, Bethesda, MD 20892 **[189]**

Cornelius Knabbe, Medical Breast Cancer Section, Medicine Branch, National Cancer Institute, Bethesda, MD 20892 **[1]**

Hilary Koprowski, The Wistar Institute of Anatomy and Biology, Philadelphia, PA 19104 **[65]**

M.H. Kraus, Laboratory of Cellular and Molecular Biology, National Cancer Institute, Bethesda, MD 20892 **[189]**

Henry C. Krutzsch, Laboratory of Experimental Carcinogenesis, Division of Cancer Etiology, National Cancer Institute, Bethesda, MD 20892 **[55]**

Alain E. Lagarde, Mount Sinai Hospital Research Institute, Division of Cancer and Cell Biology, and Department of Medical Genetics, University of Toronto, Toronto, Ontario M5G 1X5, Canada **[97]**

Anne-Marie Lebacq-Verheyden, NCI-Navy Medical Oncology Branch, National Cancer Institute, Bethesda, MD 20814 **[85]**

Yuri Lemeshev, Wadley Institutes of Molecular Medicine, Dallas, TX 75235 **[121]**

M. Linder, Department of Human Biological Chemistry and Genetics, The University of Texas Medical Branch, Galveston, TX 77550 **[221]**

Marc E. Lippman, Medical Breast Cancer Section, Medicine Branch, National Cancer Institute, Bethesda, MD 20892 **[xvii,1]**

George R. Martin, Laboratory for Developmental Biology and Anomalies, National Institute of Dental Research, National Institutes of Health, Bethesda, MD 20892 **[137]**

Timothy C. Meeker, The Wistar Institute of Anatomy and Biology, Philadelphia, PA 19104 **[31]**

John Mendelsohn, Department of Medicine, Memorial Sloan-Kettering Cancer Center and Cornell University Medical College, New York, NY 10021 **[169]**

Charles D. Mitchell, Division of Virology, Office of Biologics Research and Review, Center for Drugs and Biologics, Food and Drug Administration, Bethesda, MD 20892 **[137]**

S. Mohanam, Laboratory of Tumor Immunology and Biology, National Cancer Institute, Bethesda, MD 20892 **[145]**

Muriel Morisset, Unité d'Endocrinologie Cellulaire et Moléculaire, INSERM and University of Montpellier, Montpellier, France **[17]**

Lalitha Nagarajan, The Wistar Institute of Anatomy and Biology, Philadelphia, PA 19104 **[31]**

Sonia Paris, Centre de Biochemie, CNRS, Université de Nice, Parc Valrose, 06034 Nice, France **[97]**

Sathit Pichyangkul, Wadley Institutes of Molecular Medicine, Dallas, TX 75235 **[121]**

J.H. Pierce, Laboratory of Cellular and Molecular Biology, National Cancer Institute, Bethesda, MD 20892 **[189]**

Jacques M. Pouysségur, Centre de Biochemie, CNRS, Université de Nice, Parc Valrose, 06034 Nice, France **[97]**

Janet E. Price, Department of Cell Biology, The University of Texas, M.D. Anderson Hospital and Tumor Institute, Houston, TX 77030 **[205]**

Gerald V. Quinnan, Division of Virology, Office of Biologics Research and Review, Center for Drugs and Biologics, Food and Drug Administration, Bethesda, MD 20892 **[137]**

Ann Richmond, Veterans Administration Medical Center, Department of Medicine, Division of Endocrinology, Emory University School of Medicine, Atlanta, GA 30322 **[71]**

Henri Rochefort, Unité d'Endocrinologie Cellulaire et Moléculaire, INSERM and University of Montpellier, Montpellier, France **[17]**

Ulrich Rodeck, The Wistar Institute of Anatomy and Biology, Philadelphia, PA 19104 **[65]**

Neal Rosen, Medical Breast Cancer Section, Medicine Branch, National Cancer Institute, Bethesda, MD 20892 **[1,39]**

Michael G. Rosenfeld, Department of Medicine, Division of Endocrinology and Metabolism, University of California-San Diego, La Jolla, CA 92093 **[157]**

D.S. Salomon, Laboratory of Tumor Immunology and Biology, National Cancer Institute, Bethesda, MD 20892 **[145]**

B. Sanfilippo, Laboratory of Tumor Immunology and Biology, National Cancer Institute, Bethesda, MD 20892 **[145]**

P. Sassone-Corsi, Molecular Biology and Virology Laboratory, The Salk Institute, San Diego, CA 92138 **[175]**

Alexandra Schläfli, Ludwig Institute for Cancer Research, Inselspital, CH-3010 Bern, Switzerland **[213]**

Gregory Schultz, Department of Biochemistry, University of Louisville, Louisville, KY 40292 **[109]**

Ruth Seeman, Division of Virology, Office of Biologics Research and Review, Center for Drugs and Biologics, Food and Drug Administration, Bethesda, MD 20892 **[137]**

Shoshana Segal, NCI-Navy Medical Oncology Branch, National Cancer Institute, and Department of Medicine, Uniformed Services University of the Health Sciences, National Navy Medical Center, Bethesda, MD 20814 **[85]**

O. Segatto, Laboratory of Cellular and Molecular Biology, National Cancer Institute, Bethesda, MD 20892 **[189]**

Elaine Sonnenfeld, Department of Biochemistry, University of Louisville, Louisville, KY 40292 **[109]**

Arno Spatola, Department of Chemistry, University of Louisville, Louisville, KY 40292 **[109]**

H. Greg Thomas, Veterans Administration Medical Center, Department of Medicine, Division of Endocrinology, Emory University School of Medicine, Atlanta, GA 30322 **[71]**

E.B. Thompson, Department of Human Biological Chemistry and Genetics, The University of Texas Medical Branch, Galveston, TX 77550 **[221]**

Erik W. Thompson, Laboratory for Developmental Biology and Anomalies, National Institute of Dental Research, National Institutes of Health, Bethesda, MD 20892 **[137]**

Snorri S. Thorgeirsson, Laboratory of Experimental Carcinogenesis, Division of Cancer Etiology, National Cancer Institute, Bethesda, MD 20892 **[55]**

Richard M. Torczynski, Wadley Institutes of Molecular Medicine, Dallas, TX 75235 **[121]**

Daniel Twardzik, Oncogen, Seattle, WA 98121 **[109]**

I.M. Verma, Molecular Biology and Virology Laboratory, The Salk Institute, San Diego, CA 92138 **[175]**

Françoise Vignon, Unité d'Endocrinologie Cellulaire et Moléculaire, INSERM and University of Montpellier, Montpellier, France **[17]**

Lewis T. Williams, Department of Medicine, Cardiovascular Research Institute, and Howard Hughes Medical Institute, University of California, San Francisco, CA 94143 **[151]**

Alec E. Wittek, Laboratory for Developmental Biology and Anomalies, National Institute of Dental Research, National Institutes of Health, Bethesda, MD 20892 **[137]**

Philip Woost, Department of Biochemistry, University of Louisville, Louisville, KY 40292 **[109]**

Y.-S. Yuh, Department of Human Biological Chemistry and Genetics, The University of Texas Medical Branch, Galveston, TX 77550 **[221]**

Preface

Enormous progress has been made during the past few years toward understanding the growth regulation of human cancer. A remarkable synthesis of somewhat diverse fields, including cell biology, endocrinology, molecular virology, and molecular genetics, has provided confluent results that have enhanced understanding of fundamental events that control both neoplastic cell growth and the malignant process as characterized by invasion and metastasis.

This volume represents critical contributions presented at the Ortho-UCLA Symposium on Growth Regulation of Cancer held in Park City, Utah, January 17–23, 1987. Presentations at this meeting were geared toward synthesizing the varied disciplines at work in the study of growth regulation of cancer. Particular emphasis was placed on the cellular and molecular biology of growth factors and their receptors, which contribute to mitogenesis. Mechanisms of signal transduction by which those receptors evoke phenotypic effects were also explored. Specific aspects of the malignant process, including angiogenesis and critical host interactions regulating the metastatic process, were also given substantial attention, as the communications between normal and malignant tissue are critical for neoplastic progression. Other presentations described the role of oncogenes in the malignant process, with particular attention to those oncogenes that are, or interact with, growth factors and their receptors.

An alternative view of malignant progression reflects the loss of negative or repressive influences. This area was also explored in depth, with major focus on the areas of transforming growth factor beta and tumor necrosis factor and the interferons.

Finally, the role of steroid hormones as critical regulatory molecules of hormone-dependent neoplasia was examined. Work was presented on systems stimulated by steroids, as in human breast cancer, and systems in which steroid hormones function as negative regulators of cell proliferation, as in the leukemias and lymphomas.

We wish to thank the Ortho Pharmaceutical Corporation for generous sponsorship of this meeting. We also gratefully acknowledge gifts from Stuart Pharmaceuticals, Division of ICI Americas, Inc.; Pfizer Central Research, Pfizer, Inc.; and Meloy Laboratories. Additional financial support was received from USHHS grant R13 CA44065-01.

A special acknowledgment of appreciation goes to the members of the UCLA Symposia staff, who provided major input into every aspect of the planning and implementation of this meeting, as well as the preparation of this volume. Robin Yeaton provided coordination for every aspect of the meeting, with substantial help from Sara Abelson, Ed Burgess, and Hank Harwood.

Marc E. Lippman

Journal of Cellular Biochemistry 35:1–16 (1987)
Growth Regulation of Cancer 1–16

Growth Regulation of Human Breast Carcinoma Occurs Through Regulated Growth Factor Secretion

Marc E. Lippman, Robert B. Dickson, Edward P. Gelmann, Neal Rosen, Cornelius Knabbe, Susan Bates, Diane Bronzert, Karen Huff, and Attan Kasid

Medical Breast Cancer Section, Medicine Branch, National Cancer Institute, Bethesda, Maryland 20892

We describe studies on human breast cancer in which it is shown that specific growth factors (IGF-I, TGFα, PDGF) are secreted by human breast cancer cells and likely to be involved in tumor growth and progression. These activities are regulated by estradiol in hormone-dependent breast cancer and secreted constitutively by hormone-independent cells. These growth factor activities can induce the growth of hormone-dependent cells in vivo in athymic nude mice. Hormone-dependent breast cancer cells also secrete TGFβ, a growth-inhibitory substance, when treated with antiestrogens. TGFβ functions as a negative autocrine growth regulator and is responsible for some of the growth-inhibitory effects of antiestrogens.

Key words: breast cancer, growth factors, estrogen, IGF-I, TGF, PDGF

Estrogens play a central role in growth regulation of both normal and neoplastic breast tissue. At puberty and throughout menstrual life including pregnancy-lactation, estrogen exerts mitogenic, anabolic, and secretory effects on mammary epithelium. Estrogen treatment of males will induce breast development at any age. Breast cancer occurs in women who have never had functional ovaries with only 1% of the frequency of that in women with intact ovaries. Thus estrogens play a critical role, at least initially, in nearly all breast cancers. Metastatic breast cancer growth is strongly regulated in about one-third of clinical cases by therapies which alter concentrations or activities of estrogens [1]. This hormonal component of growth control appears to be a remnant of the normal control of epithelial proliferation. While estrogen is a proximate mitogen for either normal or malignant breast epithelium, the hypothalamus-pituitary axis is indirectly in control of ovarian estrogen secretion by virtue of GnRH and gonadotropin stimulation [2]. In addition, the pituitary gland (or other

Received February 13, 1987; revised and accepted May 19, 1987.

organs) may secrete as-yet-undefined direct- or indirect-acting mitogens. Such hypothetical, estrogen-induced, endocrine-acting mitogens have been termed estromedins [3,4]. The hormonal control of cancer cell proliferation has recently received an additional potential regulatory component with the proposal of autocrine or self-stimulating polypeptide growth factors [5].

Our laboratory has devoted itself to studies on the biochemical and molecular events, induced by estrogen, which are associated with direct stimulation of proliferation of human breast cancer cell lines in vitro and of breast cancer in vivo. Using clonal lines of cells, usually derived from pleural or ascites fluid of patients, we have succeeded in demonstrating receptors for and direct proliferative responses to physiologic doses of 17β estradiol (E_2) (a result which has subsequently been confirmed in numerous other laboratories) [6–9]. Several estrogen-responsive human breast cancer cell lines exist, including MCF-7, T47D, MDA-MB-134, ZR-75-1, and CAMA-1 [10]. MCF-7 is probably the best characterized of these. We will review the hormonal responses of these cell lines and the mechanisms by which such cells respond to estrogens and examine some recent experiments whereby the tumorigenic properties of MCF-7 cells are enhanced by v-ras[H] oncogene transfection, bypassing estrogen controls. We will also examine another aspect of growth regulation—the fact that growth inhibitors exert their negative effects on cell proliferation, at least in part, by secretion of growth-inhibitory substances which fulfill negative autocrine loops.

RESPONSES OF HUMAN BREAST CANCER TO ESTROGENS AND ANTIESTROGENS

Because mitogenic effects are a central part of regulation by estrogens, many enzymes involved in macromolecular synthesis have been examined. A systematic search in MCF-7 and other breast cancer cells has led to observations that E_2 induces a large number of enzymes involved in nucleic acid synthesis, including DNA polymerase, thymidine and uridine kinases, thymidylate synthetase, carbamyl phosphate synthetase, asparate transcarbamylase, dihydroorotase, and dihydrofolate reductase [11,12]. Physiologic concentrations of E_2 stimulate DNA synthesis through both scavenger and de novo biosynthetic pathways. In two instances recently reported, estrogen regulates thymidine kinase and dihydrofolate reductase at the mRNA level [13,14]. Regulation of thymidine kinase mRNA occurs, at least in part, at the transcriptional level [14]. Estrogens appear to modulate many enzyme activities involved in growth. Whether growth is induced by generalized induction of numerous genes or by pleiotropic or cascade mechanisms is not known. The existence of "second message" regulatory systems in this process is possible and any of the data to be reviewed here are supportive of such a pathway. We have also recently observed that E_2 stimulates the turnover of phosphatidyl inositol in MCF-7 cells [15]. In a variety of other model systems, this metabolic effect is quite rapid and tightly coupled to growth control by proteases and hormones, particularly the polypeptide growth factors [16,17]. In breast cancer cells, induction of phosphatidyl inositol turnover is slower. Estrogen induction of growth factors (to be described below) could explain the delayed time course of the phospholipid effects. Thus, phosphatidyl inositol turnover, with its associated stimulation of protein kinase C and Ca^{++} fluxes, could be a fundamental metabolic mediator of mitogenic effects of E_2.

Others have identified the progesterone receptor [18] as an additional protein induced by estrogen. However, progesterone is apparently not directly growth modulatory of human breast cancer at least in vitro and physiologic concentrations of progestins do not exert major effects on breast cancer growth in patients. The presence of the progesterone receptor does, however, appear tightly coupled to functional growth regulation by estrogen. Thus progesterone receptor content of human breast tumors is used (alone with the estrogen receptor) as a marker for estrogen and antiestrogen responsiveness of tumors in clinical therapy [1].

In addition to regulation of these essential growth-controlling enzymes and the progesterone receptor, estrogens (and antiestrogenic compounds) alter the cellular or secreted activity of several other proteins whose function in growth control remains less well characterized. These include tissue plasminogen activator and other collagenolytic enzymes [19], several relatively abundant secreted proteins, including a 24-kDa protein described by McGuire and colleagues [20], 52- and 160-kDa glycoproteins described by Rochefort and colleagues [21], a 39-kDa glycoprotein complex [22], a 7-kDa protein initially identified by Chambon and colleagues by detection of an estrogen-induced mRNA species (termed pS2) [23], and the cytoplasmic enzyme LDH [24]. Tissue plasminogen activator (along with other proteases) is thought to contribute to tumor progression and growth by allowing the tumor to digest and traverse encapsulating basement membrane [25]. While this is likely, it is conceivable that proteases may serve additional role such as facilitating release of mitogenic growth factors like IGF-I (somatomedin C) from carrier proteins, or processing inactive precursor growth factor and proteases to active species [26]. Interestingly, one of the major secreted proteins, the 52-kDa glycoprotein, is also reported to have biologic activity in purified form—it is mitogenic for MCF-7 cells when tested in vitro [27]. These investigators have recently discovered that purified 52 kDa has cathepsin D–like proteolytic activity and thus its mitogenic effects may be linked to cell-surface proteolysis. The activities of the 160-, 39-, 24-, and 7-kDa proteins are unknown at present. It is of note that at least the induction of the 160-, 52-, and 7-kDa secreted proteins may apparently be dissociated from estrogen and antiestrogen modulation of MCF-7 cells growth by using two MCF-7 clonal variants aberrant in their growth response to these hormones [28–30]. These three protein species are decreased by antiestrogen to the same extent in MCF-7 and LY2, a stable, antiestrogen-resistant variant of MCF-7. This suggests that a significant reduction in secretion of these proteins has no impact on in vitro growth in the case of LY2. In I-13, an MCF-7 clonal variant which is growth arrested by physiologic concentrations of E_2, the same three proteins are induced to the same extent as in MCF-7.

In summary, while estrogens may exert a considerable number of influences in vivo which may indirectly alter breast cancer progression, direct effects of estrogens on isolated breast cancer cells in vitro are also well established. These effects includes growth regulation itself as well as modulation of enzymes and other activities thought to mediate mitogenic and metastatic events. Later we will consider estrogenic influences on a class of secreted proteins which although relatively minor in abundance are very active biologically—the polypeptide growth factors. These factors, along with some of the above-mentioned major secreted proteins, are likely candidates as "second messengers" in the actions of estrogen on breast cancer. Milk is an abundantly rich source of growth factor activities [31,32]. These factors in milk may be important in neonatal development and nutrition or may have additional actions on the mammary gland. Since breast cancer cells produce and respond to these growth factors, it seems possible that growth factor secretion either by itself or in the presence of some as-yet-undefined transforming event may play a critical factor in neoplastic progression.

The triphenylethylene antiestrogen prototype known as tamoxifen has become a mainstay in adjuvant breast cancer therapy of postmenopausal women as well as in advanced disease for all estrogen-receptor-positive women and is effective either by itself or when used in combination with cytotoxic chemotherapy. In contrast to cytotoxic agents, antiestrogens appear to be cytostatic rather than cytocidal and have a remarkably low incidence of significant side effects. Many investigators have noted the close correlation between the clinical response to antiestrogens and the presence of the estrogen receptor (and its induced product—the progesterone receptor). Since antiestrogens and their active metabolites have a high affinity for the estrogen receptor, the most likely explanation of antiestrogen action appears to be simple antagonism of the growth-promoting effects of estrogen [33,34]. However, alternate views involving other microsomal binding sites for antiestrogen have been presented [35]. The failure to observe antiestrogen responses in estrogen-receptor-negative cells [7,11,12] is the strongest argument in favor of the centrol role of estrogen receptor in antiestrogen action.

Antiestrogen treatment of estrogen-dependent breast cancer leads to cell-cycle blockade (early G_1) of most of the cells in vitro and to arrest of tumor growth in vivo [33,36–38]. It had been initially observed that MCF-7 cells responded in vitro (though oppositely) to estrogens and antiestrogens under cell culture conditions in which estrogens were not thought to be present [39]. While these experiments could be interpreted to suggest that antiestrogens could act (to arrest growth) independently of an occupied estrogen-receptor complex, recent work by Katzenellenbogen and co-workers has clearly shown that high concentrations of phenol red present in the culture medium of the cells in these studies provided a significant estrogenic stimulus [39]. Removal of phenol red, whose structure resembles that of certain nonsteroidal estrogens, abrogated antiestrogen action on MCF-7 cells and dramatically enhanced the responsiveness of the cells to estrogen induction of cell growth and progesterone receptor. There remains little compelling evidence at present that antiestrogens act in any fashion other than by direct antagonism of the initiation of signals generated by an agonist-occupied receptor. These studies provide strong evidence for the direct estrogen responsivity of human breast cancer cells.

The principle limitation with respect to the clinical utility of antiestrogens is the gradual resistance which develops in tumors treated with these agents. While in some cases antiestrogen-resistant tumors lack the estrogen receptor, it is not likely that loss of the estrogen receptors explains the majority of instances of in vivo loss of antiestrogen sensitivity during treatment. If the cell requires estrogen action through the receptor for growth, then loss of receptor will be accompanied by slowing of growth. Clearly estrogen independence must come first and loss of receptor is either random or results from hormone independence. It is of interest that in a model system for acquired resistance—a stable clone of MCF-7 cells stepwise selected in vitro for antiestrogen resistance—high levels of the estrogen receptor and estrogen responsivity for some functions not apparently directly involved in growth are still maintained [29]. These data suggest that positive and negative growth control elements lie distal to the estrogen receptor; data supporting this contention follow.

GROWTH REGULATION OF EPITHELIAL CELLS

In order to study growth regulation of human breast cancer by polypeptide growth factors we used previous work to identify likely starting points. A well-established system in the study of polypeptide growth factor action has been the growth of rodent fibroblasts in vitro. Studies were initially carried out in cell monolayers on plastic surfaces. Smith, Scher, and Todaro, among others, identified "restriction points" in the cell cycle of "normal" (but immortalized) fibroblasts. Various growth factors abrogated these restriction points, allowing the cell cycle to progress [40]. Platelet-derived growth factor (PDGF), a "competence" growth factor, allowed cells to pass a restriction point in early G_1, epidermal growth factor (EGF or the related transforming growth factor α, TGFα) acted later, while insulinlike growth factor-I (IGF-I or somatomedin C) acted still later in G_1 [41]. EGF and IGF-I are "progression" growth factors. Malignant transformation was proposed to result from production of autostimulatory growth factors, abolishing both competence and progression restriction points in a cell's own cycle. One consequence of autocrine growth factors appears to be the serum-independent growth of some cancer cells [42–44].

Factors inducing "anchorage-independent" growth were also studied by using agar or agarose suspensions of cells. It had been observed that the ability of cells to grow in colonies under anchorage-independent conditions was correlated with their tumorigenicity or state of malignant "transformation" [45]. Research from a number of laboratories over the past few years had identified at least four growth factor activities which together can reversibly induce the transformed phenotype in murine fibroblasts. These studies have identified PDGF, EGF (or TGFα), IGF-I (or IGF-II), and an additional growth factor, transforming growth factor β (TGFβ) [40,46,47]. These growth factors are considered likely to be involved in cancer growth control for this reason. However, it should be emphasized that the murine fibroblast model system may not apply to cancers of other tissues or species of origin.

The principle restriction points for epithelial cell growth are unknown. A major departure from the fibroblast model, however, is the fact that TGFβ is a growth inhibitor for many types of primary and malignant epithelial cells [48,49]. Therefore, it is likely that while some of the same growth factors may facilitate traverse of the cell cycle in fibroblasts and epithelial cells, control of anchorage-independent growth may involve another less well-defined growth factor(s). A candidate for such a growth factor is provided by the work of Halper [50]. Basic pituitary FGF can fulfill such a function in cloning of an adrenal carcinoma cell line (SW13), and epithelial cancers produce a related activity which remains relatively uncharacterized at present [50]. A variety of other growth factors have been described [5,41,45].

GROWTH FACTOR PRODUCTION AND GROWTH REGULATION BY HUMAN BREAST CANCER CELLS

Notwithstanding the unknown features of cell-cycle control in breast cancer, we have begun the analysis of its secreted growth factors with study of representative members of all of the above-mentioned activity classes: PDGF, TGFα, IGF-I, TGFβ, and an epithelial transformation factor. We have placed special emphasis on the regulatory effects of estradiol in the activities of these growth factors.

We and others have shown growth regulation of MCF-7 cells in monolayer culture by a variety of lipid-soluble trophic hormones other than estradiol. These include glucocorticoids, iodothyronines, androgens, and retinoids. MCF-7 cells have receptors but very little growth response to progesterone and vitamin D. Additional studies have demonstrated receptors for and responses to the polypeptides, insulin, EGF, and IGF-I. Receptors, but little mitogenic response, have been demonstrated for other hormones, such as prolactin and calcitonin [51]. The multiplicity of growth-stimulating hormones for breast cancer cell culture systems in vitro has several interpretations. Obviously, multiple hormones may influence breast cancer growth. Alternatively, serum borne factors induced by E_2 (estromedins) may play important contributory roles in vivo [52]. Finally, growth factors with a similar spectrum of activities could be elaborated by the breast cancer cells themselves. E_2 is an absolute tumor growth requirement for two human cell lines, MCF-7 and T47D, and a growth stimulator for a third cell line, ZR-75-1, in vivo in the nude (athymic) mouse model system [19,37,53]. McGrath and his colleagues have further defined this system by showing that E_2 need not enter the systemic circulation in nude mice to promote sufficient MCF-7 tumorigenesis; elevation of local E_2 concentration near the tumor sufficed [54]. This suggests that if estrogen acts by inducing changes in the host which permit tumor growth, the production and action of such factors is probably restricted to the local area of the tumor. The mammary stroma is, however, likely to provide an as-yet-unidentified contributory factor(s) in vivo for full mitogenicity of estrogen [55]. Other human breast cancer cell lines, such as Hs578T and MDA-MB-231, lack estrogen receptors and form rapidly growing, estrogen-independent tumors in the nude mouse [10,53,56]. Hs578T is derived from a carcinosarcoma and not a true epithelial tumor. These five human cell lines (MCF-7, ZR-75-1, T47D, Hs578T, MDA-MB-231) have been studied in detail by our laboratory in an attempt to better understand growth regulation of breast cancer in vivo and in vitro.

Our attention was directed to the possible involvement of secreted growth factors in growth control of breast cancer by an observation made with MCF-7 cells plated at various densities. We found that initial growth rate was proportional to number of cells plated [57]. While multiple interpretations of these data are possible, they are consistent with the production of autostimulatory growth factors by the MCF-7 cells. In preliminary experiments we found that conditioned medium harvested from MCF-7 cells treated with E_2 (CME_2) was capable of stimulating thymidine incorporation and proliferation of other MCF-7 cells. The residual E_2 was removed from CME_2 prior to its use as a mitogen. This kind of result had also been obtained by Vignon and Rochefort and their colleagues [58], who had noticed that MCF-7 cells grew faster with less frequent medium exchanges as compared to cells in which medium was changed every other day. They had also noted that CME_2 was directly capable of stimulating other MCF-7 cells.

GROWTH FACTOR PRODUCTION—TRANSFORMING GROWTH FACTOR ALPHA

We therefore began the fractionation and purification of CM from MCF-7 and other breast cancer cell lines to identify the growth factors present. These cell lines secrete stimulatory activity for MCF-7 and 3T3 fibroblast monolayer cultures as well as "transforming growth activity" (TGF) for anchorage-independent growth of NRK and AKR-2B fibroblasts in soft agar culture [53,59,60]. In initial studies using acid Biogel P60 and P150 chromatography we identified a 30-kDa apparent molecular weight peak of transforming activity for NRK fibroblasts. This peak also coincided with a peak of MCF-7-stimulating activity and the principle species of EGF receptor-competing activity [53,59]. This peak of activity was also identified by an antibody specific for TGFα species but not cross reacting with EGF. Thus, this activity may be related to TGFα, but it appears to be larger than the cloned and sequenced 6-kDa species from transformed fibroblasts [61]. The 30-kDa TGFα-like species is induced by E_2 treatment of MCF-7, T47D, and ZR-75-1 cells two to eightfold depending on cell type and culture conditions. This observation is consistently seen with bioassays of transforming activity, EGF radioreceptor assays, radioimmunoassays, and assays of TGFα mRNA [53]. Current experiments are focused on regulation, purification, and characterization of this activity. The expected 4.8-kb TGFα mRNA species has been detected by Derynck and co-workers in MCF-7 and some other human breast cancer cell lines [61,62]. It is of interest that all estrogen-independent epithelial breast cancer cells secrete high levels of the TGFα -like activity [53]. Hs578T, which is hormone independent but not epithelial, does not secrete TGF α. Preliminary experiments in which cell growth is inhibited by using EGF-receptor-blocking antibodies (kindly supplied by J. Kudlow) and anti-TGFα antibodies (generously supplied by J. Tam) are strongly consistent with the hypothesis that TGFα secretion is part of an autocrine loop.

Both EGF and TGFα can act via the EGF receptor on both diploid and immortalized cell lines. Many groups of investigators have detected the EGF receptor in human and rodent mammary tumor biopsies and malignant cell lines [63,64]. The apparent molecular size in breast cancer cells is 170 kDa and the kinase domain is unaltered as determined by S1 ribonuclease analysis [63]. At the present time little work has addressed the state of phosphorylation or the tyrosine kinase activity of the receptor.

GROWTH FACTOR PRODUCTION—INSULINLIKE GROWTH FACTOR I

Using radioimmunoassay, we and others have noted that a second potential autostimulatory mitogen, IGF-I, is also secreted by all human breast cancer cells examined to date [65,66]. This species, partially purified from MCF-7 cells, comigrates with authentic serum-derived IGF-I after acid ethanol extraction. IGF-I mRNA species were also detected with Northern blot analysis [68] by using a DNA probe to authentic IGF-I [67]. One of these, a 600-bp mRNA, corresponded to the smallest of three RNA transcripts observed in poly A selected RNA from human liver in the same study. We initially observed no E_2 induction of secreted IGF-I in standard culture conditions employing phenol-red-containing medium although antiestrogens inhibited IGF-1 secretion. Subsequent studies, utilizing the more substantially estrogen-depleted phenol-red-free medium, have observed a fivefold IGF-I induction with E_2 treatment [67]. IGF-I secretion is inhibited by growth-inhibitory antiestrogens (in phenol-red-containing medium) and glucocorticoids. Current work is focussed on the mechanism of IGF-I induction and its possible biological role(s). Interestingly, two highly malignant estrogen-receptor-negative breast cancer cell lines (MDA-MB-231 and Hs-578T) secrete high levels of IGF-I and have low responsiveness to exogenous IGF-I [66].

IGF-I mitogenesis is mediated by its receptor, a close homologue of the insulin receptor. The receptor in a variety of cell types consists of a 450-kDa complex (two

α chains of 130 kDa and two β chains of 85 kDa) [5]. The receptor has tyrosine kinase activity [5]. Its mechanism of action is largely unknown but is thought to stimulate growth by some as-yet-undefined posttranscriptional mechanism [69]. IGF-I receptors of the expected size have been reported on several human breast cancer cell lines [70]. The quantities of IGF-I secreted into the medium are more than sufficient to saturate the IGF-I receptors found on all of the breast cancer cell lines we have thus far studied. We conclude that IGF-I is a hormonally regulated autocrine growth stimulator. This is further substantiated by nude mouse data to be described later. We are currently performing an extensive series of experiments attempting to prove that IGF-I secretion is part of an autocrine loop. These experiments involve use of antibodies against IGF-I and antibodies against the IGF-I receptor. In addition, we have performed a series of transfections involving the introduction of antisense cDNA for IGF-I in a regulatable expression vector. These experiments preliminarily suggest that IGF-I secretion is required for continued cell growth.

GROWTH FACTOR PRODUCTION—PLATELET-DERIVED GROWTH FACTOR

In addition to IGF-I and the TGFα species previously mentioned, all breast cancer cell lines which we have examined to date secrete a PDGF-related activity detected by anchorage-dependent growth stimulation of 3T3 fibroblasts in the presence of platelet-poor plasma [71,72]. Immunoprecipitation of metabolic labeled MDA-MB-231 breast cancer cell extracts and medium detected the expected 28-kDa and 14-kDa species [71]. The secretion of the PDGF-like species is estrogen regulated by biologic, immunologic, and nucleic acid assays. PDGF acts through its 185-kDa tryosine kinase receptor on a variety of mesenchymal cell types [5]. The receptor has recently been purified, cloned, and sequenced [73]. Human breast cancer cells are not known to be growth regulated by PDGF and we do not have detectable PDGF receptors [71]. Therefore, PDGF may have a paracrine role in nature. Interestingly, the highly tumorigenic MDA-MB-231 cell line produces the most PDGF of the cell lines examined so far [71].

A NOVEL ANCHORAGE-INDEPENDENT EPITHELIAL GROWTH FACTOR

The hormonal controls on the cell cycle for epithelial cells are only poorly understood. While it is known that EGF and IGF-I are commonly mitogenic and TGFβ commonly growth inhibitory for epithelial cells, the corresponding restriction points in the cell cycle where these growth factors might act is largely unknown. In addition, the controls for anchorage-independent growth are also mysterious. Halper [50] has established a model system with human SW-13 adrenal carcinoma cells in soft agar culture. These cells clone poorly unless basic fibroblast growth factor (FGF) or conditioned medium from certain epithelial cancers such as SW-13 is applied. No other growth factors are known to be active. This activity has been only partially characterized from kidney but appears to be 40–42 kDa in size.

We have begun to purify a related activity by using a previously described assay [50] from human breast cancer cells [74]. The most tumorigenic lines MDA-MB-231 and Hs578T produce high levels of the activity, while estrogen-receptor-containing lines produce much lower levels. The activity from MDA-MB-231 cells is very acidic in its isoelectric point, and approximately 60 kDa in size by gel filtration and gel electrophoresis. It has been extensively purified by an acid-ethanol extraction, isoelectric focussing, and HPLC sizing. Current work is directed toward complete purification and characterization of this activity and examination of its regulation [74]. This activity has some similarities to a growth factor described by Kidwell [13] but preliminary data suggest that they are distinct.

In summary, we have observed that estrogen regulation of MCF-7 cells is associated with inductions of TFGα and IGF-I and repression of TGFβ, to be discussed later. It is possible that estrogen-antiestrogen regulation of MCF-7 cells is at least partly mediated by coordinant effects on growth-stimulatory and growth-inhibitory growth factor "second messengers." Future studies with blocking antibodies against growth factors and these receptors should help evaluate this hypothesis. Two other growth factors are also secreted by MCF-7 cells—PDGF and a partially characterized epithelial transforming factor purified to near homogeneity. These two activities are produced in very large amounts by estrogen-receptor-negative, highly tumorigenic lines. Estrogen-independent cancers are associated with increased output of a large number of growth factor activities. The critical growth factors in this type of cancer will undoubtably require extensive future study. In the next section we will further evaluate growth factor secretion as it relates to malignant status in a nude model system for tumor progression.

TUMORIGENESIS IN ATHYMIC NUDE MICE

Previous work has shown that MCF-7 cells were absolutely dependent upon estrogen supplementation for tumor formation in nude mice [19,37,53]. We wanted to determine if CM proteins induced by estrogen were capable of acting humorally in vivo in the nude mouse to stimulate MCF-7 tumorigenesis, thus replacing the requirement for estradiol [75]. For this purpose we developed a serum-free culture system which has supported cell growth for all five above–mentioned cell lines for up to 1 wk. The medium consists of Richter's IMEM + 2 mg/liters transferring + 2 mg/liters fibronectin. MCF-7 cells $\pm$ E$_2$ pretreatment (10^{-9}M, 4 days) were used to condition serum-free medium, collected over a subsequent 2-day period (CM and CME$_2$). Media were dialyzed extensively against 1 M acetic aid, lyophilized, reconstituted in phosphate-buffered saline, and the precipitated protein was removed. This extraction also removed 99.98% of the residual E$_2$. Reconstituted CM and CME$_2$ were infused into athymic female oophorectomized mice via Alzet minipumps. The equivalent of 10 ml of CM or CME$_2$ per day for 4 wk was infused from a mid-dorsal, subcutaneous location. MCF-7 cells were injected (2–5×10^6 cells/injection) at four different mammary fat pad locations in each mouse. Small tumors (up to 0.5 cm diameter) appeared at MCF-7 sites within 2 wk. Tumors in CME$_2$-infused animals appeared with two to threefold greater frequency than in CM-infused animals; animals innoculated with only MCF-7 cells and sham pump implantations did not have tumors. CM- and CME$_2$-supported tumors reached maximum size in 2–3 wk of treatment, usually declining in size thereafter, whereas E$_2$-pellet-implanted animals have continuously growing tumors for at least 4 wk and they do not regress. CM- and CME$_2$-induced tumors were verified as adenocarcinoma by histologic analysis. While the CME$_2$ supported tumor growth, uterine weight was unaffected. In addition, CME$_2$ activity was decreased by treatment with trypsin, a reducing reagent, or heating to 56°C for 1 hr. Therefore the tumor growth-promoting substance(s) in CME$_2$ was unlike E_2 and likely to be similar to a polypeptide growth factors(s). These data suggest that cultured human breast cancer cells under estrogenic stimulation release a tumor-promoting factor(s) which can act in vivo after release into the general circulation of the athymic mouse. We do not know why the tumors induced by CM regress. There appear to be four potential explanations. First, during the process of growth factor purification and concentration one or more essential activities are lost. Second, it should be recalled that these growth factor activities infused via minipump are acting via an endocrine route. Thus any of a large number of pharmacologic explanations may explain our failure to induce sustained tumor growth. Third, it remains reasonable that estrogens do exert systemic effects which their induced growth factors do not. Thus estrogen effects on the immune system, etc, are possible. Finally, estrogens may induce many effects of tumor cells themselves which cannot be induced secondarily by secreted growth factors.

As an independent line of investigation to evaluate the possibility of autoregulatory growth factors, we have also utilized the MCF-7 cells grown as xenografts in the nude mouse to study the activity of individual growth factors. As previously above, conditioned medium extracts from E_2-treated MCF-7 cells stimulate limited growth of MCF-7 tumor in the absence of E_2 itself. As a test of the hypothesis that E_2-induced growth factors may mediate this effect, we have directly infused human EGF (1 μg/day), human IGF-I (0.6 μg/day) into female oophorectomized nude mice injected at four mammary fat pad locations (2–5 $\times$ 10^6 cells/injection site) with MCF-7 cells. These concentrations correspond to those observed in the conditioned medium extracts utilized in the previous studies. As before, growth factors were infused with Alzet minipumps, and the experiment was carried out for 2 wk. Both growth factors induced tumors, but EGF induced more than twice the tumor incidence as IGF-I. EGF supported development of tumors to 0.5 cm in diameter. As expected, E_2-pellet-implanted control animals had a high incidence of continously growing tumors to 0.8 cm over the time of the experiment [75]. Thus, based on these experiments with authentic growth factors, it is likely that breast-cancer-produced and closely related IGF-I and TGF-like species have some autostimulatory actions on tumor growth in vivo. In addition, the TGFα species induced by E_2 may be relevant in E_2-stimulated tumor growth. Greater availability of TGFα, TGFβ, PDGF, and epithelial-transforming activity in the future should facilitate the testing of these activities in this in vivo reconstitution system.

In other studies [76] investigating mouse mammary carcinogenesis, Oka and co-workers have recently demonstrated a likely role of EGF in both mammary tumor onset and subsequent growth support. Using a mouse strain highly susceptible to spontaneous mammary tumors, removal of the submandibular glands (sialoadenectomy) dramatically reduced the incidence of tumor formation and/or the rate of growth of the breast tumors allowed to form. The submandibular gland is a major source of EGF in mice and reinfusion of EGF into such sialoadenectomized mice returned tumor incidence and growth rate of tumors to their normally high level. TGFα- and EGF-like activities thus may have endocrine functions in tumor support. As the data with MCF-7 cells show, one mechanism of tumor progression might involve local production (estrogen regulated) of TGFα by the tumor. Clearly, TGFα- or EGF-like growth factors are likely to be important regulators of mammary tumor progression by a variety of possible mechanisms. A large body of literature already exists demonstrating that EGF has both tumor promotional and immunosuppressive activities [77].

Interestingly, at least some of the growth factor products of breast cancer appear related to growth factors in milk [31,32,78]. One example is TGFα. The function of such factors may be related to offspring growth rather than parental mammary growth, since TGFα (and EGF) can promote eyelid opening in mice (ref). Though growth factors such as IGF-I and TGFα may be capable of autocrine stimulation of tumor cells, they and other growth factors may also subserve paracrine functions on surrounding non-neoplastic tissue. PDGF promotes fibroblast growth and chemotaxis and its secretion may contribute to the marked stromal proliferation characteristically surrounding breast carcinoma [79]. In addition, TGFα and TGFβ stimulate bone resorption and hypercalcemia, also characteristic of breast cancer [80]. Other effects of paracrine growth factors might be immunomodulatory in nature. Finally but potentially the most important paracrine function secreted by cancer is angiogenesis factor(s). Though many activities may contribute, both growth factors and proteolytic degradation products of basement membranes are likely candidates [81–83]. The principle components secreted by breast cancer leading to vascular infiltration of the tumor have not yet been identified. However, Vallee and co-workers have recently isolated, sequenced, and cloned an angiogenic protein secreted by human colon carcinoma cells [84]. Substantial additional work is required to sort out which growth factor activities are growth related and which, if any, directly contribute to the malignant phenotype.

EFFECTS OF RAS GENE TRANSFECTION IN HUMAN BREAST CANCER CELLS

Recent studies carried out in rodent systems have implicated specific genetic alterations leading to malignant transformation and tumor progression. In the carcinogen-treated rat model system, activation of the oncogene known as the Harvey ras (c-ras[H]) occurs by point mutation [85]. At the present time, no such unifying statements can be made about human breast cancer. Rather, diverse observations of oncogene activation suggest a plethora of mechanisms at work in malignant progression. In one human breast cancer cell line, Hs578T, an activated c-ras[H] oncogene has been observed, as predicted based on the rat model system [86]. However, this potential mechanism appears far from universal. Second, a whole series of cellular proto-oncogenes is observed to be expressed in diverse studies employing cell lines and tumor specimens [64,87]. These oncogenes (all members of the ras family, as well as myc, myb, fms, fos, fes) include those localized in plasma membrane, nucleus, and cytoplasm. Two other oncogenes, c-erb b (the EGF receptor) and neu (or c-erb b$_2$), are closely related to the EGF receptor and have also been detected in breast cancer cell lines and tumor biopsies [64,88]. Interestingly, c-erb b (the EGF receptor) is expressed to the greatest extent in estrogen-receptor-negative cell lines and tumor biopsies [63,89]. It may represent a new marker for dedifferentiation or increased malignant potential in breast cancer. It is not yet known whether over-expression of c-erb b in cancer directly contributes to the transformed phenotype or indirectly mediates the effects of EGF (or TGF) produced in an autocrine-type loop. Finally, as previously mentioned, PDGF, partially the product of the c-sis protoon-cogene, is expressed by a variety of breast cancer cell lines [71,72]. Though PDGF itself is not generally growth stimulatory of epithelial cells it may contribute in other ways to the transformed phenotype (such as through paracrine actions). It is possible that additional oncogene activities will be observed in breast cancer by using different techniques in the future. One such possibility is that an epithelial cell test system will detect transforming genes which go unrecognized by the well-established NIH 3T3 fibroblast test system.

The diversity in observations of activated oncogenes and expressed cellular proto-oncogenes may suggest that many mechanisms or steps exist in the malignant progression of breast cancer. Alternatively, observations of expression of some of these cellular protoonocogenes could reflect malignant status rather than induce it. Clearly, to test hypotheses concerning oncogene activity in breast cancer it is necessary to directly insert the oncogene of interest into a relevant cell test system. This objective may recently have been approached by using normal diploid human mammary epithelium first immortalized with brief benzo[a] pyrene treatment and then transfected with oncogenes [90]. Stampfer has observed that treatment of normal mammary epithelial cells in culture with benzo[a]pyrene achieved immortalized but nontumorigenic lines. These lines appear nearly normal by several criteria. Subsequently, using retroviral vectors, Clarke has inserted various oncogenes into one of these lines to determine the phenotype effects [91]. Insertion of v-ras^H, v-mos, and SV40 T antigen rendered the cells capable of growth in high levels of serum but did not confer tumorigenicity. Transfectants containing SV40 T plus either v-ras or v-mos were strongly tumorigenic in nude mice. Interestingly, in unpublished studies, we find that all of these cell lines including the diploid human mammary epithelium secretes biologically active TGFα.

While estrogens are critical in the pathogenesis of nearly all breast cancer it is unfortunate that by the time metastases are clinically apparent at least 50% of all breast cancer is hormone independent and after selective pressure with endocrine therapy all breast cancer becomes hormone independent. In order to be able to study this process in detail we attempted to convert hormone-dependent breast cancer to a hormone-independent phenotype.

For this purpose we chose to permanently transfer DNA from the tumor-causing retrovirus Harvey sarcoma virus to MCF-7 cells. The tumor-inducing portion of this viral DNA (the oncogene) is called v-ras^H, the most commonly detected activated oncogene in highly malignant human cancers. MCF-7 cells did not initially contain this oncogene, but one estrogen-independent cell line, Hs578T, does [86]. We transferred the v-ras^H oncogene to MCF-7 cells by the calcium phosphate method [92].

MCF-7 cells containing stably integrated v-ras^H genes in their DNA (MCF-7$_{ras}$) had five to eight times the level of ras mRNA as in control cells, and had detectable phosphorylated p21 (the protein which is the ras gene product). The cellular p21 is not a substrate for phosphorylation. MCF-7$_{ras}$ cells displayed unaltered growth rate under control conditions in vitro but had resistance to growth inhibition by antiestrogens. The transfected cells were tumorigenic in the absence of estrogen in 85% of inoculated female oophorectomized nude mice [92]. Interestingly, the MCF-7$_{ras}$ cells also exhibited increased rates of turnover of phosphatidyl inositol, analogous to E_2 treatment of MCF-7 cells [15]. In addition, these cells also expressed increased levels of the laminin receptor on their surfaces and increased invasiveness [93].

We next assayed for secreted growth factors by MCF-7$_{ras}$ cells. CM prepared from MCF-7$_{ras}$ cultures as compared with control cultures contained three to fourfold-elevated levels of radioreceptor assayable TGFα and bioactive TGFα as assayed by anchorage-independent growth of NRK fibroblasts. A single peak of TGFα -like activity was eluted at an apparent MW of 30 kDa from acid gel chromatography of MCF-7$_{ras}$ CM. Also, secretion of immunoreactive IGF-I and TGFα was augmented three to fourfold in MCF$_{ras}$ cells, but PDGF secretion was further not elevated. MCF-7$_{ras}$ tumors in the nude mouse were able to induce the development of small tumors derived from MCF-7 cells separately implanted at a distant site in the nude mouse [94]. That is, when MCF-7$_{ras}$ cells were inoculated on one side of a nude mouse and wild-type cells on the other, tumors appeared nearly 100% of the time on the MCF-7$_{ras}$ side and about 40% of the time on the wild-type side. These do not represent metastases. They do not contain v-ras sequences. When removed from the animal and growth in culture they are still hormone dependent. We can repeat this experimental result with an entirely in vitro model system in which MCF-7$_{ras}$ cells are used as a feeder layer. Thus, the presence of MCF-7$_{ras}$ tumor is able to temper growth of previously hormone-dependent cells without permanently altering their phenotype. Ras gene activation could bring about phenotypic and tumorigenic changes in human breast cancer cells, some of which may also be induced by estrogens. However, the cells retained the capacity to bind estrogen and respond to estrogens as shown by E$_2$ induction of the progesterone receptor. Thus ras gene transfection bypasses estrogen activation of the transformed phenotype but induces that phenotype via a pathway which appears to be similar but not identical to the E$_2$ induction pathway. Future studies will more clearly define the similarities and differences between E$_2$- and v-ras^H-induced malignant progression of MCF-7 cells.

GROWTH INHIBITION BY TRANSFORMING GROWTH FACTOR BETA

We will now address one last hypothesis—that growth inhibition (for example by antiestrogens) not only occurs by a down regulation of growth-stimulatory activities, but in addition by enhanced production of growth-inhibitory substances. Our attention was drawn to this possibility for two reasons. First, in work with glucocorticoid-sensitive lymphoblasts evidence has been presented that effects occur through positive induction of gene products capable of inducing cell lysis. Second in preliminary experiments we found that conditioned media derived from antiestrogen-treated MCF-7 cells was capable of inducing growth inhibition of estrogen-receptor-negative, antiestrogen-resistant MDA-MB-231 cells. Based on apparent molecular weight of some of this activity, we considered TGFβ as one potential negative regulator.

Breast cancer cells secrete a TGFβ-related activity [95]. A major peak of radioreceptor-competing and AKR-2B-fibroblast-transforming activity comigrates with authentic platelet-derived TGFβ on acid Biogel chromatography. In contrast to its transforming effects on some fibroblasts, authentic TGFβ is growth inhibiting for many breast cancer (and other epithelial-derived lines) [48,49]. All breast cancer cells examined expressed the expected 2.5-kb mRNA species. Though estrogen deprivation can induce TGFβ secretion more than 30-fold there are no changes in mRNA concentration for TGFβ. Interestingly, TGFβ secretion is inhibited by treatment of MCF-7 cells with growth-stimulatory E$_2$ and insulin. Growth-inhibitory antiestrogens and glucocorticoids strongly stimulate its secretion. Intracellular TGFβ did not appear to be modulated. TGFβ from antiestrogen-induced MCF-7 cells strongly inhibits the growth of another estrogen-receptor-negative cell line, MDA-MB-231. This growth inhibitor was reversed in the presence of a polyclonal antibody directed against native TGFβ. Interestingly, in the antiestrogen, but not TGFβ-resistant, resistant MCF-7 variant LY2, antiestrogens do not significantly induce TGFβ secretion. These cells contain identical amounts of TGFβ mRNA to wild-type MCF-7 cells. Current work is further addressing the mechanism of TGF regulation [96].

TGFβ acts through a high molecular weight (615 kDa) receptor complex. The receptor subunits have been reported as identical 330-kDa species. This receptor has not yet been purified, cloned, or sequenced, but it is not reported to have tyrosine kinase activity [5]. High-affinity binding sites for TGF have been reported on responsive (growth inhibited) human breast cancer cell lines. Taken together we believe that these data suggest that growth regulation of some breast cancers (and as a speculation in normal mammary cell(s)) may be modulated by secretion of potent growth inhibitors.

REFERENCES

1. Lipsett MB, Lippman ME: In Williams RH (ed): "Textbook of Endocrinology." Philadelphia: WB Saunders, 1981, pp 1213–1226.
2. Ross GT, Vande Wiele RL, Frantz AG: In Williams RH (ed): "Textbook of Endocrinology." Philadelphia: WB Saunders, 1981, pp 355–411.
3. Eidne KA, Flanagan CA, Miller RP: Science 229–989, 1985.
4. Ikeda T, Danielpour D, Sirbasku BA: In Bresciani F, King RJB, Lippman ME, Namer M, Raynaud JP (eds): "Progress in Cancer Research and Therapy" New York: Raven Press, Vol. 31 1983, pp 171–186.
5. Goustin AS, Leof EB, Shipley GD, Moses HL: Cancer Res 46:1015, 1986.
6. Brooks SC, Locke ER, Soule HD: J Biol Chem 248:6251, 1973.
7. Lippman ME, Bolan G, Huff K: Cancer Res 43:1244, 1983.
8. Page MJ, Field JK, Everett NP, Green CD: Cancer Res 43:1244, 1983.
9. Soule HD, McGrath CM: Cancer Lett 10:177, 1980.
10. Engle LW, Young NW: Cancer Res 38:4327, 1978.
11. Aitken SC, Lippman ME: Cancer Res: 4681, 1983.
12. Aitken SC, Lippman ME: Cancer Res 45:1611, 1985.
13. Cowan K, Levine R, Aitken S, Goldsmith M, Douglass E, Clendennin N, Nienhius A, Lippman ME: J Biol Chem 257:15079, 1982.
14. Kasid A, Davidson N, Gelmann E, Lippman ME: J Biol Chem 261:5562, 1986.
15. Freter CE, Lippman ME, Gelmann EP: Proc AACR Los Angeles, CA 1986.
16. Carney DH, Scott DL, Gordon EA, LaBelle EF: Cell 42:479, 1985.
17. Nishizuka Y: Trends Biochem Sci 9:163, 1984.
18. Horwitz KB, McGuire WL: J Biol Chem 253:2223, 1978.
19. Butler WB, Kirkland WL, Jorgensen TL: Biochem Biophys Res Comm 90:1328, 1978.
20. Ciocca DR, Adams DJ, Edwards DP, Bjerke RJ, McGuire WL: Cancer Res 43:1204, 1983.
21. Westley B, Rochefort H: Cell 20:353, 1980.
22. Bronzert DA, Silverman S, Lippman ME: Cancer Res 47:1234, 1987.
23. Jakolew SB, Breathnach R, Jeltsch J, Chambon P: Nucleic Acids Res 12:2861, 1985.
24. Burke RE, Harris SC, McGuire WC: Cancer Res 38:2773, 1978.
25. Liotta L: Proc AARC 26:385, 1985.
26. Kaufman U, Zapf J, Torretti B, Froesch ER: Clin Endocrinol Metab 44:160, 1977.
27. Vignon F, Capony F, Chambon M, Freiss L, Garcia M, Rochefort H: Endocrinology 118:1537, 1986.
28. Bronzert DA, Triche TJ, Gleason P, Lippman ME; Cancer Res 44:3942, 1984.
29. Bronzert DA, Greene GL, Lippman ME: Endocrinology 117:1409, 1985.
30. Davidson NE, Bronzert DA, Chambon P, Gelmann EP, Lippman ME: Cancer Res 46:1904, 1986.
31. Buno M, Salomon DS, Kidwell WR: J Biol Chem 260:5745, 1985.
32. Zwiebel JA, Buno M, Nexo E, Salomon P, Kidwell WR: Cancer Res 46:933, 1986.
33. Jordan VC: Pharmacological Reviews 36:245, 1984.

34. Lippman ME, Buzdar A, Tormey DC, McGuire WL: Breast Cancer Res Treat 4:251, 1985.

35. Watts CKW, Murphy LC, Sutherland RL: J Biol Chem 259:4223, 1984.

36. Osborne CK, Boldt DH, Clark GM, Trent JM: Cancer Res 43:3583, 1983.

37. Osborne CK, Hobbs K, Clark GM: Cancer Res 45:584, 1985.

38. Sutherland RL, Hall RE, Taylor IW: Cancer Res 43:3998, 1983.

39. Berthois Y, Katzenellenbogen JA, Katzenellenbogen BS: Proc Natl Acad Sci USA 83:2496, 1986.

40. Smith HS, Scher CD, Todaro GJ: Virology 44:359, 1971.

41. Heldin CH, Westermark B: Cell 37:9, 1984.

42. Delarco JE, Todaro GJ: Proc Natl Acad Sci USA 75:4001, 1978.

43. Pastan I: Adv Metab Dis 8:7, 1975.

44. Sporn MB, Todaro GJ: N Engl J Med 303:878, 1980.

45. Freedman VH, Shin S: Cell 3:355, 1974.

46. Assoian RK, Grotendorst GR, Miller DM, Sporn, MB: Nature 309:804, 1984.

47. Massague J, Kelly B, Mottola C: J Biol Chem 260:4551, 1985.

48. Roberts AB, Anzano MA, Wakefield LM, Roche NS, Stern DF, Sporn MB: Proc Natl Acad Sci USA 82:119, 1985.

49. Tucker RF, Shipley GD, Moses HL, Holley RW: Science 226:705, 1984.

50. Halper J: Cancer Res 43:1972, 1983.

51. Lippman ME: In Barnes DW, Sirbasku DA, Sato GH (eds): "Methods for Serum-Free Culture of Cells of the Endocrine System." New York: Alan R. Liss, 1984, Vol 2, pp 183–200.

52. Ikeda T, Sirbasku DA: J Biol Chem 259:4049, 1984.

53. Dickson RB, Bates SE, McManaway ME, Lippman ME: Cancer Res 46:1707, 1986.

54. Huseby RA, Maloney TM, McGrath CM: Cancer Res 44:2654, 1984.

55. McGrath CM: Cancer Res 43:1355, 1983.

56. Hackett AJ, Smith HS, Springer EL, Owens RB, Nelson-Rees WA, Riggs JL, Gardner MB: J Natl Cancer Inst 58:1795, 1977.

57. Jakesz R, Smith CA, Aitken S, Huff K, Schuette W, Shackney S, Lippman ME: Cancer Res 44:619, 1984.

58. Vignon F, Derocq DF, Chambon M, Rochefort H: CR Acad Sci Paris Endocrinol 296:151, 1983.

59. Dickson RB, Huff KK, Spencer EM, Lippman ME: Endocrinology 118:138, 1986.

60. Salomon DS, Zwiebel JA, Bano M, Losonczy I, Felnel P, Kidwell WR: Cancer Res 44:4069, 1984.

61. Derynck R, Roberts AB, Winkler ME, Chen EY, Goeddel DV: Cell 38:287, 1984.

62. Derynck R, Roberts AB, Eaton DH, Winkler MC, Goeddel: In Feramisco J, Oznne B, Stiles C (eds): "Cancer Cells 3: Growth Factors and Transformation." Cold Spring Harbor, New York: Cold Spring Harbor Laboratory, 1985, pp 79–86.

63. Davidson NE, Gelmann EP, Lippman ME, Dickson RB: Mol Endocrinol 1:216, 1987.

64. Fitzpatrick SL, Brightwell J, Wittliff JL, Barrows GH, Schultz GS: Cancer Res 44:3448, 1984.

65. Baxter RC, Maitland JE, Raisur RL, Reddel R, Sutherland RL: In Spencer EM (ed): "Insulin-like Growth Factors/Somatomedins." Berlin: Walter deGruyter, 1983, pp 615–618.

66. Huff KK, Kaufman D, Gabbay KH, Spencer EM, Lippman ME, Dickson RB: Cancer Res 46:4613, 1986.

67. Huff, KK, Knabbe C, Kaufman D, Gabbay KH, Dickson RB: Mol Endocrinol submitted, 1987.

68. Jansen M, Van Schaik FMA, Ricker AT, Bullock B, Woods PE, Gabbay KH, Nussbaum AL, Sussenback JS, Vander Branch JR: Nature 306:609, 1983.

69. Campisi J, Pardee AB: Mole Cell Biol 4:1807, 1984.

70. Furlanetto RW, DiCado JN: Cancer Res 44:2122, 1984.

71. Bronzert D, Davidson N, Pantazis P, Antoniades H: Proc Natl Acad Sci USA, in press, 1987.

72. Rozengurt E, Sinnett-Smith J, Taylor-Papadimitriou J: Int J Cancer 36:247, 1985.

73. Williams LT, Daniel TO, Escobedo JA, Fried UA, Coughlin SR: ICSU Short Reports 4:168, 1986.

74. Swain S, Dickson RB, Lippman ME: "Proc AACR Annual Meeting." Los Angeles, CA, 1986.

75. Dickson RB, McManaway M, Lippman ME: Science 232:1540, 1986.

76. Kurachi H, Okamoto S, Oka T: Proc Natl Acad Sci USA 81:5940, 1985.

77. Stoscheck CM, King LE: Cancer Res 46:1030, 1986.

78. Shing YW, Klagsbran M: Endocrinology 115:273, 1984.

79. Kao RT, Hall J, Engel L, Stern R: Am J Pathol 115:109, 1984.

80. Tasjian AH, Voelkel EF, Lazzaro M, Singer FR, Roberts AB, Derynck R, Winkler ME, Levine L: Proc Natl Acad Sci USA 82:4535, 1985.

81. Gospodarowicz D, Greenburg G, Bialecki H, Zetter BR: In vitro 14:85, 1978.
82. Schreiber AB, Kenney J, Kowalski J, Thomas KA, Gimenez-Gallego G, Rios-Candelore M, DiSalvo J, Bamitault D, Courty J, Courtois Y, Moemer M, Loret C, Burgess WH, Mehlman T, Friesel R, Johnson W, Maciag T: J Cell Biol 101:1623, 1985.
83. West DC, Hampson IN, Arnold F, Kumar S: Science 228:1324, 1985.
84. Kurachi K, Davie EW, Strydom DJ, Riordan JF, Vallee BL: Biochemistry 24:5494, 1986.
85. Zarbl H, Sukumar S, Arthur AV, Martin-Zanea D, Barbacid M: Nature 315:382, 1985.
86. Kraus MH, Yuasa Y, Aaronson SA: Proc Natl Acad Sci USA 81:5384, 1984.
87. Slamon DJ, deKernion JB, Verma IM, Cline, MJ: Science 224:256, 1984.
88. King CR, Kraus MH, Aaronson S: Science 229:974, 1986.
89. Gainsbury JRC, Farndon JR, Sherbert GV, Harris AL: Lancet 16:364, 1985.
90. Stampfer MR, Bartley JC: Proc Natl Acad Sci USA 82:2394, 1985.
91. Clark R, Milleg R, O'Rouke E, Trahey M, Stampfer M, Kreigler M, McCormick F; "Proc First Annual Meeting on Oncogenes." Frederick, MD, 1985.
92. Kasid A, Lippman ME, Papgeorge AG, Lowy DR, Gelmann EP: Science 228:725, 1985.
93. Albini A, Graf JO, Kleinman HK, Martin GR, Veillette A, Lippman ME; Proc Natl Acad Sci USA 83: in press, 1987.
94. Kasid A, Dickson R, Huff K, Bates S, Lowy D, Lippman M, Gelmann E: Mole Endocrinol, in press, 1987.
95. Derynck R, Jarrett JA, Chen EY, Eaton DH, Bell JR, Assoian RK, Roberts AB, Sporn, Goeddel DV: Nature 316:701, 1985.
96. Knabbe C, Huff K, Wakefield L, Lippman ME, Dickson RB: Cell 48:417, 1987.

Journal of Cellular Biochemistry 35:17–29 (1987)
Growth Regulation of Cancer 17–29

Estrogen-Induced Lysosomal Proteases Secreted by Breast Cancer Cells: A Role in Carcinogenesis?

Henri Rochefort, Françoise Capony, Marcel Garcia, Vincent Cavaillès, Gilles Freiss, Monique Chambon, Muriel Morisset, and Françoise Vignon

Unité d'Endocrinologie Cellulaire et Moléculaire, INSERM and University of Montpellier, Montpellier, France

In an attempt to understand the mechanism by which estrogens stimulate cell proliferation and mammary carcinogenesis, metastatic human breast cancer cell lines (MCF7, ZR75-1) were found to secrete a 52,000 dalton (52K) protein under estrogen stimulation. Following its purification to homogeneity, the 52K protein was identified as a secreted procathepsin-D-like aspartyl protease bearing mannose-6-phosphate signals. This precursor displays an in vitro autocrine mitogenic activity on estrogen-deprived MCF7 cells and is able to degrade basement membrane and proteoglycans following its autoactivation. The total protease (52K + 48K and 34K) was detected and assayed by monoclonal antibodies and was found to be highly concentrated in proliferative and cystic mastopathies. In breast cancer, its cytosolic concentration appears to be correlated more to tumor invasiveness than to hormone responsiveness. The mRNA of the 52K protease accumulates rapidly following estradiol treatment, as was shown by Northern blot analysis with cloned cDNA. The 52K cathepsin-D-like protease is the first example of a lysosomal protease induced by estrogens in cancer cells. Results obtained using different approaches suggest that two cysteinyl cathepsins are also related to cell transformation and invasiveness. It has been proposed that cathepsin-B is involved in breast cancer and metastatic melanoma, and its regulation by estrogen has been shown in the rat uterus. Cathepsin-L corresponds to the major excreted protein (MEP) whose synthesis and secretion are markedly increased by transformation of NIH 3T3 cells with Ki ras and are regulated by several growth factors. In addition to secreted autocrine growth factors and to other proteases (plasminogen activator, collagenase), lysosomal cathepsins may therefore play an important role in the process of tumor growth and invasion as long as their precursor is secreted abundantly.

Key words: cell proliferation, tumor invasion, MCF7 cells, cathepsin-B, -D, -L, breast cancer, lysosomal proteases

Received February 19, 1987; accepted April 13, 1987.

The role of estrogens in stimulating the growth of estrogen receptor-positive breast cancer is well established [1]. However, the way in which these hormones act on tumor cells is poorly understood. It has been proposed that their action might be directly triggered by interactions of receptors with nuclear machinery, such as the nuclear matrix, to stimulate DNA replication or might be indirectly mediated by estromedins coming from other organs [2]. Recent studies showing that estrogens are able to stimulate directly the growth of breast cancer cell lines in vitro [3–5] after inducing the synthesis of several proteins suggest a third type of mechanism mediated by estrogen-induced factors or proteins directly secreted by breast cancer cells. The study of hormone-regulated proteins in cancer cell lines helps us to understand the mechanism of hormone action on gene expression [6–8], and we illustrate here that it can also guide us in understanding the control of cancer growth and invasion.

ESTROGEN-INDUCED AUTOCRINE MITOGENS

Steroid hormones regulate specific gene expression within minutes following their interaction with specific nuclear receptors [8]. In contrast, the mitogenic effect of sex steroids is observed only after a lag of approximately 1 day; during this time, the transcription of several genes has been stimulated, and different proteins have been induced. Among them, the proteins secreted by breast cancer cells are good candidates for mediating the effect of estrogens by interacting in turn on the plasma membrane of the same cells via an estrogen-regulated autocrine mechanism [9]. An autocrine mechanism has been proposed for cancer cells that acquire the ability to make and to respond to their own growth factors [10]. This concept has been applied to breast cancer cells, which remain under the control of sex-steroid hormones during the first steps of tumor progression [9].

One way to define growth factors and other mitogens involved in this autocrine mechanism is to characterize the proteins and peptides that are secreted by hormone-dependent human breast cancer cells and induced by estrogens, since estrogens are the only steroids with mitogenic activity in these cells [3–5]. This hypothesis was supported by the demonstration that glycoprotein fractions prepared from serum-free media conditioned by estrogen-stimulated MC57 cells increase the growth of resting MCF7 cells, whereas similar fractions from the conditioned media of estrogen-stripped MCF7 cells are inactive [11]. A mitogenic activity of estrogen-induced conditioned media has been confirmed by different groups [12,13]. Following the labeling of newly synthesized proteins by ^{35}S-methionine or ^{35}S-cysteine and analysis of the labeled proteins by SDS-PAGE, several estrogen-regulated proteins have been detected [for review, see 6,7,14]. In addition to the 52K protein [15], a 160K protein has been described, and a 65K protein has recently been identified as being α_1-antichymotrypsin [16], as has a 6–7K protein coded by cloned pS2 mRNA [8]. More classical growth factors such as EGF, IGF, and PDGF-like peptides are also secreted by these cells [17–18] (Fig. 1). One of the major challenges in the field of hormone-dependent cancer research is to define the protein(s) or peptide(s) responsible for the control of proliferation and invasion by these cancers.

Two strategies have been followed. The first was to characterize classical growth and transforming factor activities and to show that some of these growth factors were induced by estrogens in breast cancer cell lines [17,18]. The second was to purify and to identify the major proteins that were actually found to be regulated

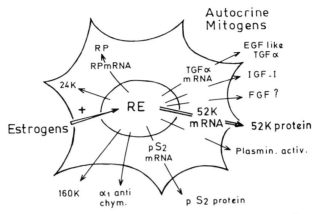

Fig. 1. Estrogens-regulated proteins and peptides in a human breast cancer cell. Estrogens stimulate the synthesis of several proteins via their nuclear receptor (RE). Some of the proteins whose functions are unknown were first identified by labeling and SDS-PAGE analysis and were designated by their molecular weight under denaturing conditions. The corresponding mRNAs have also in some cases been found to accumulate. Several of the secreted proteins and peptides recovered in culture media conditioned by estradiol-treated MCF7 cells are suspected of being the agent that stimulates cell proliferation and tumor invasion. RP progesterone receptor, α_1 antichymotrypsin. (Reproduced from Morisset et al [27] with permission of the publisher.)

by estrogens in these cells. This second approach lead us to identify a lysosomal protease with mitogenic and invasive potential.

REGULATION AND PURIFICATION OF THE 52K PROTEIN

The 52K protein, which we first described in 1979 [19], is secreted in small amounts into the culture medium by estrogen-treated MCF7 cells (5 ng/10^6 cells/hr) and by other ER-positive breast cancer cells under estrogen control (T47D, ZR75-1). It is constitutively produced without requiring the influence of estrogen in ER-negative cell lines (MDA-MB231, BT20) [20]. In ER-positive cells, the protein is specifically regulated by hormones (estrogens and high doses of androgens) that can bind to and activate the estrogen receptor, but not by glucocorticoids, progestins, or androgens at low concentrations [15]. The effects of the antiestrogens tamoxifen and hydroxytamoxifen suggested that this protein was in some way related to the mitogenic activity of estrogens. In wild-type MCF7 cells, the antiestrogens totally inhibited the synthesis of the protein, whereas they partially stimulated the synthesis of the progesterone receptor. In contrast, in the antiestrogen-resistant variants of MCF7 cells (R27 and RTx6) cloned for their ability to grow in 1 μM tamoxifen, the antiestrogens became able, like estrogens, to increase the production of the 52K protein but remained unable, as in wild-type MCF7 cells, to stimulate the production of the estrogen-regulated 160K secreted protein and of pS2 mRNA [21] (Table I). In these cell lines, the 52K protein was therefore a better candidate for being a mitogen than the pS2 and 160K proteins. A possible mechanism for the antiestrogen resistance was that cells had acquired a growth advantage resulting from the tamoxifen-induced increased production of autocrine growth factors such as the 52K protein.

We applied a three-step strategy to purify the 52K glycoprotein. Using concanavalin-A-Sepharose chromatography, we partially purified it from 22 liters of conditioned medium from MCF7 cell cultures. From this partially purified fraction, we

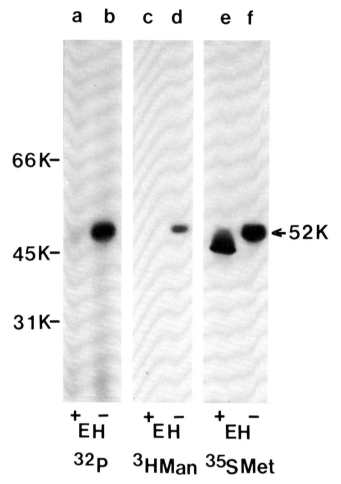

Fig. 2. Estrogen-treated MCF7 cells were labeled with ^{35}S-methionine, ^{32}P-H₃PO₄, or ^{3}H-mannose. Media were immunoprecipitated with the M1G8 antibody to the 52K protein and were analyzed by SDS-PAGE. The immunoprecipitated secreted 52K protein was (+) or was not (−) digested with endoglycosidase H (EH) and the TCA-precipated proteins were electrophoresed. (Reproduced from Morisset et al [29] with permission of the publisher.)

TABLE I. Effect of Tamoxifen on Three Estrogen Receptor-Positive Cell Lines*

Cell line	R_P	pS2 mRNA	160K protein	52K protein	Cell proliferation
MCF7	+	−	−	−	Inhibition
R27 RTx6	+	−	−	+	Resistance

*Summary of the effect of tamoxifen on five estrogen-regulated responses in the antiestrogen-sensitive (MCF7) and -resistant (R27 and RTx6) cell lines showing that only the 52K secreted protein behaves differently in the antiestrogen-resistant variants, in which it acquires the ability to be induced by antiestrogens. Results are detailed in Westley et al [21].

obtained several mouse monoclonal antibodies [22]. Finally, using an immunoaffinity column, we purified the 52K protein to apparent homogeneity (1,000-fold purification) in both its secreted and its cellular form [23]. The purification of 52K protein made it possible to study its activity on cell growth, to determine its structure and identity, and finally to clone its corresponding cDNA sequences.

By immunopurification without detergent, a homogeneous secreted 52K protein was obtained, which was shown to stimulate the growth of estrogen-deprived recipient MCF7 cells [24]. This stimulation was dose-dependent and occured at concentrations (1–10 nM) similar to those found in the culture medium. However, time-course experiments indicated that both estradiol and the 52K protein required the same (18 hr) lag before stimulating ^{3}H-thymidine incorporation. Like estradiol, the 52K protein was also able to stimulate the number and length of microvilli on the cell surface. This mitogenic activity of the purified 52K protein could be intrinsic or could be due to a contaminant not visible by silver staining overloaded gels. However, ^{35}S-cysteine-labeling experiments have excluded the possibility that the activity could be produced by newly synthesized peptides incorporating cysteine residues such as TGFα, pS2 protein, or IGF1 [24]. The in vitro mitogenic activity of the purified 52K protein was in agreement with an estrogen-regulated autocrine mechanism.

STRUCTURE AND IDENTIFICATION AS A LYSOSOMAL PROTEASE

Study of the co- and posttranslational modifications of the 52K protein helped us to define its structure and enzymatic activity. After exposure of cultured MCF7 cells to ^{32}P, the 52K protein is intensely labeled. Most of this label can be removed by endoglycosidase-H treatment, which deletes two N-glycosylated chains of the protein (Fig. 2). Mannose-6-P signals have been identified on these chains [25]. Pulse-chase experiments and Western blot analysis show that the 52K protein is the precursor of a lysosomal enzyme that accumulates in lysosomes as a stable 34K protein. About 40% of the cellular 52K precursor is secreted, whereas about 60% is successively processed into a 48K and a 34K + 14K protein [23,26] (Fig. 3). Part of

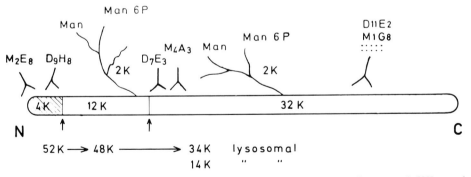

Fig. 3. Structure and processing of the 52K protein of MCF7 cells. The secreted 52K protein corresponds to a lysosomal procathepsin. In the cell, it is successively processed into a 48K active enzyme and a 34K + 14K enzyme, which normally function in the lysosomes. Two N-glycosylated oligosaccharide chains are represented bearing an accessible mannose-6-P signal (Man-6-P). The sugar composition of each chain and number of man-6-P sites per chain are not known. The overall structure is similar to that of procathepsin-D. Sequencing of cloned cDNAs is in progress [27].

the secreted 52K protein can be taken up and processed by MCF7 cells, but this binding is specifically inhibited by mannose-6-P [25] (Fig. 4).

The presence of mannose-6-P signals indicated that the protein is normally routed to lysosomes, where it exerts its usual function [28]. In testing several enzymatic activities corresponding to lysosomal hydrolases of similar molecular weight, we found that both the purified secreted 52K protein and the corresponding cellular proteins (52K, 48K, 34K + 14K) displayed a strong proteolytic activity at acidic pH, which was mostly inhibited by pepstatin [25,29]. There are similarities with the previously described cathepsin-D [30]. Antibodies to the 52K protein interact with liver cathepsin-D, and anticathepsin-D immunoprecipitates the 52K protein. The pH and inhibitor sensitivities of the two proteases are very similar, as are their

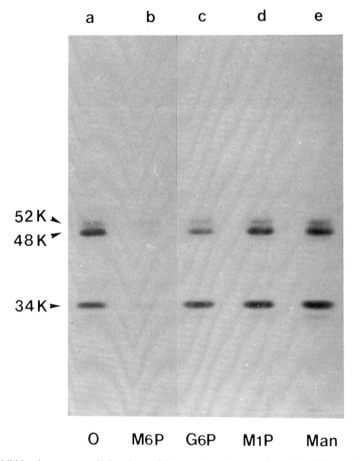

Fig. 4. Inhibition by mannose-6-phosphate of the uptake and processing of the 52K protein by MCF7 cells. Confluent MCF7 cells (1×10^6 cells) maintained in F12/DEM containing 1% FCS/DCC were rinsed twice in R12/DEM plus 0.1% BSA. They were then incubated with 400 μl of conditioned medium containing ^{35}S-methionine-labeled proteins secreted by MCF7 cells (300,000 TCA-precipitable counts) for 24 hr in F12/DEM with **(lane a)** 0.1% BSA alone (O), or **(lane b)** 10 mM mannose-6-phosphate or **(lane c)** 10 mM glucose-6-phosphate (G6P), or **(lane d)** 10 mM mannose-1-phosphate, or **(lane e)** 10 mM mannose (Man). The labeled cells were then washed three times in F12/DEM plus 0.1% BSA, and the cell lysate proteins were immunoprecipitated with the M1G8 anti-52K monoclonal antibody. The immunoprecipitates of each series were analyzed by SDS-PAGE and revealed by fluorography. (Reproduced from Capony et al [25] with permission of the publisher.)

molecular weights [25]. In addition, the first 15 amino acids as determined by microsequencing the N-terminal of the molecules are identical (P. Ferrara, unpublished data).

However, there are some differences compared to normal cathepsin-D [30]. 1) The tissue distribution appears to be different from that reported for cathepsin-D [31]; immunoperoxidase staining is mostly positive in breast cancer, melanoma, and liver but not in endometrium or other tissues [32]. This may be due to a markedly higher concentration of the protease in proliferative mammary cells compared to other cells. 2) Its secretion is tenfold greater in breast cancer cells than in normal mammary cells in culture (Capony, unpublished data). 3) The endo-H sensitivities of the oligosaccharide chain are different; the breast cancer 52K protein is fully endo-H-sensitive, unlike cathepsin-D from liver or placenta [25]. Available cDNA clones [27] will allow us to determine the complete coding sequences of the MCF7-52K cathepsin-D, and to detect any alteration in the structure of the protease, compared to the normal cathepsin-D sequence [33]. The study of gene promoter may also show differences related to its regulation by estrogens in cancer.

This secreted protein may be regulated by estrogens at a different level. Using a cloned 52K-cDNA probe and Northern blot analysis of poly-A+ RNA of the MCF7 breast cancer cell line, we have recently shown that estradiol rapidly induces the accumulation of a 2.2 kb 52K mRNA [27] (Fig. 5). The degree of stimulation was six to ten fold, and there was a basal level of the 52K-mRNA in the absence of estrogens. It is therefore likely that, in the case of other estrogen-regulated genes [8], the cathepsin-D-like enzyme is transcriptionnaly regulated by estrogens.

POTENTIAL ROLE OF THE 52K-CATHEPSIN-D PROTEASE IN MAMMARY CARCINOGENESIS

Some of the characteristics of the 52K protease, ie, its high concentration in proliferative and tumoral cells, its induction by estrogen, and the large proportion of its secreted form, suggest that it has a major function(s) in mammary carcinogenesis related to stimulating tumor growth and/or invasion via its proteolytic activity (Fig. 6). The mechanism of the mitogenic action of the 52K cathepsin-D-like enzyme is not yet understood, but it can be approached using specific inhibitors and several monoclonal antibodies [24,34]. Proteases are known to be potential mitogens. Several mechanisms are possible; they may act indirectly by releasing growth factors from precursors or the extracellular matrix via their enzymatic activity and/or by activating growth factor receptors. In this respect, proteolytic cleavages are needed to detach the TGFα precursor from the plasma membrane [35] and to activate the secreted TGFβ precursor [36]. The proteases responsible for these cleavages are unknown. Proteases may also act more directly via specific receptors, as in the case of thrombin [37], and they do in fact contain sequences analogous to growth factors.

Clinical studies indicate an association between high cellular concentrations of the 52K protease and cell proliferation of ductal mammary tissue [32,38]. These findings are consistent with a mitogenic activity, but the high 52K protein level may be a consequence rather than a cause of cell proliferation.

The major normal functions of cathepsins occur in lysosomes at very low pH, where they degrade endogenous proteins [39]. Since a procathepsin-D enzyme is secreted in large amounts at the periphery of cancer cells, the enzyme may acquire

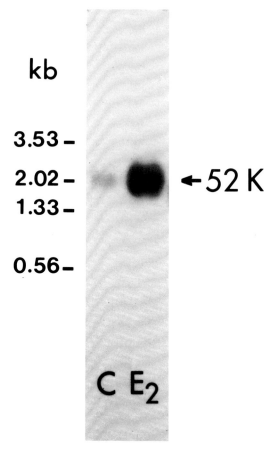

Fig. 5. Effect of estradiol on the 52K protease mRNA in MCF7 cells. Six hours following addition of estradiol (E₂) or solvent (C) to MCF7 cells, 10 μg of total RNA as analyzed in each track by 1% agarose gel electrophoresis. The 52K mRNA was detected by hybridization with a cloned cDNA isolated from a λgt11 cDNA library of estrogen-treated MCF7 cells (a gift of Dr. P. Chambon). The molecular weight of markers is shown in kilobases [27] (also see Cavaillès et al, in preparation).

abnormal functions, such as facilitating cancer cell migration and invasion by digesting basement membrane, extracellular matrix, and connective tissue. Cathepsin-D is secreted as an inactive proenzyme, but, at acidic pH, it can be autoactivated by the removal of a small part of the N-terminal profragment [40]. The same is true of breast cancer 52K protein [25]. Culture media conditioned under serum-free conditions by estradiol-treated MCF7 cells contain potential proteolytic activities that can digest methemoglobin [30] and extracellular matrix prepared from bovine corneal endothelial cells [25,41]. This activity appears to be due entirely to the 52K procathepsin-D since it is inhibited by pepstatin [25]. Between pH 5 and 6, and following its activation, the 52K protease can then digest the extracellular matrix of bovine corneal cells and human proteoglycans [25,41]. It is conceivable that breast cancer cells develop a sufficiently acidic microenvironment close to the extracellular matrix, where the secreted cathepsin-D-like 52K then behaves as a protease [41].

Clinical studies have recently supported the hypothesis of a role of the 52K protease in mammary carcinogenesis. Using different monoclonal antibodies to the

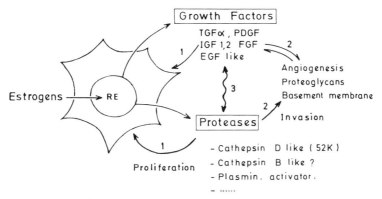

Fig. 6.   Putative functions of estrogen-regulated secreted proteins and peptides secreted by breast cancer cells. Estrogens, via their nuclear receptors (RE), induce several proteins and factors that are secreted by breast cancer cells. One category (growth factors) may act as autocrine factors that stimulate the growth of the same cells [17]. Other proteins, such as proteases, can potentially act as mitogens and may also facilitate cancer cell migration, invasion, and possibly metastasis. The 52K protein is the precursor of a cathepsin-D-like protease, and its secretion, as well as that of cathepsin-B, appears to be increased in mammary cells following their transformation.

total 52K protein and its precursor, we were able to detect the protein in the cytoplasm of cancer tissue by immunoperoxidase staining of frozen sections and to assay total 52K protein (52K + 48K + 34K) or only its precursor in the cytosol of breast cancers [for review, see 42].

In a prospective study of 183 patients, high concentrations of the 52K protein ($\geqslant$700 U/mg protein) were found to be correlated with axillary lymph node involvement but not with estrogen receptor content [43]. A retrospective study involving a 5 year follow-up of 150 postmenopausal patients [44] indicated that the patients had a significantly shorter disease-free interval when the 52K protein concentrations in primary tumors were superior to 400 U/mg cytosol protein than when the concentrations were lower. The bad prognostic significance of high concentrations of the protease may be related to a subsequent increase in its secretion.

OTHER LYSOSOMAL PROTEASES IN CARCINOGENESIS

Three types of cathepsins have most often been studied in relation to cancer. Cathepsin-D-like enzymes have also been shown to be secreted by pancreatic [45] and ovarian [46] cancers. No steroid hormone regulation has previously been demonstrated in cancer tissue, but cathepsin-D has been reported to be induced by progesterone in the rat uterus [47].

It has been proposed that cathepsin-B-like enzymes are involved in breast carcinogenesis [48]. They are thiol proteinases with an optimal pH of 5–6. Cathepsin-B activity and antigenicity are greater in mammary cancer cells than in normal cells [48,49]. The proenzyme (40K) is secreted in cancer cells, but it is inactive and requires a pepsine-like enzyme to be activated by removal of the profragment. A regulation by prolactin has been suggested [49] but not confirmed in the T47D cell line [50]. Cathepsin-B was also proposed to be correlated with the potential metastatic activities of human melanoma cells [51] and with the mitogenic activity of human mammary tumors. The relationship between estrogen and lysosomal enzymes has long been suggested by the pioneering work of Clara Szego and her colleagues [52]. Cathepsin-B was shown to be stimulated by estrogens in the rat uterus and was proposed to be related to the mitogenic activity of estradiol [53].

Using a totally different approach, another lysosomal protease, the major excreted protein (MEP), has been extensively studied and characterized by Gottesman and colleagues [54]. MEP is specifically secreted by mouse NIH 3T3 transformed fibroblasts but not by normal untransformed cells [54,55]. It is a cysteinyl proteinase, mostly active at pH 4–5, recently identified as a cathepsin-L by its substrate specificity [56] and by cDNA sequencing [57]; its synthesis and secretion are stimulated by several mitogens (phorbol ester, PDGF. . .) [58].

In these three examples, cathepsins (-D, -B, or -L) appear to be secreted in higher proportions in cancer cells than in normal cells. Their synthesis and secretion appear to be stimulated by mitogens, and they are secreted by cancer cells as higher-M_r proenzymes, which can be auto activated by partial proteolysis at acidic pH [25,55]. The reason for this greater secretion of lysosomal protease by cancer cells is not known but may be important in explaining invasiveness of cancer cells.

CONCLUSIONS AND PERSPECTIVES

It has often been proposed that proteases are involved in the process of invasion and metastasis by cancer cells [for review, see 59,60]. Collagenases [60] and plasminogen activator [61] have been the most extensively studied and have been considered to be involved in the process of metastasis. However, clinical data have not confirmed a correlation between plasminogen activator activity and the prognosis of breast cancer [62]. Tissue plasminogen activator appears to be correlated with estrogen and progesterone receptor sites more than with prognosis [63,64]. In contrast, evidence is converging favoring the idea that cathepsins are closely related to the metastatic and invasive processes in cancer. Cell transformation and several mitogens have been shown to stimulate the secretion of the precursors of MEP-cathepsin-L, cathepsin-B, and 52K procathepsin-D-like protease. Moreover, our first clinical results indicate that high concentrations of the cathepsin-D-like antigen in breast cancer cytosol are associated with rapidly developing breast cancers. These results strongly support the idea that secreted lysosomal proteases are involved in the process of tumor growth and invasion. As has been suggested in the case of secreted proteases in several cancer cells [59], we propose that the increased synthesis and secretion of 52K cathepsin-D by estrogens may facilitate the invasion of basement membrane, connective tissue, and blood vessels by breast cancer cells and consequently increase the frequency of metastasis [25,65]. In support of this hypothesis, estradiol appears to stimulate the migration of MCF7 cells through a reconstituted basement membrane [66]. Other cancers may also be controlled by the enzyme, but immunoperoxidase staining has revealed high concentrations of the protein mostly in breast cancer cells and melanoma [34], suggesting that it acts more specifically in these two types of cancer, which frequently result in metastases. The regulation of lysosomal enzymes by sex-steroid hormones may have similar consequences in other hormone-regulated cancers (prostate, endometrium). The involvement of proteases in the control of cancer growth has important therapeutical implications [59]. Since the 52K protease, like other autocrine growth factors, is produced by both hormone-dependent and

-independent breast cancer cells, the neutralization of its activity (by antibodies, analogs, enzyme inhibitors, etc) could be of considerable importance in treating breast cancer and melanoma and in preventing metastasis, in the same way that small-cell lung cancer is treated by neutralizing bombesin-like growth factors [67]. These antimitogenic treatments would be of more general use than antihormone therapy, whose efficacy is restricted to hormone-dependent cancers. Further studies are needed to prove the biological function of these proteases in carcinogenesis and to discover how to inhibit their putative destructive effects.

ACKNOWLEDGMENTS

We thank members of our laboratory and of CLIN-MIDY SANOFI Laboratory (B. Pau; grant INSERM/SANOFI No. 81039.3) who have contributed to several parts of this work; and E. Barrié and E. Egéa for their skillful preparation of the manuscript. We are grateful to CLIN-MIDY SANOFI Laboratory (B. Pau, F. Paolucci) for monoclonal antibodies, P. Chambon (Strasbourg) and F. Rougeon (Pasteur, Paris) for 52K-cDNA cloning, P. Ferrara and P. Louisot for protein structure studies, and several scientists (Drs. M. Lippman, M. Rich, I. Keydar, and the Mason Research Institute) for their gifts of mammary cell lines. Clinical studies were performed with the help of several clinical centers in Montpellier (Prs. Pujol, J.L. Lamarque, F. Laffargue) and in Copenhagen (Finsen Institute, Dr. S. Thorpe). This work was supported by the "Institut National de la Santé et de la Recherche Médicale," the Faculty of Medicine of Montpellier, and the "Association pour la Recherche sur le Cancer."

REFERENCES

1. Pike MC, Siiteri PK, Welsch CW (eds): "Banbury Report 8. Hormones and Breast Cancer." Cold Spring Harbor, NY: Cold Spring Harbor Laboratory, 1981.
2. Sirbasku DA, Benson RH: In Sato JH, Ross R (eds): "Hormones and Cell Culture." Cold Spring Harbor, NY: Cold Spring Harbor Laboratory, 1979, Vol 6, p 477.
3. Lippman ME, Bolan G, Huff K: Cancer Res 36:4595–4601, 1976.
4. Chalbos D, Vignon F, Keydar I, Rochefort H: J Clin Endocrinol Metab 55:276–283, 1982.
5. Darbre P, Yates J, Curtis S, King RJB: Cancer Res 43:349–354, 1983.
6. Adams DJ, Edwards DP, McGuire WL; Biomembranes 11; 389, 1983.
7. Rochefort H, Chalbos D, Capony F, Garcia M, Veith F, Vignon F, Westley B: In Gurpide E, Calandra R, Levy C, Soto RJ (eds): "Hormones and Cancer." New York: Alan R. Liss, Inc., 1984, pp 37–51.
8. Chambon P, Dierich A, Gaub MP, Jakowlew S, Jongstra J, Krust A, Lepennec JP, Oudet P, Reudelhuber T: Rec Prog Horm Res 40: 1–42, 1984.
9. Rochefort H, Coezy E, Joly E, Westley B, Vignon F: In Iacobelli S, et al (eds): "Hormones and Cancer," New York: Raven Press, 1980, pp 21–29.
10. De Larco JE, Todaro GJ: Proc Natl Acad Sci USA 75:4001–4005, 1978.
11. Vignon F, Derocq D, Chambon M, Rochefort H: CR Acad Sci 296:151–156, 1983.
12. Dickson RB, Huff KK, Spencer EM, Lippman ME: Endocrinology 118:138–142, 1986.
13. Manni A, Wright C, Feil P, Baranao L, Demers L, Garcia M, Rochefort H: Cancer Res 46:1594–1599, 1986.
14. Vignon F, Rochefort H: In Hollander VP (ed): "Hormone Responsive Tumors," New York: Academic Press, 1985, pp 135–153.
15. Westley W, Rochefort H: Cell 20:352–362, 1980.
16. Massot O, Baskevitch PP, Capony F, Garcia M, Rochefort H: Mol Cell Endocrinol 42:207–214, 1985.

17. Lippman ME, Dickson RB, Bates S, Knabbe C, Huff K, Swain S, McManaway M, Bronzert D, Kasid A, Gelmann EP: Breast Cancer Res Treat 1:59–70, 1986.
18. Salomon DS, Zwiebel JA, Bano M, Lasonczy L, Fehnel P, Kidwell WR: Cancer Res 44:4069–4077, 1984.
19. Westley W, Rochefort H: Biochem Biophys Res Commun 90:410–416, 1979.
20. Garcia M, Contesso G, Duplay H, Cavailles V, Derocq D, Delarue JC, Krebs B, Sancho-Garnier H, Richer G, Domergue J, Namer M, Rochefort H: J Steroid Biochem (in press).
21. Westley B, May FEB, Brown AMC, Krust A, Chambon P, Lippman ME, Rochefort H: J Biol Chem 259:10030–10035, 1984.
22. Garcia M, Capony F, Derocq D, Simon D, Pau B, Rochefort H: Cancer Res 45:709–716, 1985.
23. Capony F, Garcia M, Capdevielle J, Rougeot C, Ferrara P, Rochefort H: Eur J Biochem 161:505–512, 1986.
24. Vignon F, Capony F, Chambon M, Freiss G, Garcia M, Rochefort H: Endocrinology 118:1537–1545, 1986.
25. Capony F, Morisset M, Barrett AJ, Capony JP, Broquet P, Vignon F, Chambon M, Louisot P, Rochefort H: J Cell Biol 104:253–262, 1987.
26. Morisset M, Capony F, Rochefort H: Endocrinology 119:2773–2783, 1986.
27. Augereau P, Garcia M, Cavailles V, Chalbos D, Capony F, Rochefort H: In: "Program and Abstracts of the Endocrine Society 69th Annual Meeting." Abstract 953, p. 259, The Endocrine Society, Besthesda, MD, 1987.
28. Von Figura K, Hasilik A: Annu Rev Biochem 55:167–193, 1985.
29. Morisset M, Capony F, Rochefort H: Biochem Biophys Res Commun 138:102–109, 1986.
30. Barrett AJ: Biochem J 117:601–607, 1970.
31. Barrett AJ: Fed Proc 39:9–14, 1980.
32. Garcia M, Salazar-Retana G, Pages A, Richer G, Domergue J, Pages AM, Cavalie G, Martin JM, Lamarque JL, Pau B, Pujol H, Rochefort H: Cancer Res 46:3734–3738, 1986.
33. Faust PL, Kornfeld S, Chirgwin JM: Proc Natl Acad Sci USA 82:4910–4914, 1985.
34. Freiss G, Vignon F, Rogier H, Duporté J, Rochefort H: In preparation.
35. Derynck R, Roberts AB, Winkler ME, Chen EY, Goeddel DV: Cell 38:287–297, 1984.
36. Lawrence DA, Pircher R, Jullien P: Biochem Biophys Res Commun 133:1026–1034, 1985.
37. Low DA, Wiley HS, Cunningham DD: In Feramisco J, Ozanne B, Stiles B (eds): "Cancer Cells 3. Growth Factors and Transformation." Cold Spring Harbor NY: Cold Spring Harbor Laboratory, 1985, pp 401–408.
38. Rochefort H, Capony F, Cavalié-Barthez G, Chambon M, Freiss G, Garcia M, Morisset M, Touitou I, Vignon F: In Nunez J, et al (eds): "Hormone and Cell Regulation." London, Paris: Colloque INSERM/John Libbey Eurotext Ltd., 1986, Vol 139, pp 15–26.
39. De Duve C (ed): "A Guided Tour of the Living Cell." New York: Scientific American Books, Inc., 1984, Vol 1.
40. Hasilik A, Von Figura K, Conzelmann E, Nehrkorn H, Sandhoff K: Eur J Biochem 125:317–321, 1982.
41. Briozzo P, Morisset M, Capony F, Rochefort H: In preparation.
42. Rochefort H, Cavailles V, Freiss G, Derocq D, Salazar G, Maudelonde T, Khalaf S, Rogier H, Paolucci F, Pau B, Garcia M: In Ceriani R (ed): "Immunological Approaches to the Diagnosis and Therapy of Breast Cancer," New York: Plenum Press, (in press).
43. Maudelonde T, Khalaf S, Cavalié G, Frances D, Freiss G, Benatia M, Rogier H, Paolucci F, Simony J, Pujol H, Rochefort H: Submitted for publication.
44. Thorpe S, Rochefort H, Garcia M, Freiss G, Christensen IJ, Khala ES, Propucci F, Rasmussen BB, Rose C: Submitted for publication.
45. Yamaguchi N, Kawai K: Cancer Res 46:5353–5359, 1986.
46. Esumi H, Sato S, Sugimura T, Okasaki N: Biochim Biophys Acta 523:191–197, 1978.
47. Elangovan S, Moulton BC: J Biol Chem 255:7474–7479, 1980.
48. Recklies AD, Mort JS, Poole AR: Cancer Res 42:1026–1032, 1982.
49. Poole AR: In Dingle, Fell (eds): "Lysosomes in Biology and Pathology." New York: American Elsevier, 1979, Vol 29, pp 304–337.
50. Yee C, Shiu RPC: Cancer Res 46:1835–1839, 1986.
51. Sloane BF, Dunn JR, Honn KV: Science 212:1151–1153, 1981.
52. Szego CM: Rec Prog Horm Res 30:171–233, 1974.
53. Pietras RJ, Szego CM: J Cell Biol 81:649–663, 1979.
54. Gal S, Willingham MC, Gottesman MM: J Cell Biol 100:535–544, 1985.

55. Gal S, Gottesman MM: J Biol Chem 261:1760–1765, 1986.
56. Gal S, Gottesman MM: Biochem Biophys Res Commun 139:156–162, 1986.
57. Denhardt DT, Hamilton RT, Parfett CLJ, Edwards DR, Pierre RS, Waterhouse P, Nilsen-Hamilton M: Cancer Res 46:4590–4593, 1986.
58. Rabin MS, Doherty PJ, Gottesman MM: Proc Natl Acad Sci USA 83:357–360, 1986.
59. Goldfarb RH: In Honn KV, Powers WE, Sloane BF (eds): "Mechanisms of Cancer Metastasis." Boston: Martinus Nijhoff Publishing, 1986, pp 341–375.
60. Liotta LA, Tryggvason K, Garbisa S, Hart I, Foltz CM, Shafie S: Nature 284:67–68, 1980.
61. Reich E: In Berlin RD, Herrman M, Lepow IH, Tanzer JM (eds): "Molecular Basis of Biological Degradative Processes." New York: Academic Press, 1978, pp 155–169.
62. O'Grady P, Lijnen HR, Duffy MJ: Cancer Res 45:6216–6218, 1985.
63. Thorsen T: Eur J Cancer Clin Oncol 18:129–132, 1982.
64. Magdelenat H, Bieth J, Coppey J, Durand JC: Breast Cancer Res Treat 3:383–384, 1983.
65. Rochefort H, Capony F, Cavalié G, Chambon M, Freiss G, Garcia M, Morisset M, Vignon F: In Klijn JGM (ed): "Hormonal Manipulation of Cancer." New York: Raven Press Vol. 18, pp 407–414, 1987.
66. Albini A, Graf J., Kitten GT, Kleinman HK, Martin GR, Veillette A, Lippman ME: Proc Natl Acad Sci USA 83:8182–8186, 1986.
67. Cuttitta F, Carney DN, Mulshine J, Moody TW, Fedorko J, Fischler A, Minna JD: Nature 316:823–826, 1985.

Journal of Cellular Biochemistry 35:105–112 (1987)
Growth Regulation of Cancer 31–38

Cloning and Characterization of the Human PIM-1 Gene: A Putative Oncogene Related to the Protein Kinases

Timothy C. Meeker, Lalitha Nagarajan, Abbas ar-Rushdi, and Carlo M. Croce

The Wistar Institute of Anatomy and Biology, Philadelphia, Pennsylvania 19104

The mouse PIM-1 gene has been implicated in the evolution of retrovirus-associated mouse lymphomas. We have initiated a study of the human PIM-1 gene because of its potential importance as a human oncogene. We have isolated genomic and cDNA clones for this gene and characterized this locus in detail. The predicted PIM-1 protein is 313 amino acids in length. It has homology to a number of the protein kinases but does not have a transmembrane region. The amino acid corresponding to tyrosine-416 of pp60v-src is a tyrosine (position 198), which is consistent with the hypothesis that PIM-1 is a tyrosine kinase rather than a serine-threonine kinase. The PIM-1 gene was found to have six exons and five introns derived from 5 kb of genomic DNA. The site of transcription initiation was localized by S1 nuclease protection studies which indicated that the mature PIM-1 mRNA was approximately 2.7 kb in length. The promotor of this gene had no TATA or CAAT box but did have multiple GC boxes (CCGCCC) that might bind the Sp1 protein. The PIM-1 gene was expressed in myeloid and B lymphoid cell lines, but not in T lymphoid and nonhemopoietic lines. This initial characterization of PIM-1 will allow us to define its role in normal and malignant hematolymphoid differentiation.

Key words: human PIM-1 gene, protein kinase, oncogene, hematolymphoid genes

Tumor-associated retroviruses in animals frequently activate cellular proto-oncogenes by integrating adjacent to them. Examples of activation by retroviral insertion include c-myc by avian leukosis virus, erb-B by avian leukosis virus, c-myc by Abelson and Moloney retrovirus, and int-1 and int-2 by mouse mammary tumor virus [1–5]. The PIM-1 gene has recently been added to this list [6]. Murine leukemia retroviruses frequently integrate in the PIM-1 locus in mouse T cell lymphomas [7]. The increased levels of PIM-1 mRNA that result apparently have a role in the evolution of these lymphomas. It is interesting that abnormalities of *c-myc* and PIM-1 are often found in the same tumor, suggesting that these genes might cooperate in oncogenesis.

Received February 10, 1987; accepted May 27, 1987.

Because of our interest in the genes associated with human leukemia and lymphoma, we began to investigate the human PIM-1 gene. We have previously reported the cloning of a genomic fragment for the human PIM-1 gene and the use of this clone to map the human PIM-1 gene to chromosome band 6p21 [8]. In this report we describe the isolation of cDNA clones for this gene, the complete characterization of the cDNA and genomic clones, and our studies of the expression of the PIM-1 gene.

MATERIALS AND METHODS

Isolation of RNA and Northern Blotting

The following cell lines were used for RNA isolation: B lineage—380, 697, Alli, Daudi, BL2, ST486, JD38, Manca, CA46, PA682, SB, LY67, LY91, GM607, GM1056, GM2471, GM2669, GM1500, RPMI 8226; T lineage—Jurkat, HUT78, Molt4, SUPT1, CEM, JM; myeloid lineage—K562, ML3, KG1, HL-60, WEH1-3B (the only mouse line studied); nonhemopoietic—BR3, BR5, Colo320, 2102E, JAR, WM793, A424, TERA1 and WM373 [9–12].

RNA was isolated from cell lines by previously published methods. For Northern blots RNA was fractionated in formaldehyde gels and transferred to nitrocellulose as published [13].

cDNA Libraries

Two K562 cDNA libraries were screened. The first has been previously described [14]. The second library was constructed in lambda gt10 by using published methods [15,16].

Nucleic Acid Sequencing

All sequencing was performed in the M13 system by using the chain termination technique [17]. Data represent information from both strands.

RESULTS

Cloning

Our group has previously reported the cloning of a 13-kb genomic fragment containing the human PIM-1 gene from the 380 cell line [8]. With the aid of a probe from this fragment, the K562 cDNA libraries were screened. Approximately, 0.02% of the clones were positive. Upon detailed restriction mapping, two of these clones were found to cover approximately 2.6 kb of the PIM-1 transcriptional unit. The cDNA clones and appropriate regions from the genomic clone were sequenced. Our goal was to define the nature of the PIM-1 protein, promotor region, and intron/exon structure.

Deduced PIM-1 Protein Structure

The K562 cDNA clones covered 2514 bp of the mature PIM-1 transcript as noted in Figure 1. The major protein-coding region defined a protein of 313 amino acids. This protein-coding region initiates translation at the first ATG codon in the cDNA clones. Because of our concern about possible additional upstream translation initiation sites we defined the site of transcription initiation by S1 mapping and

```
TCCTGCCCCGCGGCGGCTGCCGCACGAGCCCCACGAGCCGCTCACCCCGCCGTTCTCAGCGCTGCCCGACCCCGCTGGCGC

GCCCTCCCGCCGCCAGTCCCGGCAGCGCCCTCAGTTGTCCTCCGACTCGCCCTCGGCCTTCCGCGCCAGCCGCAGCCACA

GCCGCAACGCCACCCGCAGCCACAGCCACAGCCACAGCCCCAGGCATAGCCTTCGGCACAGCCCCGGCTCCGGCTCCTGC
```

```
                                                          M   L   L   S   K   I   N   S
GGCAGCTCCTCTGGGCACCGTCCCTGCGCCGACATCCTGGAGGTTGGG ATG CTC TTG TCC AAA ATC AAC TCG

  L   A   H   L   R   A   A   P   C   N   D   L   H   A   T   K   L   A   P   G
CTT GCC CAC CTG CGC GCC GCG CCC TGC AAC GAC CTG CAC GCC ACC AAG CTG GCG CCC GGC

  K   E   K   E   P   L   E   S   Q   Y   Q   V   G   P   L   L   G   S   G   G
AAG GAG AAG GAG CCC CTG GAG TCG CAG TAC CAG GTG GGC CCG CTA CTG GGC AGC GGC GGC

  F   G   S   V   Y   S   G   I   R   V   S   D   N   L   P   V   A   I  |K|  H
TTC GGC TCG GTC TAC TCA GGC ATC CGC GTC TCC GAC AAC TTG CCG GTG GCC ATC|AAA| CAC

  V   E   K   D   R   I   S   D   W   G   E   L   P   N   G   T   R   V   P   M
GTG GAG AAG GAC CGG ATT TCC GAC TGG GGA GAG CTG CCT AAT GGC ACT CGA GTG CCC ATG

  E   V   V   L   L   K   K   V   S   S   G   F   S   G   V   I   R   L   L   D
GAA GTG GTC CTG CTG AAG AAG GTG AGC TCG GGT TTC TCC GGC GTC ATT AGG CTC CTG GAC

  W   F   E   R   P   D   S   F   V   L   I   L   E   R   P   E   P   V   Q   D
TGG TTC GAG AGG CCC GAC AGT TTC GTC CTG ATC CTG GAG AGG CCC GAG CCG GTG CAA GAT

  L   F   D   F   I   T   E   R   G   A   L   Q   E   E   L   A   R   S   F   F
CTC TTC GAC TTC ATC ACG GAA AGG GGA GCC CTG CAA GAG GAG CTC GCC CGC AGC TTC TTC

  W   Q   V   L   E   A   V   R   H   C   H   N   C   G   V   L   H   R   D   I
TGG CAG GTG CTG GAG GCC GTG CGG CAC TGC CAC AAC TGC GGG GTG CTC CAC CGC GAC ATC

  K   D   E   N   I   L   I   D   L   N   R   G   E   L   K   L   I   D   F   G
AAG GAC GAA AAC ATC CTT ATC GAC CTC AAT CGC GGC GAG CTC AAG CTC ATC GAC TTC GGG

  S   G   A   L   L   K   D   T   V  |Y|  T   D   F   D   G   T   R   V   Y   S
TCG GGG GCG CTG CTC AAA GAC ACC GTC|TAC| ACG GAC TTC GAT GGG ACC CGA GTG TAT AGC

  P   P   E   W   I   R   Y   H   R   Y   H   G   R   S   A   A   V   W   S   L
CCT CCA GAG TGG ATC CGC TAC CAT CGC TAC CAT GGC AGG TCG GCG GCA GTC TGG TCC CTG

  G   I   L   L   Y   D   M   V   C   G   D   I   P   F   E   H   D   E   E   I
GGG ATC CTG CTG TAT GAT ATG GTG TGT GGA GAT ATT CCT TTC GAG CAT GAC GAA GAG ATC

  I   R   G   Q   V   F   F   R   Q   R   V   S   S   E   C   Q   H   L   I   R
ATC AGG GGC CAG GTT TTC TTC AGG CAG AGG GTC TCT TCA GAA TGT CAG CAT CTC ATT AGA

  W   C   L   A   L   R   P   S   D   R   P   T   F   E   E   I   Q   N   H   P
TGG TGC TTG GCC CTG AGA CCA TCA GAT AGG CCA ACC TTC GAA GAA ATC CAG AAC CAT CCA

  W   M   Q   D   V   L   L   P   Q   E   T   A   E   I   H   L   H   S   L   S
TGG ATG CAA GAT GTT CTC CTG CCC CAG GAA ACT GCT GAG ATC CAC CTC CAC AGC CTG TCG

  P   G   P   S   K   *
CCG GGG CCC AGC AAA TAG CAGCCTTTCTGGCAGGTCCTCCCCTCTCTTGTCAGATGCCCGAGGGAGGGGAAGCT

TCTGTCTCCAGCTTCCCGAGTACCAGTGACACGTCTCGCCAAGCAGGACAGTGCTTGATACAGGAACAACATTTACAACT

CATTCCAGATCCCAGGCCCCTGGAGGCTGCCTCCCAACAGTGAGGAAGAGTGACTCTCCAGGGGTCCTAGGCCTCAACTC

CTCCCATAGATACTCTCTTCTTCTTCATAGGTGTCCAGCATTGCTGGACTGCTGAAATATCCCGGGGGTGGGGGTGGGGG

TGGGTCAGAACCCTGCCATGGAACTGTTTCCTTCATCATGAGTTCTGCTGAATGCCGCGATGGGTCAGGTAGGGGGGAAA

CAGGTTGGGATGGGATAGGACTAGCACCATTTTAAGTCCCTGTCACCTCTTCCGACTCTTTCTGAGTGCCTTCTGTGGGG

ACTCCGGCTGTGCTGGGAGAAATACTTGAACTTGCCTCTTTTACCTGCTGCTTCTCCAAAAATCTGCCTGGGTTTTGTTC

CCTATTTTTCTCTCCTGTCCTCCCTCACCCCCTCCTTCATATGAAAGGTGCCATGGAAGAGGCTACAGGGCCAAACGCTG

AGCCACCTGCCCTTTTTTCTGCCTCCTTTAGTAAAACTCCGAGTGAACTGGTCTTCCTTTTTGGTTTTTACTTAACTGTT

TCAAAGCCAAGACCTCACACACAGAAAAAATGCACAAACAATGCAATCAACAGAAAAGCTGTAAATGTGTGTACAGTTGG

CATGGTAGTATACAAAAAGATTGTAGTGGATCTAATTTTTCAGAAATTTTGCCTTTAAGTTATTTTACCTGTTTTTGTTT

CTTGTTTTGAAAGATGCGCATTCTAACCTGGAGGTCAATGTTATGTATTTATTTATTTATTTATTTGGTTCCCTTCCTAT

TCCAAGCTTCCATAGCTGCTGCCCTAGTTTTCTTTCCTCCTTTCCTCCTCTGACTTGGGGACCTTTTGGGGGAGGGCTGC

GACGCTTGCTCTGTTTGTGGGGTGACGGGACTCAGGCGGGACAGTGCTGCAGCTCCCTGGCTTCTGTGGGGCCCCTCACC

TACTTACCCAGGTGGGTCCCGGCTCTGTGGGTGATGGGGAGGGGCATTGCTGACTGTGTATATAGGATAATTATGAAAAG

CAGTTCTGGATGGTGTGCCTTCCAGATCCTCTCTGGGGCGTGTGTTTTGAGCAGCAGGTAGCCTGGCTGGTTTTATCTGAG

TGAAATACTGTACAGGGGAATAAAAGAGATCTTATTTTT
```

Fig. 1. Amino acid sequence. The amino acid sequence of the PIM-1 protein is deduced from the cDNA clones. The single-letter amino acid code indicates the region of the predicted protein of 313 amino acids. Boxes identify Lys 67 and Tyr 198. The poly A signal is underlined. The cDNA clones contained a 289-bp 5′ untranslated region rich in G and C with a single termination codon (underlined). A 3′ AT-rich repeat is also indicated.

genomic sequencing. We found no alternative translation initiation sites upstream in the transcribed region of the PIM-1 gene. An analysis of the deduced PIM-1 amino acid sequence did not reveal a transmembrane region. The human PIM-1 protein was found to be highly homologous to the mouse PIM-1 protein; 94% of the sequence was identical [18].

A search of the Bionet protein sequence data base revealed that PIM-1 was homologous to a number of the protein kinases, including c-mos from rat, mouse, and man, bovine cGMP-dependent protein kinase, phosphorylase kinase b, gamma subunit, v-ros, v-erb-B, v-kit, v-fes, and v-fps [19–29]. This homology to the protein kinases was most obvious in several regions within the catalytic domain. These regions are indicated in Figure 2. The region from amino acid 44 to 67 is the region of ATP binding [30]. Specifically, the motif LGXGXXG is highly conserved among protein kinases. It is suspected that this sequence aligns with the ribose ring of deoxynucleotide triphosphates [30]. Lysine-67 of PIM-1 is homlogous to lysine-71 of cAMP-dependent protein kinase and lysine-295 of pp60v-src, both of which can be modified by 5′-p-fluorosulphonylbenzoyladenosine (FBSA), the ATP analog [31,32].

The region from amino acid 165 to 204 is also highly conserved among protein kinases (Fig. 2). Specifically, Tyr-198 appears to be homologous to Tyr-416 of pp 60 v-src. It is this tyrosine in the v-src protein that can be autophosphorylated. A tyrosine in a homologous location is present in all tyrosine kinases described to date [30]. The homology that PIM-1 shows to the tyrosine-kinase family in this region would be

```
           *  *    *       *    *                       *  *   *
HU PIM-1   L G S G G F G S V Y S G I R V S D N L P . V A I K   (44-67)
HU MOS     L G A G G F G S V Y K A T Y R G V P . . . V A I K   (44-65)
v-SRC      L G Q C F G E V W M G T W N D T T R . . V A I K     (274-296)
GKIN       L G V G G F G R V E L V Q L K S E E S K T F A M K   (365-389)
PKb        L G R G V S S V V R R C I H K E E P T C K E Y A V K (24-48)
v-FES      I G R G N F G E V F S G R L R A D N T L . V A V K   (699-722)
v-FPS      I G R G N F G E V F S G R L R A D N T P . V A V K   (923-946)
A
```

```
           *  *  *       *   *              *     *  *  *                       +              *
HU PIM-1   H R D I K D E N I L I D L N R G E L K L I D F G S G A L . . . . . L K D T V Y T D F D G T   (165-204)
HU MOS     H L D L K P A N I L I S E Q D . V C K I S D F G C S E K L E D L L C R Q T P S Y P L G G T   (177-220)
v-SRC      H R D L R A A N I L V G E N L . V C K V A D F G L A R L . . . . . I E D N E Y T A R Q G A   (385-423)
GKIN       Y R D L K P E N L I L D H R G . Y A K L V D F G F A K K I . . . . . G F G K K T W T F C G T (482-521)
PKb        H R D L K P E N I L L D D D M . N I K L T D F G F S C Q L . . . . D P G E K L R E V C G T   (132-171)
v-FES      H R D L A A R N C L V T E K N . V L K I S D F G M S R E . . . . . . E A D G V Y A A S G G L (814-852)
v-FPS      H R D L A A R N C L V T E K N . T L K I S D F G M S R Q . . . . . E E D G V Y A S T G G M   (1038-1076)
B
```

Fig. 2. Homology of PIM-1 with other protein kinases. **A:** The region of PIM-1 from amino acid 44 to 67 is compared to homologous regions of human mos, v-src, G kinase, phosphorylase kinase B-γ subunit, v-fes, and v-fps. This region is the ATP binding region. Asterisks denote highly conserved amino acid positions. Homologous bases are boxed and the amino acid positions used for comparison are noted in parentheses. The lysine at position 67 is highly conserved among all protein kinases. **B:** The central part of the kinase region of PIM-1 is compared to homologous regions of other protein kinases. Homologous bases are boxed and asterisks identify highly conserved amino acids as in Figure 2A. The tyrosine at position 198 (+) is homologous to that of v-src position 416. This tyrosine is conserved in all tyrosine kinases. Note that mos, which is a serine-threonine kinase, does have a tyrosine in this region but without adjacent homologous bases. All alignments are similar to those of Hunter and Cooper [30]. (For sequences, see [21–24, 26, 48–50].)

consistent with the hypothesis that PIM-1 is a tyrosine kinase and Tyr-198 can be autophosphorylated. Further experiments will clarify this issue.

The carboxy-terminal part of the PIM-1 protein has several regions which are homologous to the protein kinases. However, the carboxy-terminus of PIM-1 does not have a tyrosine as do some of the other tyrosine kinases [33,34]. It has been suggested that phosphorylation of a tyrosine in this region negatively regulates these kinases. Furthermore, elimination of the terminal tyrosine by truncation of the protein is directly related to oncogenicity in a number of tyrosine kinases. Therefore, if it can be shown that PIM-1 codes for a tyrosine kinase, the lack of a carboxy terminal tyrosine in the PIM-1 sequence might have important implications for the possible mechanisms of activation and regulation of this proto-oncogene.

Although there are regions of PIM-1 that are highly homologous to the other protein kinases, the overall homology throughout the entire sequence is low. A comparison of the PIM-1 sequence with that of several other protein kinases revealed less than 20% identical amino acids over the full length of the protein. This suggests that PIM-1 has some unique functional role among the protein kinases.

Transcriptional Unit

A schematic of the PIM-1 transcriptional unit is indicated in Figure 3. We defined the site of transcription initiation by S1 nuclease analysis by using mRNA from K562 and GM607. There are six exons and five introns. There are two polyadenylation signals at the 3' end of the gene, but only one polyA signal is present in our cDNA clones. Apparently the second polyA signal is most frequently used. We predict that the processed mRNA is approximately 2.7 kb in length.

The striking feature about the PIM-1 promotor is the high GC content (greater than 75% from nucleotide -1 to -300). The promotor region does not contain a TATA or CAAT box. However there are seven GC boxes which may be capable of binding the Sp-1 protein [35]. Additionally, the sequence (ATGCAGAT) is present starting at position -248. This sequence is very similar to an octamer found in immunoglobulin enhancer and promotor regions (ATGCAAAT) [36]. This octamer sequence may be important for the regulation of PIM-1 expression.

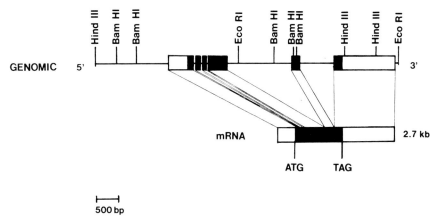

Fig. 3. PIM-1 gene structure. This figure shows the intron/exon structure of PM-1. The mature transcript arises from 5.0 kb of genomic DNA. Boxes indicate the genomic regions represented in the mature transcript and shaded regions represent the protein-coding regions.

Expression in Human Cell Lines

We analyzed over 38 human cell lines for expression of the PIM-1 transcript by Northern blotting. These included four myeloid lines, 19 B lymphocytic lines, seven T lymphocytic lines, and a number of nonhemopoietic lines. Two of the myeloid lines, K562 and KG-1, had the highest levels of PIM-1 mRNA (see Fig. 3). Among the other myeloid lines, ML3 had moderate levels and HL-60 had undetectable levels. Fourteen of 19 B lymphocytic lines were positive. Surprisingly, none of the seven T cell lines and only one of nine nonhcmopoietic lines expressed PIM-1. Therefore the PIM-1 gene is expressed selectively in myeloid and B lymphoid lines, perhaps in a manner dictated by the stage of differentiation of these lineages.

We additionally compared the mouse and human PIM-1 mRNA to confirm that the size of the transcript was conserved. The transcript from WEHI-3B, a mouse myeloid line, was the same size as the human PIM-1 transcript (Fig. 4).

DISCUSSION

In this report we describe the cDNA cloning of the human PIM-1 gene and the characterization of the gene locus. The human PIM-1 gene was found to code for a 313 amino acid protein in the K562 cell line. This protein showed significant homology to a number of the protein kinases. This protein has a tyrosine at position 198 which may be homlgous to Tyr-416 of pp60 v-src. This finding is consistent with the hypothesis that PIM-1 is a tyrosine protein kinase rather than a serine-threonine kinase. No transmembrane region was identified.

The mature PIM-1 mRNA was found to be approximately 2.7 kb in length. The gene consisted of six exons and five introns. The promotor region was unusual in that no TATA or CAAT box was identified. The promotor is therefore similar to a small number of genes that include hydroxy-methyl glutaryl coenzyme A reductase (HMG CoA reductase), adenosine deaminase (ADA), hypoxanthine phosphoribosyl transferase (HPRT), adenosine phosphoribosyl transferase (APRT), 3-phosphoglycerate kinase (PGK), and dihydrofolate reductase (DHRF) [37–42]. The reason that this family of genes has this unusual promotor structure will be an area of future investigation.

The expression of the PIM-1 gene is unusual because it is primarily restricted to myeloid and B lymphoid cell lineages. In the mouse it has been shown that normal T cells and T cell tumors express pim-1 [7,43]. Our data show that human T cell lines do not express PIM-1 in appreciable amounts. This discrepancy in lineage expression is surprising for a gene that is so highly conserved. Further study of this issue is in progress.

One of our primary interests in the human PIM-1 gene locus relates to its disruption by chromosomal abnormalities or viral insertions. Chromosomal abnormalities of chromosome 6p have been reported in myeloid and undifferentiated leukemia, T cell lymphoma, and malignant melanoma [44–47]. Certainly, a number of tumor-associated viruses (HIV, HTLVI, HBLV, etc) might integrate in this region, as occurs in retroviral infection in mouse leukemogenesis. In our studies of a small number of human cancer samples to date, we have been unable to find abnormalities of this locus by Southern blotting. Nonetheless, we suspect that such abnormalities exist and plan to study a larger number of patients with probes that span the entire PIM-1 gene locus and, if necessary, to employ reversed-field gel electrophoresis to identify cancer samples with abnormalities of this gene.

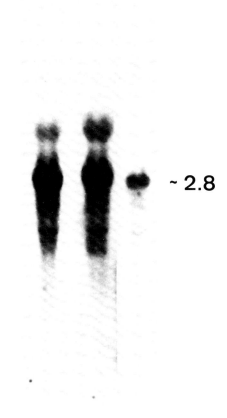

Fig. 4. Expression of the PIM-1 gene. Expression of the PIM-1 gene was analyzed by Northern blotting. A band of approximately 2.8 kb was found in K562 (**lane 1**), KG-1 (**lane 2**), and WEHI-3B (a mouse myeloid line, **lane 3**).

REFERENCES

1. Payne GS, Bishop JM, Varmus HE: Nature 295:209, 1982.
2. Nilsen TW, Maroney PA, Goodwin RG, Rottman FM, Crittenden LB, Raines MA, Kung H-J: Cell 41:719, 1985.
3. Nusse R, van Ooyen A, Cox D, Fung YKT, Varmus H: Nature 307:131, 1984.
4. Peters G, Brookes S, Smith R, Dickson C: Cell 33:369, 1983.
5. Sheng-Ong GLC, Polter M, Mushinski JF, Lavu S, Reddy EP: Science 226:1077, 1984.
6. Cuypers HT, Selten G, Quint W, Zijlstra M, Maandag ER, Boelens W, van Wezenbeek P, Melief C, Berns A: Cell 37:141, 1984.
7. Selten G, Cuypers HT, Berns A: EMBO J 4:1793, 1985.
8. Nagarajan L, Louie E, Tsujimoto Y, ar-Rushdi A, Huebner K, Croce CM: Proc Natl Acad Sci USA 83:2556, 1986.
9. Warner NL, Moore MAS, Metcalf D: J Natl Cancer Inst 43:963, 1969.
10. Minowada J: In Gunz E, Hendersen E (eds): "Leukemia." New York: Grune and Stratton, 1983, pp 119–139.
11. Nishikura K, ar-Rushdi A, Erikson J, Watt R, Rovera G, Croce CM: Proc Natl Acad Sci USA 80:4822, 1983.

12. Pegoraro L, Palumbo A, Erickson J, Falda M, Giovanazzo B, Emanuel BS, Rovera G, Nowell PC, Croce CM: Proc Natl Acad Sci USA 81:7166, 1984.
13. ar-Rushdi A, Tan KB, Croce CM: Somatic Cell Genet 8:151, 1982.
14. Watt R, Stanton LW, Marcu KB, Gallo RC, Croce CM, Rovera G: Nature 303:725, 1983.
15. Huynh TV, Young RA, Davis RW: In Glover (ed): "DNA Cloning, a Practical Approach." Oxford: IRL Press, 1984.
16. Gubler U, Hoffman B: Gene 25:263, 1983.
17. Messing J: In Wu R, Grossman L, Moldave K (eds): "Methods in Enzymology 101." New York: Academic Press, 1983, pp 20–27.
18. Selten G, Cuypers HT, Boelens W, Robanus-Maandag E, Verbeek J, Domen J, van Beveren C, Berns A: Cell 46:603, 1986.
19. Van Beveren C, Galleshaw JA, Jonas V, Berns AJM, Doolittle RF, Donoghue DJ, Verma IM: Nature 289:258, 1981.
20. Van der Hoorn FA, Firzlaff J: Nucleic Acids Res 12:2147, 1984.
21. Watson R, Oskarsson M, Vande Woude GF: Proc Natl Acad Sci USA 79:4078, 1982.
22. Takio K, Wade RD, Smith SB, Krebs EG, Walsh KA, Titani K: Biochemistry 23:4207, 1984.
23. Reimann EM, Titani K, Ericsson LH, Wade RD, Rischer EH, Walsh KA: Biochemistry 23:4185, 1984.
24. Hashimoto E, Taio K, Krebs EG: J Biol Chem 257:727, 1982.
25. Neckameyer W, Wang LH: J Virol 53:879, 1985.
26. Hampe A, Laprevotte I, Galibert F, Fedele LA, Sherr CJ: Cell 30:775, 1982.
27. Besmer P, Murphy JE, George PC, Qiu F, Bergold PJ, Lederman L, Snyder HW, Jr, Brodeur D, Zuckerman EE, Hardy WD: Nature 320:415, 1986.
28. Yamamoto T, Nishida T, Mijajima N, Kawai S, Doi T, Toyoshima K: Cell 35:71, 1983.
29. Huang C, Hammond C, Bishop JM: J Virol 50:125, 1984.
30. Hunter T, Cooper JA: Annu Rev Biochem 54:897, 1985.
31. Zother M, Nelson N, Taylor S: J Biol Chem 256:10837, 1981.
32. Kamps M, Taylor S, Sefton B: Nature 310:589, 1984.
33. Sefton B, Hunter T: Cancer Surveys 5:159, 1986.
34. Coussens L, Van Beveren C, Smith D, Chen E, Mitchell RL, Isacke CM, Verma IM, Ullrich A: Nature 320:277, 1986.
35. Dynan WS, Tjian R: Nature 316:774, 1985.
36. Staudt LM, Singh H, Sen R, Wirth T, Sharp PA, Baltimore D: Nature 323:640, 1986.
37. Reynolds GA, Basu SK, Osborne TF, Chin DJ, Gil G, Brown MS, Goldstein JL, Luskey KL: Cell 38:275, 1984.
38. Melton DW, Konecki DS, Brennand J, Caskey CT: Proc Natl Acad Sci USA 81:2147, 1984.
39. Dush MK, Sikela JM, Sohaib AK, Tischfield JA, Stambrook P: Proc Natl Acad Sci USA 82:2731, 1985.
40. Valerio D, Duyvesteyn MGC, Dekker BMM, Weeda G, Berkvens TM, van der Voorn L, van Ormondt H, van der Eb AJ: EMBO J 4:437, 1985.
41. Singer-Sam J, Keith DH, Tani K, Simmer RL, Shively L, Lindsay S, Hyoshida A, Riggs AD: Gene 32:409, 1984.
42. Crouse GF, Leys EJ, McEwan RN, Frayne EG, Kellems RE: Mol Cell Biol 1985:1847, 1985.
43. Mally JI, Vogt M, Swift SE, Haas M: Virology 144:115, 1985.
44. Carbonell F, Kratt E, Neuhaus K: Cancer Genet Cytogenet 2:139, 1980.
45. Carroll AJ, Castleberry RP, Prchal JT, Finley WH: Cancer Genet Cytogenet 18:303, 1985.
46. Mecucci C, Michaux J-L, Tricot G, Louwagie A, van den Berghe H: Leuk Res 9:1139, 1985.
47. Vermaelen K, Michaux J-L, Louwagie A, van den Berghe H: Cancer Genet Cytogenet 10:125, 1983.
48. Shibuja M, Hanafusa H: Cell 30:787, 1982.
49. Czernilofsky AP, Levinson D, Varmus HE, Bishop JM, Tischler E, Goodman HM: Nature 287:198, 1980.
50. Schwarz D, Tizard R, Gilbert W: Cell 32:853, 1983.

Journal of Cellular Biochemistry 35:113–128 (1987)
Growth Regulation of Cancer 39–54

Analysis of pp60$^{\text{c-src}}$ Tyrosine Kinase Activity and Phosphotyrosyl Phosphatase Activity in Human Colon Carcinoma and Normal Human Colon Mucosal Cells

Virginia DeSeau, Neal Rosen, and Joseph B. Bolen

Laboratory of Tumor Virus Biology (V.D., J.B.B.) and Medicine Branch (N.R.), National Cancer Institute, Bethesda, Maryland 20892

We have compared the level of phosphotyrosyl phosphatase activity in lysates from normal human colon mucosal cells and human colon carcinoma cells and analyzed the effect of incubating these cells with sodium orthovanadate, an inhibitor of phosphotyrosyl phosphatase activity, on the relative abundance of acid-stable phosphotyrosine and on in vitro protein kinase activity of pp60$^{\text{c-src}}$. Additionally, we compared the effect of lysing these cells in buffer containing only nonionic detergents with RIPA buffer, which contains both sodium dodecyl sulfate and deoxycholate, on the in vitro kinase activity of pp60$^{\text{c-src}}$. Our results show that the level of detectable phosphotyrosyl phosphatase activity in lysates derived from normal colon cells and colon carcinoma cells is very similar. Additionally, the abundance of acid-stable phosphotyrosine in these cells cultured in the absence or presence of vanadate is not significantly different. However, incubation of these cells with vanadate significantly stimulates the activity of pp60$^{\text{c-src}}$ derived from the normal colon cells in immune-complex kinase assays, while having no detectable effect on the activity of pp60$^{\text{c-src}}$ from the colon tumor cells. The in vitro protein kinase activity of pp60$^{\text{c-src}}$ derived from RIPA buffer lysates of colon carcinoma cells was found to be elevated five- to sevenfold when compared with pp60$^{\text{c-src}}$ from these same cells lysed in buffer containing only Nonidet-P 40 as a detergent. The type of lysis buffer did not effect the activity of pp60$^{\text{c-src}}$ from normal colon mucosal cells. These results provide additional evidence that the activity of pp60$^{\text{c-src}}$ may be regulated differently in colon carcinoma and normal colon mucosal cells.

Key words: pp60$^{\text{c-src}}$, tyrosine kinase, phosphotyrosyl phosphatase, human colon carcinoma, normal human colon mucosal cells

The *c-src* proto-oncogene encodes a 60,000-dalton membrane-associated phosphoprotein which possesses endogenous tyrosine-specific protein kinase activity [reviewed in 1 and 2]. The transforming potential of *c-src* mutants appears to be related

Received February 7, 1987; revised and accepted May 20, 1987.

to the specific activity of the mutated *c-src*-encoded pp60^{c-src} protein phosphotransferase [3–7]. The specific activity of pp60^{c-src} is currently thought to be negatively regulated in cells by the phosphorylation of tyrosine residues in the carboxyterminal portion of the molecule [4,8,9]. Recently, this site of tyrosine phosphorylation on avian pp60^{c-src} molecules has been localized to tyrosine residue 527 [10].

The critical role phosphorylation of tyrosine residue 527 plays in governing the specific activity and transforming potential of pp60^{c-src} has been demonstrated by site-specific mutation of tyrosine 527 to phenylalanine which results in transformation-competent pp60^{c-src} molecules possessing elevated protein kinase activity [11–13]. Since pp60^{c-src} does not appear to autophosphorylate tyrosine 527 residues at a significant rate in in vitro protein kinase assays [9,14], it is thought that phosphorylation of this amino acid within cells represents a function of cellular tyrosine kinases distinct from pp60^{c-src}. Thus, regulation of pp60^{c-src} tyrosine kinase activity in cells can apparently be controlled by cellular phosphotyrosyl phosphatases which function to stimulate kinase activity and cellular tyrosine kinases which act to inhibit pp60^{c-src} protein kinase activity.

Recently, we reported that the tyrosine-specific protein kinase activity of pp60^{c-src} molecules isolated from human colon carcinoma tissues and tumor-derived cell lines is consistently elevated over that from normal colon tissues and cultures of normal colon mucosal cells [15]. Analysis of the tumor tissues and cell lines showed that the elevation of pp60^{c-src} kinase activity did not correlate with a proportional increase in the synthesis rate or abundance of pp60^{c-src}, suggesting that the specific activity of the *c-src*-encoded phosphotransferase might be enhanced. Additional comparison of pp60^{c-src} molecules from colon carcinoma cells lines and normal colon mucosal cells reveals that they possess indistinguishable sites and quantities of phosphorylated serine and tyrosine residues and are not stably complexed with other cellular proteins [14]. However, the elevated protein kinase activity of pp60^{c-src} from the colon carcinoma cell lines was found to be associated with an increase in the apparent turnover rate of phosphate groups from carboxy-terminal tyrosine residues in vivo. These observations were interpreted to suggest that the level of phosphotyrosyl phosphatase activity in the colon carcinoma cell lines may be elevated [14].

In the present study, we have compared the phosphotyrosyl phosphatase activity in lysates from representative colon carcinoma cells with that from cultures of normal colon mucosal cells. Our results demonstrate that the level of detectable phosphotyrosyl phosphatase activity in these lysates is not significantly different. However, incubation of colon carcinoma cells and normal colon mucosal cells with sodium vanadate, an inhibitor of cellular phosphotyrosyl phosphatase function [16–18], stimulates the kinase activity of pp60^{c-src} isolated from the normal colon cells but has no effect on the activity of pp60^{c-src} from the colon carcinoma cells. Additionally, our results demonstrate that the level of pp60^{c-src} kinase activity detected in immune-complex protein kinase assays can be substantially influenced by the type of buffer used for cell lysis.

MATERIALS AND METHODS
Cell Culture

Normal human colon mucosal cells (CCL 239) and human adenocarcinoma cell lines HT29 and WiDr were obtained from the American Type Culture Collection

(Rockville, MD). NIH 3T3 cells. Rous sarcoma virus-transformed NIH 3T3 cells (RSV 3T3), and NIH 3T3 (pMcsrc/cos)A cells, which are NIH 3T3 cells that over-express normal avian pp60[c-src] [4], were obtained from David Shalloway (Pennsylvania State University).

Cell Lysis and Protein Kinase Assays

Culture cells were lysed in either a modified RIPA buffer (20 mM morpholine-propanesulfonic acid pH 7.0, 150 mM NaCl, 1% (w/v) deoxycholate, 1% (v/v) Nonidet P-40, 0.1% (w/v) sodium dodecyl sulfate, and 2 mM ethylenediaminetetraa-cetic acid) or MNNE buffer (100 mM morpholinepropanesulfonic acid, pH 7.0, 100 mM NaCl, 1% (v/v) Nonidet P-40, and 1 mM ethylenediaminetetraacetic acid) containing 10 μg/ml each of the following protease inhibitors—aprotinin, leupeptin, N-tosyl-L-phenylalanine chloromethyl ketone, N-p-tosyl-L-lysine chloromethyl ke-tone, and phenylmethylsulfonyl fluoride, as previously described [14]. The protein concentration of the cellular lysates was adjusted to the indicated level and immuno-precipitation of pp60[c-src] was conducted as previously described [14] following addi-tion of MAb 327, a monoclonal antibody that recognizes avian and mammalian pp60[c-src] [19], or EC10, a monoclonal antibody that recognizes only avian pp60[c-src] [20]. Immune-complex protein kinase assays were performed on the washed immu-noprecipitates by the addition of kinase buffer (20 mM morpholinepropanesulfonic acid pH 7.0, 5mM MgCl$_2$) containing 20 μCi gamma ^{32}P ATP (3,000 Ci/mmol, New England Nuclear, Boston, MA) and 10 μM unlabeled ATP. The reactions were allowed to proceed for 10 min at 23°C with constant shaking. Casein and enolase phosphorylation in immune-complex protein kinase assays was conducted by addition of either 1 mg/ml alpha-casein (Sigma, St. Louis, MO) or 100 μg/ml rabbit muscle enolase (Sigma) to the kinase buffer. The samples were analyzed on 8% sodium dodecyl sulfate (SDS) polyacrylamide gels, the radioactive bands were detected by autoradiography, and the radioactivity was quantitated as previously described [14].

Metabolic Labeling and Immunoblot Analysis

Metabolic labeling of cells with either ^{35}S methionine or ^{32}P orthophosphate has been previously described [14]. Immunoblot analysis of pp60[c-src] using MAb 327/273 has also been described previously [14,21].

Peptide Mapping and Phosphoamino Acid Analysis

Determination of the phosphorylated amino acid products of immune-complex protein kinase reactions was conducted as previously described [22]. Analysis of the ^{32}P-labeled proteins by limited proteolysis using *Staphylococcus aureus* V8 protease (Pierce, Rockford, IL) has been described [23]. Total cellular phosphoamino acid analysis was conducted as described by Cooper et al [22].

RESULTS

Comparison of Total Cellular Phosphoamino Acids

Previously we reported that the activity of pp60[c-src] isolated from HT29 and WiDr colon carcinoma cells is elevated approximately 50- to 60-fold over that of pp60[c-src] isolated from normal colon mucosal cells [14,15]. To determine whether the elevation in tumor-derived pp60[c-src] kinase activity in in vitro immune-complex protein kinase assays is potentially reflected in vivo by elevation of phosphorylated proteins within the tumor cells, we conducted total cellular phosphoamino acid analysis. For these experiments HT29, WiDr, and CCL 239 cells were labeled for 18 hr with ^{32}P orthophosphate and the relative abundance of acid-stable phosphoserine, phosphothreonine, and phosphotyrosine was determined as described by Cooper et al [22]. We also conducted this analysis in parallel on NIH 3T3 and RSV NIH 3T3 cells. The results of these experiments are shown in Figure 1. As previously described by others [24], our results demonstrate that transformation of NIH 3T3 (Fig. 1C) cells with RSV (Fig. 1B) elevates the abundance of cellular phosphotyrosine. The increase was determined to be approximately tenfold, raising the relative abundance of phosphotyrosine in the NIH 3T3 cells from 0.1% to 0.96% in the RSV NIH 3T3 cells. The ratio of acid-stable phosphoamino acids in HT29 (Fig. 1D), WiDr (Fig. 1E), and CCL 239 (Fig. 1F) cells was found to be indistinguishable with phosphotyrosine representing approximately 0.07 to 0.12% of the detectable ^{32}P-labeled phosphoamino acids. Similar results were obtained when shorter labeling times were used (data not shown). Addition of 50 μM sodium vanadate to the cell culture medium during the 18-hr incubation with ^{32}P orthophosphate resulted in elevating the relative level of phosphotyrosine to approximately 0.25 to 0.35% in these cells. Significant differences in the response of the colon tumor cells and normal colon mucosal cells to the addition of vanadate were not detected.

Analysis of Phosphatase Activity in Immune-Complexes

The results obtained from phosphoamino acid analysis of normal and tumor-derived cells suggest that if pp60^{c-src} kinase activity is elevated in the tumor cells, the activity of cellular phosphotyrosyl phosphatases in these cells in the absence of vanadate may be sufficiently high so that no detectable elevation in cellular phosphotyrosine is evident. These observations could also indicate that the number of potential pp60^{c-src} substrates in the colon cells is limited. Alternatively, these results can be interpreted to suggest that pp60^{c-src} kinase activity in the colon tumor cells may not be elevated in vivo and becomes activated subsequent to cellular lysis. One obvious possibility is that cellular phosphatases might be nonspecifically coprecipitated in the immune-complexes derived from the tumor cell lysates thereby stimulating the activity of pp60^{c-src} in the immune-complex kinase assays by dephosphorylation of tyrosine residues.

To evaluate whether our immunoprecipitates contained phosphatase activity, CCL 239 and HT29 cells were labeled with ^{32}P orthophosphate or ^{35}S methionine for 8 hr prior to cell lysis and immunoprecipitation with MAb 327. The immune-complexes were washed according to our standard protocol; the samples were then divided into two equal aliquots and an immune-complex protein kinase assay using unlabeled ATP was conducted on one of the aliquots. The results of this experiment (Fig. 2) demonstrate that no detectable ^{32}P was lost from the normal or tumor-derived pp60^{c-src} samples which participated in the kinase assays (Fig. 2A), nor was there any detectable loss of ^{35}S-labeled pp60^{c-src} protein (Fig. 2B). In parallel experiments we observed that addition of 50 μM or 100 μM vanadate to the kinase buffer did not affect either the level of ^{32}P-labeled pp60^{c-src} or pp60^{c-src} protein kinase activity in the immune-complexes (data not shown).

To examine the possibility that ^{32}P corresponding to phosphoserine and phosphotyrosine could have been differentially lost from the ^{32}P in vivo labeled pp60^{c-src}

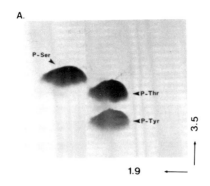

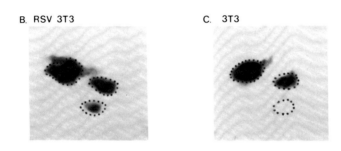

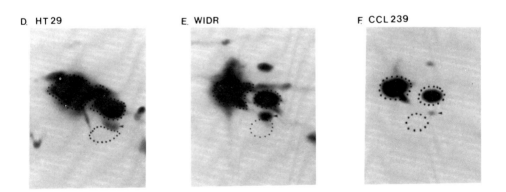

Fig. 1. Total cell phosphoamino acid analysis. Cell lines were labeled for 18 hr with ^{32}P orthophosphate and prepared for analysis of acid-stable phosphoamino acids as described in Materials and Methods. (A) Pattern of ninhydrin-stained phosphoamino acid standards following two-dimensional electrophoresis. The direction of electrophoresis at either pH 1.9 or pH 3.5 is shown. Autoradiograms of the resolved ^{32}P-labeled phosphoamino acids from RSV transformed NIH 3T3 cells (**B**), NIH 3T3 cells (**C**), HT29 cells (**D**), WiDr cells (**E**), and CCL 239 cells (**F**). The arrowheads in panels D–F show the position of a phosphorylated species described by Cooper et al [19] that contains exclusively phosphoserine upon further acid hydrolysis. The positions of ninhydrin-stained phosphoamino acid standards are indicated by the dotted lines on the autoradiograms.

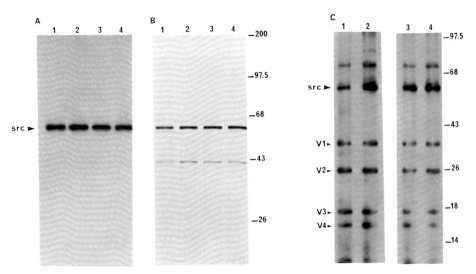

Fig. 2. Effect of immune-complex kinase assays on the level of ^{32}P orthophosphate-and ^{35}S methionine-labeled pp60[c-src] from normal colon cells and colon carcinoma cells; ^{32}P orthophosphate (**A**) and ^{35}S methionine (**B**) labeled CCL 239 cells (lanes 1, 2) or HT 29 cells (lanes 3,4) were lysed in RIPA buffer and immunoprecipitated by MAb 327. The amount of lysate from each cell was adjusted so that approximately equal amounts of ^{32}P or ^{35}S counts were present in the pp60[c-src] bands. Immune-complex protein kinase assays using 10 μM unlabeled ATP were conducted on the immunoprecipitates represented in lanes 2 and 4. (**C**) The ^{32}P-labeled pp60[c-src] bands shown in panel A analyzed by limited proteolysis using V8 protease. The samples represented in each lane are the same as given in panel A. The position of pp60[c-src] (src), various V8 phosphopeptides (VI–V4), and prestained molecular mass markers (BRL, Gaithersburg, MD) are indicated.

molecules, partial V8 proteolytic peptide analysis of the ^{32}P pp60[c-src] bands was conducted. The results of this analysis (Fig. 2C) show that the amount of amino-terminal phosphoserine contained in the V1, V3, and V4 V8 phosphopeptides and carboxy-terminal phosphotyrosine contained in the V2 V8 phosphopeptides was similar regardless of the immune-complex reaction conditions. These results demonstrate that phosphatase activity capable of significant dephosphorylation of either phosphoserine or phosphotyrosine residues from pp60[c-src] is not present in the MAb 327 immune-complexes.

Effect of Lysis Buffer Conditions and Vanadate on pp60[c-src] Kinase Activity

To determine whether incubation of the cells with vanadate would alter immune-complex pp60[c-src] kinase activity, CCL 239, HT29, and WiDr cells were cultured in the presence of 50 μM vanadate for 4 hr prior to lysis in RIPA buffer containing 50 μM vanadate. MAb 327 immune-complex protein kinase assays conducted with equal amounts of cellular protein from the lysates (500 μg/ml/reaction) show that incubation with vanadate does not significantly affect the kinase activity of pp60[c-src] derived from either the HT29 or WiDr colon carcinoma cells (Fig. 3, lanes 3–6). However, incubation of the normal colon mucosal cells with vanadate stimulates immune-complex pp60[c-src] protein kinase activity approximately fivefold (Fig. 3, lanes 1, 2). In parallel experiments, we also analyzed the effect of lysing the cells in MNNE buffer containing 100 μM vanadate in the presence and absence of 1 mM ATP and

RIPA

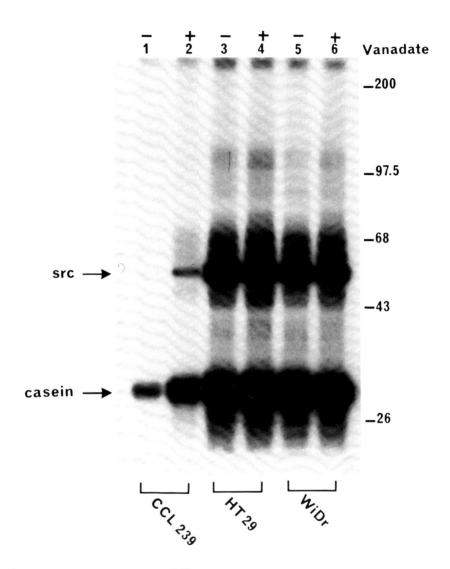

Fig. 3.   Protein kinase activity of pp60^{c-src} from vanadate-treated and untreated cells lysed in RIPA buffer. CCL 239 (**lanes 1, 2**), HT29 (**lanes 3, 4**), and WiDr cells (**lanes 5,6**) were cultured with (**lanes 2,4, 6**) or without (**lanes 1,3, 5**) 100 μM vanadate for 4 hr prior to lysis in RIPA buffer and MAb 327 immune-complex protein kinase assays were conducted as described in Materials and Methods. The positions of pp60^{c-src} (src), casein, and prestained molecular mass markers are indicated.

5 mM MgCl$_2$ on pp60^{c-src} immune-complex protein kinase activity. The results of this experiment demonstrate that addition of ATP and Mg^{2+} to the MNNE lysis buffer decreases the activity of pp60^{c-src} derived from in both the HT29 and WiDr cells (Fig. 4, lanes 3–6), while having no detectable effect on the activity of pp60^{c-src} derived from the normal colon mucosal cells (Fig. 4, lanes 1, 2).

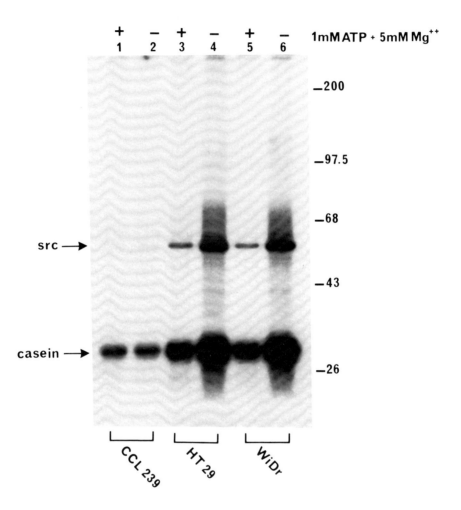

Fig. 4.   Effect of ATP and Mg^{2+} on the protein kinase activity of pp60^{c-src} from cells lysed in MNNE buffer. CCL 239 (**lanes 1, 2**), HT29 (**lanes 3, 4**), and WiDr cells (**lanes 5, 6**) were lysed in MNNE buffer in the presence and absence of 1 mM ATP and 5 mM Mg^{2+} and MAb 327 immune-complex protein kinase assays were conducted as described in Materials and Methods. The positions of pp60^{c-src} (src), casein, and prestained molecular mass markers are indicated.

The results of the immune-complex kinase assays illustrated in both Figures 3 and 4 were derived from experiments conducted simultaneously with equal cellular protein concentrations and the same exposure time of the autoradiograms (4 hr). Quantitation of the resulting ^{32}P-labeled pp60^{c-src} and casein radioactivity revealed that lysis of the colon carcinoma cells in RIPA buffer yielded pp60^{c-src} molecules with five- to sevenfold-higher levels of protein kinase activity than lysis of the same cells in MNNE buffer. Interestingly, the activity of pp60^{c-src} molecules derived from the normal colon carcinoma cells was not affected by the type of lysis buffer. Immunoblot analysis of the MAb 327 immunoprecipitates revealed that the same amount of pp60^{c-src} was present in the immune-complexes obtained by using either cell lysis buffer (data not shown). It should be noted that all of the immune-complexes represented in the experiments shown in Figures 3 and 4 were washed in RIPA buffer prior to performing the immune-complex protein kinase assays.

Analysis of Phosphatase Activity in Cellular Lysates

To assess the activity of phosphotyrosyl phosphatases in cellular lysates, we utilized as substrate in vitro phosphorylated avian $pp60^{c\text{-}src}$ molecules obtained from NIH 3T3 (pMcsrc/cos)A cells following lysis in RIPA buffer, immunoprecipitation with EC10, and immune-complex kinase assays. As shown in Figure 5, addition of MNNE buffer lysates from HT29 cells to the ^{32}P-labeled $pp60^{c\text{-}src}$ molecules in the EC10 immune-complexes results in time-dependent (Fig. 5A) and concentration-dependent (Fig. 5B) loss of phosphate from tyrosine residues. The reduction in ^{32}P from the $pp60^{c\text{-}src}$ molecules in the immune-complexes is not apparently the result of protein degradation by proteases in the cellular lysates since avian $pp60^{c\text{-}src}$ molecules metabolically labeled with ^{35}S methionine and used in a parallel experiment did not reveal time- and concentration-dependent losses of ^{35}S from the immunoprecipitates (Fig. 5C,D). Additional support for this conclusion is provided by the finding that the amount of avian $pp60^{c\text{-}src}$ detected by MAb 327/273 immunoblot analysis prior to and following incubation with the HT29 cell lysates is indistinguishable (Fig. 5F).

Incubation of HT29 cell lysates with the avian $pp60^{c\text{-}src}$ molecules in the EC10 immune-complexes was found to increase the protein kinase activity of these molecules approximately four- to fivefold (Fig. 5E). These results suggest that the specific activity of the avian $pp60^{c\text{-}src}$ molecules has been increased during the course of the experiment since no additional $pp60^{c\text{-}src}$ was found associated with the EC10 immune-complexes (Fig. 5F). These observations are similar to those of Cooper and King [9], who recently demonstrated that the specific activity of $pp60^{c\text{-}src}$ molecules could be elevated in vitro following a brief treatment with potato acid phosphatase which removes phosphate from both serine and tyrosine residues.

The ability of vanadate to inhibit dephosphorylation of tyrosine on $pp60^{c\text{-}src}$ molecules in EC10 immune-complexes is shown in Figure 6A. In this experiment, 100 μM vanadate was capable of protecting 80–90% of the phosphorylated tyrosine residues during a 30-min incubation with 200 μg of HT29 MNNE buffer lysate. The ability of vanadate to inhibit phosphotyrosyl phosphatase activity in the HT29 lysates was found to be concentration dependent and the phosphatase activity was also found to be sensitive to inhibition by 10 μM zinc (Fig. 6B). No effect on HT29 phosphotyrosyl phosphatase activity was observed by the addition of either 500 μg/ml phosphotyrosine or phosphothreonine or phosphoserine (Fig. 6B).

To compare the relative phosphotyrosyl phosphatase activity in colon carcinoma and normal colon mucosal cell lysates, ^{32}P-labeled avian $pp60^{c\text{-}src}$ autophosphorylated in EC10 immune-complexes was incubated for different times with MNNE buffer lysates from HT29 (Fig. 7A) and CCL 239 (Fig. 7B) cells adjusted to 200 μg cellular protein per reaction in the presence or absence of 100 μM vanadate. The results of this analysis show that the rate of phosphate hydrolysis catalyzed by addition of the HT29 lysates was elevated approximately twofold compared to the rate observed in CCL 239 lysates. The addition of vanadate was found to inhibit greater than 95% of the loss of ^{32}P from $pp60^{c\text{-}src}$ in these assays. The results of other experiments using the same ^{32}P-labeled $pp60^{c\text{-}src}$ substrate where the protein concentration of the CCL 239 and HT29 lysates was varied also demonstrated that the maximum detectable

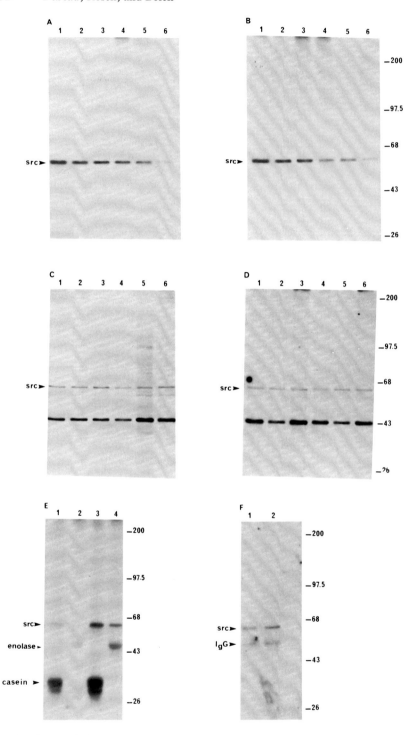

Fig. 5. Phosphotyrosyl phosphatase activity in HT29 cell lysates. (**A**) Equal amounts of in vitro phosphorylated avian pp60^{c-src} in EC10 immune-complexes were incubated for 0 (lane 1), 5 (lane 2), 10 (lane 3), 15 (lane 4), 20 (lane 5), or 30 (lane 6) min with 150 μg of HT29 MNNE cell lysate prior to analysis on SDS gels. (**B**) Equal amounts of in vitro phosphorylated avian pp60^{c-src} in EC10 immune-complexes were incubated for 15 min with 0 (lane 1), 25 (lane 2), 50 (lane 3), 100 (lane 4), 200 (lane 5), or 300 (lane 6) μg of HT29 MNNE cell lysate prior to analysis on SDS gels. (**C**, **D**) In vivo

difference in phosphatase activity from lysates of these cells was approximately twofold (data not shown).

Avian pp60[c-src] molecules autophosphorylate tyrosine residue 416 in immune-complex kinase reactions [25,26]. Thus, it is conceivable that phosphotyrosyl phosphatases that remove phosphate moieties from this tyrosine residue may be different than those which hydrolyze phosphate from tyrosine residue 527. To examine this possibility, NIH 3T3 (pMcsrc/cos)A cells were metabolically labeled with ^{32}P orthophosphate for 4 hr; the ^{32}P-labeled avian pp60[c-src] was immunoprecipitated with EC10, and the washed immune complexes were incubated for different times with equal amounts (200 μg protein/reaction) of MNNE buffer lysates from either CCL 239 (Fig. 7C) or HT29 (Fig. 7D) cells. The results of this experiment show that the initial rate of phosphate hydrolysis from the ^{32}P-labeled avian pp60[c-src] molecules

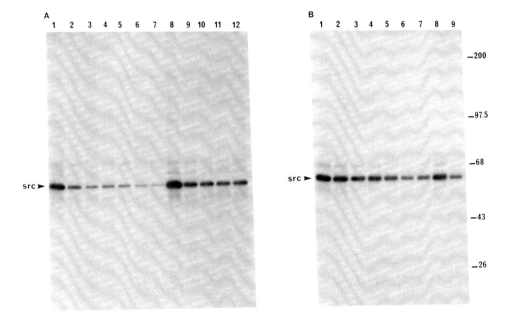

Fig. 6.   Effect of vanadate on phosphotyrosyl phosphatase activity in HT29 cell lysates. (A) Equal amounts of in vitro phosphorylated avian pp60[c-src] in EC10 immune-complexes were incubated with 200 μg of MNNE HT29 lysate for 0 (lanes 1, 8), 5 (lanes 2, 9), 10 (lanes 3, 10), 15 (lane 4), 20 (lanes 5, 11), 25 (lane 6), or 30 min (lanes 7, 12) in the absence (lanes 1–7) or presence (lanes 8–12) of 100 μM vanadate. (B) Equal amounts of in vitro phosphorylated avian pp60[c-src] in EC10 immune-complexes were incubated with 200 μg HT29 lysate for 0 (lanes 2, 4) or 15 min (lanes 1,3,5–9) in the presence of 100 μM vanadate (lane 1), 10 μM vanadate (lane 3), 1 μM vanadate (lane 5), 500 μg/ml phosphothreonine (lane 6), 500 μg/ml phosphotyrosine (lane 7), 10 μM ZnCl (lane 8), or 500 μg/ml phosphoserine (lane 9). The positions of pp60[c-src] (src) and prestained molecular mass markers are indicated.

[35]S-methionine-labeled avian pp60[c-src] in EC10 immune-complexes used in parallel experiments to those described in panels A (C) and B (D). (E) Equal amounts of unlabeled avian pp60[c-src] in EC10 immune-complexes were incubated in the absence (lanes 1, 2) or presence (lanes 3, 4) of 300 μg HT29 MNNE lysate for 15 min prior to conducting casein (lanes 1, 3) or enolase (lanes 2, 4) kinase assays. (F) MAb 327/273 immunoblot analysis of avian pp60[c-src] in EC10 immune-complexes prior to (lane 1) or following (lane 2) incubation with 300 μg HT29 MNNE lysate for 15 minutes.

DeSeau, Rosen, and Bolen

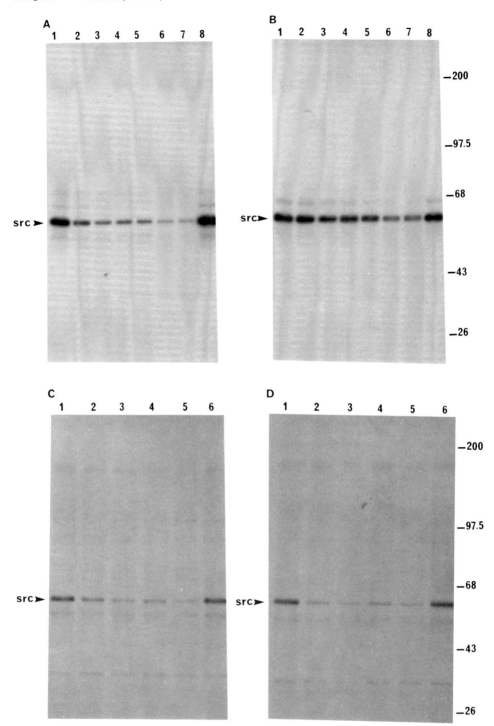

Fig. 7. Comparison of phosphatase activity in lysates of normal colon mucosal cells and colon carcinoma cells. Equal amounts of in vitro phosphorylated (**A, B**) or in vivo phosphorylated (**C,D**) avian pp60^{c-src} in EC10 immune-complexes were incubated with 200 μg of HT29 (A, C) or CCL 239 (B,D) cell lysates for 0 (lane 1), 5 (lane 2), 10 (lane 3), 15 (panels A, B, lanes 4), 20 (panels A, B, lanes 5; panels C, D, lanes 4), 25 (panels A, B, lanes 6), or 30 min (panels A, B, lanes 7, 8; panels C, D, lanes 5, 6) in the presence (panels A, B, lanes 8; panels C, D, lanes 6) or absence (all other lanes) of 100 μM vanadate. The positions of pp60^{c-src} (src) and prestained molecular mass markers are indicated.

incubated with HT29 lysates was faster than that observed with CCL 239 lysates. However, by 10 min the rate of phosphate hydrolysis by the two cell lysates was indistinguishable. Partial proteolytic V8 peptide mapping of the ^{32}P-labeled pp60^{c-src} molecules from this experiment revealed that both amino-terminal serine and carboxy-terminal tyrosine residues were being dephosphorylated at comparable rates (data not shown). Addition of 100 μM vanadate to the lysates was found to inhibit approximately 80–90% of the phosphotyrosyl phosphatase and phosphoserine phosphatase activity in the cell lysates.

The interactions of cellular phosphatases from colon cells with pp60^{c-src} in the immune-complexes could be altered by the association of pp60^{c-src} with the monoclonal antibody or other components in the immune-complexes. To examine this possibility, equal amounts of MNNE buffer lysate (50 μg protein/reaction) from ^{32}P orthophosphate metabolically labeled NIH 3T3 (pMcsrc/cos)A cells were incubated with increasing amounts of MNNE buffer lysates from CCL 239 (Fig. 8A), HT29 (Fig. 8B), or WiDr (Fig. 8C) cells for 20 min prior to addition of 100 μM vanadate and EC10 antibody. The results of this study show that the rate of phosphate hydrolysis from the avian pp60^{c-src} molecules in the lysates prior to immunoprecipitation did not differ significantly between the normal colon mucosal and colon carcinoma cell lysates. As previously observed, the addition of 100 μM vanadate to the cellular lysates protected approximately 80%–90% of the pp60^{c-src}-associated ^{32}P label.

DISCUSSION

The protein kinase activity of pp60^{c-src} derived from human colon carcinoma cell lines, such as HT29 and WiDr, has been observed to be elevated in in vitro

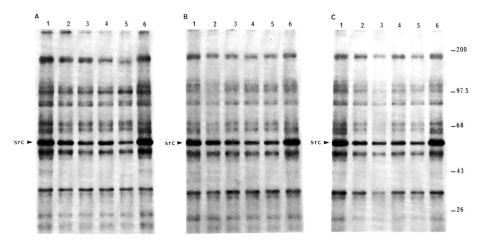

Fig. 8. Comparison of phosphatase activity in lysates of normal colon mucosal cells and colon carcinoma cells using soluble pp60^{c-src} substrate. Equal amounts (50 μg) of ^{32}P-orthophosphate-labeled (pMcsrc/cos)A NIH 3T3 MNNE cell lysates were incubated for 20 min with 0 (lane 1), 50 (lane 2), 100 (lane 3), 200 (lane 4), or 300 μg (lanes 5, 6) of MNNE lysate from CCL 239 (A), HT29 (B), or WiDr cells (C) in the presence (lane 6) or absence (all other lanes) of 100 μM vanadate prior to addition of 100 μM vanadate to all reactions and immunoprecipitation of avian pp60^{c-src} with EC10 antibody. The positions of pp60^{c-src} (src) and prestained molecular mass markers are shown.

protein kinase assays 50- to 60-fold over that of pp60^{c-src} derived from normal mucosal cells [15]. Comparison of the relative abundance of pp60^{c-src} in these cells by immunoblot analysis suggests that the apparent specific activity of pp60^{c-src} from the colon tumor cell lines is ten- to 30-fold higher than pp60^{c-src} from normal colon mucosal cells [14]. The elevated activity of pp60^{c-src} molecules from the colon tumor cells is associated with an apparent six-fold increase in the turnover rate of phosphate from tyrosine residues within the carboxy-terminal portion of the protein, suggesting that differences in the activity of phosphotyrosyl phosphatase may exist between the normal and tumor-derived cells [14].

The results presented in the report indicate that while phosphatase activity which acts to dephosphorylate pp60^{c-src} tyrosine residues may differ between normal colon mucosal cells and colon carcinoma cells in vivo by as much as sixfold or more, less than one- to twofold differences are detectable in the in vitro activity of phosphotyrosyl phosphatases in lysates prepared from these cells. These results include analysis of phosphate hydrolysis from avian pp60^{c-src} tyrosine residues 416 (Figs. 5–7) and tyrosine 527 (Fig. 7) in immune-complexes and hydrolysis of pp60^{c-src} tyrosine residue 527 in cellular lysates (Fig. 8). Similar conclusions were reached when mammalian pp60^{c-src} in MAb 327 immune-complexes was utilized in several of these assays (our unpublished result). We have also varied the lysis conditions of the normal and colon tumor cells by analyzing different combinations of detergent, pH, and salt concentrations and we varied the reaction conditions without successful demonstration of significant differences in phosphatase activity between lysates prepared from CCL 239 and HT29 cells (our unpublished results). Thus, most of our data suggest that differences in phosphatase activity do not exist between normal colon cells and colon carcinoma cells. We cannot rule out, however, the possibility that lysis of the cells using the condition tried to date has destroyed the normal cellular microenvironment which may be essential to the putative pp60^{c-src}/phosphatase interactions previously proposed [14].

Analysis of the relative abundance of stable phosphotyrosine-containing proteins in CCL 239, HT29, and WiDr cells revealed that significant differences are not evident (Fig. 1). As previously noted, these results could indicate that pp60^{c-src}-specific substrates in these cells might be limited in number. In addition, it is possible that potential protein substrates of pp60^{c-src} in these cells might have very short half-lives or are rapidly dephosphorylated. Addition of vanadate to the culture medium of these cells was found to marginally elevate the overall level of phosphotyrosine, but failed to illicit significant alterations between the normal and tumor cells. Differences in tyrosine phosphorylation of suspected pp60^{c-src} substrates such as calpactin I [27–29] were also not observed in these cells in the presence or absence of vanadate (our unpublished results). Thus, no measurable effect of vanadate on the potential in vivo activity of pp60^{c-src} could be demonstrated.

However, the presence of vanadate in the culture medium was found to significantly stimulate pp60^{c-src} in vitro kinase activity from normal colon mucosal cells while having no detectable effect on the activity of pp60^{c-src} derived from colon carcinoma cells (Fig. 3). Analysis of ^{32}P orthophosphate-labeled pp60^{c-src} molecules isolated from vanadate-treated CCL 239 and HT29 cells by V8 digestion did not reveal detectable differences in the ratio of phosphoserine to phosphotyrosine (our unpublished result). We have not conducted ^{32}P pulse-chase analysis with pp60^{c-src} molecules in the presence or absence of vanadate in these cells. While the mechanism for these observations is currently unclear, they do demonstrate differences in the response of normal colon and colon tumor cells to vanadate. Whether the observed differences are directly related to the effect of vanadate on cellular phosphatases or other cellular functions that might modulate pp60c-src kinase activity needs to be clarified. An additional possibility that could account for the differences in the observed characteristics of pp60^{c-src} molecules derived from the normal and tumor cells is that the *c-src* gene in either the tumor cells or in the cultured "normal" mucosal cells has undergone mutational alterations. We are currently analyzing other tyrosine kinases, including other members of the src "subfamily" of tyrosine kinases, in these cells to see if alterations in activity of these protein kinases or differences in phosphate turnover from these proteins can be detected.

An additional point raised by our experiments is that the in vitro kinase activity of pp60^{c-src} derived from normal colon mucosal cells and colon carcinoma cells can vary significantly depending on the cellular lysis buffer (Figs. 3,4). In this case, the alterations in pp60^{c-src} kinase activity as a function of lysis buffer conditions was limited to the colon carcinoma cells. Since the same amount of pp60^{c-src} was present in the immune-complexes derived from the colon carcinoma cells lysed by either the RIPA or MNNE buffers, these results suggest that the specific activity of these molecules was altered by postlysis events. We believe that the observed activation of pp60^{c-src} in cells lysed in RIPA buffer is independent of phosphatase interactions since 100 μM vanadate was present in both lysis buffers. The mechanism responsible for the further decrease in pp60^{c-src} kinase activity following addition of ATP and Mg^{2+} to the MNNE buffer in the tumor cell lysates is also unclear. With RIPA buffer lysates, the difference in specific activty of pp60^{c-src} between normal colon mucosal cells and colon carcinoma cells is about ten-to thirtyfold. However, with a lysis buffer which contains only Nonidet-P 40 as a detergent source, the difference in specific activity of pp60^{c-src} between normal colon and colon carcinoma cells would be less than three- to fourfold. These observations suggest that comparing of the results of pp60^{c-src} in vitro protein kinase assays in other cellular systems where only RIPA buffer lysis has been used should be interpreted with caution.

ACKNOWLEDGMENTS

We thank Joan Brugge and Sarah Parsons for providing the monclonal antibodies to pp60^{c-src}, Tony Hunter for the monoclonal antibody to human calpactin I, and David Shalloway for the various NIH 3T3 cells. We also thank Peter Howley, Joyce O'Shaughnessy, and Andre Veillette for critically reading the manuscript.

REFERENCES

1. Bishop JM: Cell 42:23, 1985.
2. Hunter T, Cooper JA: Annu Rev Biochem 54:897, 1985.
3. Iba H, Cross FR, Garber EA, Hanafusa H: Mol Cell Biol 5:1058, 1985.
4. Coussens PM, Cooper, JA, Hunter T, Shalloway D: Mol Cell Biol 5:2753, 1985.
5. Hanafusa H, Iba H, Takeya T, Cross FR: In Vande Woude G, Levine A, Topp W, Watson J (eds): "Cancer Cells II: Oncogenes and Viral Genes." New York: Cold Spring Harbor Laboratory, 1984, pp 1–17.
6. Levy JB, Iba H, Hanafusa H: Proc Natl Acad Sci USA 83:4228, 1986.
7. Kato J, Takeya T, Grandori C, Iba H, Levy JB, Hanafusa H: Mol Cell Biol 6:4155, 1986.

8. Courtneidge S: EMBO J 4:1471, 1985.
9. Cooper JA, King CS: Mol Cell Biol 6:4467, 1986.
10. Cooper JA, Gould KL, Cartwright CA, Hunter T: Science 231:1431, 1986.
11. Kmiecik TE, Shalloway D: Cell 49:65, 1987.
12. Piwnica-Worms H, Saunders KB, Roberts TM, Smith A, Cheng SH: Cell 49:75, 1987.
13. Cartwright CA, Eckhart W, Simon S, Kaplan PL: Cell 49:83, 1987.
14. Bolen JB, Veillette A, Schwartz AM, DeSeau V, Rosen N: Oncogene Res 1:149, 1987.
15. Bolen JB, Veillette A, Schwartz AM, DeSeau V, Rosen N: Proc Natl Acad Sci USA 87:2251, 1987.
16. Brautigan DL, Bornstein P, Gallis B: J Biol Chem 256:6519, 1981.
17. Foulkes JG, Erikson E, Erikson RL: J Biol Chem 258:431, 1983.
18. Nelson RL, Branton PE: Mol Cell Biol 4:1003, 1984.
19. Lipsich LA, Lewis AJ, Brugge JS: J Virol 48:352, 1983.
20. Parsons SJ, McCarley DJ, Ely CM, Benjamin C, Parsons JT: J Virol 51:272, 1984.
21. Rosen N, Bolen JB, Schwartz AM, Cohen P, DeSeau V, Israel MA: J Biol Chem 261:13754, 1986.
22. Cooper JA, Sefton BM, Hunter T: Methods Enzymol 99:387, 1983.
23. Bolen JB, Israel MA: J Biol Chem 259:11686, 1984.
24. Sefton BM, Hunter T, Beemon K, Eckhart W: Cell 20:807, 1980.
25. Patschiasky T, Hunter T, Esch FS, Cooper JA, Sefton BM: Proc Natl Acad Sci USA 79:973, 1982.
26. Smart JE, Opperman H, Czernilofsky AP, Puricho AF, Erikson RL, Bishop JM: Proc Natl Acad Sci USA 78:6013, 1981.
27. Huang KS, Wallner BP, Mattaliano RJ, Tizard R, Burne C, Frey A, Hession C, McGray P, Sinclair LK, Chow EP, Browning JL, Ramachandran KL, Tang J, Smart JE, Pepinsky RB: Cell 46:191, 1986.
28. Saris CJM, Tack BF, Kristensen T, Glenney JR, Hunter T: Cell 46:201, 1986.
29. Weber K, Johnson N: FEBS Lett 203:95, 1986.

Journal of Cellular Biochemistry 35:305–314 (1987)
Growth Regulation of Cancer 55–64

Characterization of a Hepatic Proliferation Inhibitor (HPI): Effect of HPI on the Growth of Normal Liver Cells—Comparison With Transforming Growth Factor Beta

Anthony C. Huggett, Henry C. Krutzsch, and Snorri S. Thorgeirsson

Laboratory of Experimental Carcinogenesis, Division of Cancer Etiology, National Cancer Institute, Bethesda, Maryland 20892

Improvements in the purification of a hepatic proliferation inhibitor (HPI) from adult rat liver have yielded a product that has an inhibitory activity 1,000-fold greater than previously reported. The growth inhibitory activity, which could be eluted from SDS-PAGE at 17–19 kilodaltons (kD), was compared to that of transforming growth factor beta (TGF-β). The ID_{50} of the HPI preparation in Fischer rat liver epithelial cells was 50 pg/ml (2.5 pM) compared to a value of 260 pg/ml (10.4 pM) obtained for pure human TGF-β. Both inhibitors also modulated the stimulation of DNA synthesis in primary hepatocytes by either epidermal growth factor or a growth stimulatory activity prepared from serum of hepatectomized rats. The ID_{50}s of HPI and TGF-β in these cells were 250 pg/ml and 40 pg/ml, respectively. In contrast to TGF-β the growth inhibitory activity of HPI was unaltered in the presence of an antibody raised against TGF-β. The possible mechanism of action of HPI is discussed.

Key words: growth inhibition, primary hepatocytes, liver epithelial cells

The characterization of factors that control cellular proliferation is central to the understanding of both normal and neoplastic growth. Although much progress has been made in the last few years toward the identification and characterization of polypeptide growth factors that stimulate cell proliferation, there has been much less success in the isolation and characterization of growth inhibitory polypeptides with the notable exception of transforming growth factor beta (TGF-β).

The purification of a hepatic proliferation inhibitory protein (HPI) was reported in 1982 by McMahon et al [1]. This protein, which was isolated from normal rat liver, specifically and reversibly inhibited cell division and DNA synthesis in a number of nonmalignant rat liver epithelial cell types, although it had no effect on transformed liver cells [2]. Subsequent analysis has indicated that the preparation was

Received February 19, 1987; revised and accepted June 3, 1987.

not homogeneous, the apparent single band on SDS-PAGE (26 kD) being due to a contaminant [3]. Recently, a number of improvements have been made to the purification scheme for this protein which have yielded a product that has an inhibitory activity 1,000-fold greater than that previously reported [3].

The best characterized endogenous inhibitor of normal cell proliferation is the multifunctional polypeptide TGF-β, a 25-kilodalton (kD) dimer consisting of two identical chains of 112 amino acids [4]. It has been demonstrated that TGF-β is a strong inhibitor of proliferation of many primary and secondary cell types including embryo fibroblasts [5], T and B lymphocytes [6,7], keratinocytes [8], and bronchial epithelial cells [9]. Recently, several other proteins including a growth inhibitor from the conditioned medium of monkey kidney cells (BSC-1) [10], a cartilage-inducing peptide (CIF-A) isolated from bovine bone [11], and a differentiation inhibitor (DI) secreted by Buffalo rat liver cells [12] have been shown to be similar to or identical with TGF-β. In addition, other regulatory peptides including inhibin [13] and Mullerian inhibitory substance (MIS) [14] have been found to have structural homology to TGF-β.

The wide tissue distribution of TGF-β [4], its molecular weight, and the finding that it is a potent inhibitor of DNA synthesis in primary hepatocytes [15–18] has prompted speculation that TGF-β and HPI are identical molecules [15]. The recent observation that TGF-β is produced by oval cells within the liver (personal communication, N. Fausto) has added further support to this possibility. In the present study we have further characterized HPI by means of SDS-PAGE and have utilized freshly isolated hepatocytes and a normal diploid rat liver cell line to compare the growth inhibitory activities of TGF-β and HPI.

MATERIALS AND METHODS
Cells and Materials

The cell line of normal liver epithelial cells (RLE) was maintained in culture as described previously [16] and for this study was used between the 13th and 18th passage in vitro. Primary hepatocytes were isolated from a male F344 rat (150 g) by the two-step collagenase perfusion technique of Evarts et al [19]. Waymouth MB 752/1 medium was purchased from Gibco Laboratories (Grand Island, NY); Hams F-12 medium was a product of Biofluids Inc. (Rockville, MD); and the cell culture supplements, collagen type IV, and [^{125}I]-epidermal growth factor (EGF) (122 μCi/μg) were obtained from Collaborative Research (Lexington, MA). "Defined" fetal bovine serum was from HyClone Laboratories Inc. (Alexandria, VA). Methyl-[^{3}H]-thymidine (102 μCi/μg) was purchased from Amersham Corporation (Arlington Heights, IL). Pure TGF-β, isolated from human platelets [20], and a rabbit antibody raised against human TGF-β [21], which is specific to mature 25 kD TGF-β (personal communication, A. Roberts), were gifts of Dr. Michael Sporn, NCI. HPI was purified by the method of Krutzsch et al [3]. The most highly purified form available was used for all studies except in the gel elution study where a partially purified preparation was used. All other materials were obtained from sources described previously [22].

Elution of HPI From SDS-PAGE

A crude preparation (1 μg total protein) containing HPI activity (ID$_{50}$: 500 pg/ml for RLE cells) was subjected to SDS-PAGE [23] under nonreducing conditions using a 12.5% polyacrylamide gel. Gel slices (5 mm) were excised and extracted at 4°C for 16 hr in 1 ml Ham's F-12 medium containing 10% "defined" fetal bovine serum (FBS). The extracts were then dialyzed at 4°C for 48 hr against PBS (pH 7.4) prior to the analysis of 10-μl aliquots for growth-inhibitory activity using RLE cells.

Purification of Hepatocyte Growth Factor

A crude preparation of a serum-derived hepatocyte growth factor (serum-HGF) was prepared by heparin affinity chromatography of serum obtained from F-334 rats (180 g) 24 hr after partial hepatectomy as described previously [24]. The active fraction, tested for stimulation of primary hepatocyte proliferation in serum-free cell culture, was further purified by gel filtration (Sephadex G-100), concentrated, and assayed for protein content by the method of Bradford [25] using bovine serum albumin as the standard.

Measurement of DNA Synthesis in Primary Hepatocytes

Freshly isolated hepatocytes were washed with Ham's F-12 medium containing 10% FBS supplemented with insulin (6.25 μg/ml), transferrin (6.25 μg/ml), selenium (6.25 ng/ml), and dexamethasone (20 ng/ml). The cells were seeded in 96-well microtiter plates, precoated with type IV collagen, at a density of 4.5 $\times$ 10^4 cells/ cm^2 and incubated at 37°C in a humidified atmosphere of 5% CO$_2$/95% air. The medium was replaced at 4 hr with serum-free defined medium. This consisted of Waymouth's medium supplemented with insulin (6.25 μg/ml), transferrin (6.25 μg/ ml), selenium (6.25 ng/ml), dexamethasone (20 ng/ml), bovine serum albumin (1.25 mg/ml), and linoleic acid (5.35 μg/ml). Following incubation for 16 hr, the medium was replaced with serum-free defined medium containing EGF (10 ng/ml) or HGF (50 μg/ml) together with HPI or TGF-β at various concentrations. After 4 hr methyl-[^{3}H]-thymidine (0.5 μCi) was added to each well and the cells were incubated for a further 48 hr prior to measurement of DNA content and DNA synthesis as described by Richards et al [22].

Measurement of RLE Cell Proliferation

RLE cells were seeded into 96-well microtiter plates at a density of 2.7 $\times$ 10^4 cells/cm^2. The effect of HPI and TGF-β on the extent of DNA synthesis and cell proliferation was assayed by the modification of the method of Richards et al [22] as described by McMahon et al [16].

Effect of Anti-TGF-β Antibody on Activity of Inhibitors

The effect of a rabbit antibody raised against human TGF-β on the activity of HPI and TGF-β was examined using RLE cells. Samples containing the antibody (8.3 μg/ml) and various concentrations of HPI or TGF-β in Ham's F-12 media containing 10% FBS were incubated at 37°C for 4 hr prior to their analysis for inhibitory activity. The IgG fraction (8.3 μg/ml) of normal rabbit preimmune serum [21] was used as a control.

Measurement of EGF Binding

Radioreceptor binding assays were performed using A-431 human carcinoma cells according to previously described procedures [26]. The effect of HPI pretreatment of cells on EGF-receptor binding was studied by incubating the A-431 cells for

2 hr at 37°C in a humidified atmosphere of 5% CO_2/95% air with 280 pg/ml HPI prior to the analysis of $[^{125}I]$-EGF binding.

RESULTS

The elution of growth-inhibitory activity from a polyacrylamide gel following SDS-PAGE analysis of a partially purified sample previously shown to possess HPI activity (ID_{50}:500 pg/ml) indicated a molecular weight for this activity of 17–19 kD (Fig. 1). The analysis of gel extracts from a lane in which bovine serum albumin was electrophoresed in parallel with the HPI sample indicated that this inhibitory activity was specific to the HPI sample and not due to gel contaminants.

The growth-inhibitory activities of HPI and TGF-β were initially compared using freshly isolated primary hepatocytes. These cells were stimulated to undergo DNA synthesis by the addition of either EGF (10 ng/ml) or HGF (50 μg/ml). These concentrations produced about a tenfold increase in methyl-$[^{3}H]$-thymidine incorporation over basal levels, although there was no significant change in cell number over the 48-hr time course of the experiment. Both HPI and TGF-β produced a dose-dependent decrease in the stimulation of DNA synthesis by EGF, and at the highest concentrations tested, both inhibitors were able to block completely the stimulation of DNA synthesis in these cells (Fig. 2). Essentially identical results were obtained when DNA synthesis was stimulated with HGF. The ID_{50} concentrations for the HPI- and TGF-β-dependent inhibition of DNA synthesis, 250 pg/ml and 40 pg/ml, respectively, were independent of the mitogen employed. It must be noted that the purity of

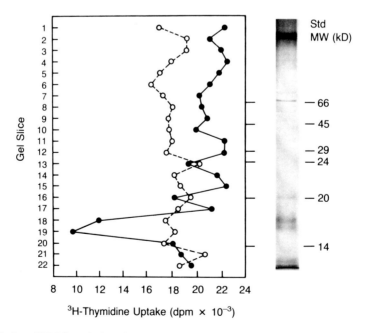

Fig. 1. Elution of HPI from SDS-PAGE. A crude preparation (1 μg total protein) containing HPI (ID_{50} = 500 pg/ml) was subjected to SDS-PAGE (12.5% acrylamide). Gel slices (5 mm) were extracted with Ham's F-12 medium containing 10% FBS. The extracts were then dialyzed against PBS (pH 7.4) prior to analysis for inhibitory growth activity using RLE cells (●). A control sample containing 1 μg albumin was analyzed in parallel (○). A silver-stained gel of the HPI preparation is also shown.

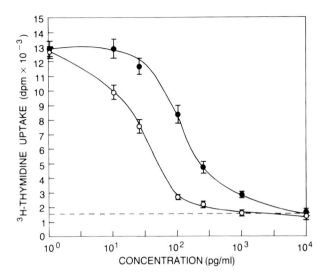

Fig. 2. The effect of HPI and TGF-β on EGF-induced DNA synthesis in primary hepatocyte cultures. EGF (10 ng/ml) together with various concentrations of HPI (●) or TGF-β (○) were added to primary hepatocyte cultures, and the incorporation of methyl-[^{3}H]-thymidine into cellular DNA was measured for 48 hr (mean $\pm$ SEM, n = 6). The dotted line indicates the basal level of DNA synthesis in the absence of EGF.

the HPI preparation is as yet unknown, and so the total protein concentration of the preparation has been used for the determination of the ID$_{50}$ concentrations for HPI.

The effect of HPI and TGF-β on DNA synthesis in RLE cells was also examined using a 96-well microtiter assay. However, as these cells proliferate during the time course of the assay, the extent of DNA synthesis, measured as incorporation of methyl-[^{3}H]-thymidine, was normalized to the cell number by dividing the [^{3}H]-dpm value with the DNA fluorescence value. Previous studies have demonstrated that this fluorescence value has a linear relationship with cell number [22]. HPI and TGF-β inhibited both DNA synthesis and cell proliferation of RLE cells in a dose-dependent manner, and the ID$_{50}$ concentrations of each were 50 pg/ml and 260 pg/ml, respectively (Fig. 3). It is of note that although the highest dose of TGF-β was almost completely able to block DNA synthesis in RLE cells, the maximal inhibition that could be obtained with HPI was about 75%.

In studies designed to distinguish the growth-inhibitory activities of HPI and TGF-β in RLE cells, it was found that the activity of HPI was essentially unchanged following its incubation with an anti-TGF-β antibody (Fig. 4A). In contrast, the dose-response curve for TGF-β inhibition of RLE cell DNA synthesis was shifted to the right following treatment of the TGF-β sample with the anti-TGF-β antibody (Fig. 4B). The ID$_{50}$ for TGF-β was increased from about 300 pg/ml to 1.6 ng/ml in the presence of the antibody.

The possibility that the inhibitory effects of HPI are mediated by an effect on EGF-receptor binding was investigated using A431 cells as only a limited degree of [^{125}I]-EGF binding was obtained using RLE cells. Preincubation of A-431 cells with HPI (280 pg/ml) for 2 hr at 37°C (5% CO_2/95% air) had no effect on the subsequent binding of EGF to its receptor (Fig. 5).

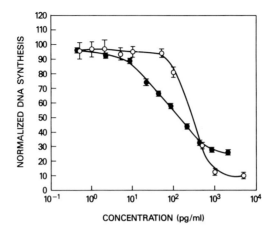

Fig. 3.   The effect of HPI and TGF-β on the proliferation of RLE cells. Various concentrations of HPI (●) or TGF-β (○) were added to proliferating RLE cell cultures. The incorporation of methyl-[^{3}H]-thymidine incorporation, normalized by cell number was then measured in a 2-hr pulse following a 48-hr incubation (mean $\pm$ SEM, n = 8).

DISCUSSION

The finding that TGF-β is a negative growth regulator in addition to being able to stimulate the proliferation of some cell types [27,28] has lent further support to the hypothesis that cellular homeostasis is the result of a delicate balance between the influence of growth factors and growth inhibitors. Although the identification of polypeptide growth factors has proceeded at an ever-increasing rate over the past few years, only a very few growth-inhibitory proteins have been isolated, and many of these have been found to be related or identical with TGF-β. This has led to the speculation that the liver-derived hepatic proliferation inhibitor is identical with TGF-β. In this paper we provide evidence that TGF-β and HPI are distinct growth inhibitors, although both produce similar effects on the growth of liver-derived normal cells in vitro.

The previously determined molecular weight and isoelectric point for HPI [1], 26 kD and 4.65, respectively, were based on the analysis by SDS-PAGE and isoelectric focusing of a preparation which was subsequently shown to contain a major contaminant responsible for the single band that was observed on staining of the gels with Coomassie blue [3]. Analysis of the present HPI preparation using chromatofocusing indicated an isoelectric point of 5.5 and elution of the activity through a gel filtration column (ACA44) was consistent with a molecular weight of about 26 kD [3]. However, the elution of growth-inhibitory activity from SDS-PAGE (Fig. 1) indicates a molecular weight for HPI in the range 17–19 kD. This apparent discrepancy may be due to the fact that the electrophoresis was performed in the presence of SDS in which reversible protein denaturation occurs, while the gel filtration elution was carried out in conditions favoring the native conformation of proteins. In addition, molecular weight data obtained from gel filtration experiments may be unreliable owing to protein-protein or protein-gel interactions. The silver-stained protein bands which appeared to comigrate with the activity on SDS-PAGE (Fig. 1) were from contaminants in the relatively crude HPI preparation used and were found to have no inhibitory activity. The elution of growth inhibitory activity from SDS-PAGE pro-

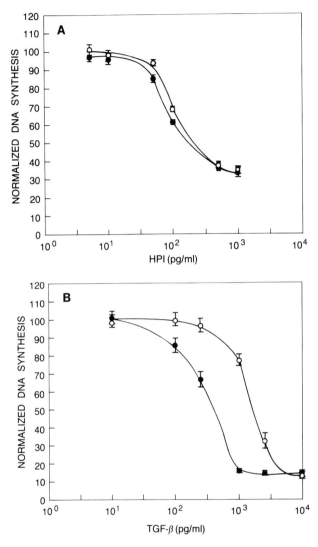

Fig. 4. The effect of anti-TGF-β antibody on the inhibition of RLE cell proliferation by TGF-β or HPI. **A:** Various concentrations of HPI were incubated for 4 hr with an anti-TGF-β antibody (8.3 μg/ml; ○) or an IgG control (●). The samples were then added to RLE cell cultures and normalized DNA synthesis was measured after 48 hr (mean ± SEM, n = 8). **B:** Various concentrations of TGF-β were incubated for 4 hr with an anti-TGF-β antibody (8.3 μg/ml; ○) or an IgG control (●). The samples were then added to RLE cell cultures, and DNA synthesis, normalized against cell number, was measured after 48 hr (mean ± SEM, n = 8).

vides further evidence that this activity is not due to TGF-β as previous experiments have demonstrated that TGF-β is eluted from SDS-PAGE at a position corresponding to a molecular weight of 25 kD [29]. Other physical/chemical studies performed on the highly purified HPI preparation also indicate that HPI and TGF-β are different polypeptides [3].

This is the first report demonstrating the inhibitory activity of HPI on growth-factor-stimulated DNA synthesis in primary hepatocyte cultures. The uptake of

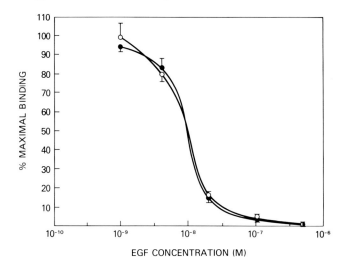

Fig. 5. The effect of preincubation with HPI on subsequent [^{125}I]-EGF binding to A431 cells. HPI (280 pg/ml) was incubated with A431 cells for 2 hr at 37°C. The cells were then washed and examined for EGF-receptor binding (●). A control experiment in which there was no preincubation of cells with HPI was performed in parallel (○) (mean ± SD, n = 4).

methyl-[^{3}H]-thymidine was studied in serum-free cell cultures plated at low cell density, conditions favoring maximal mitogen-induced DNA synthesis. The increase in methyl-[^{3}H]-thymidine uptake induced by either EGF or serum-HGF was totally abolished in the presence of the highest concentrations of HPI or TGF-β tested. Serum-HGF is a serum form of a growth-stimulatory activity for hepatocytes released by platelets which is different from platelet-derived growth factor (PDGF) and EGF [30]. Both HPI and TGF-β also inhibited DNA synthesis and cell proliferation in RLE cell cultures. However, in contrast to the results obtained with the primary hepatocyte cultures, the ID$_{50}$ for the HPI preparation was lower than that for TGF-β. In addition, the dose-response profiles for the two inhibitors were different for the RLE cells, a much steeper curve being observed for TGF-β than HPI. Although TGF-β, at the highest concentrations tested, produced almost a complete inhibition of DNA synthesis and cell proliferation, the maximal inhibition that could be achieved using HPI was about 75%. Further studies have indicated that the RLE cells become more resistant to the growth-inhibitory effects of HPI with increasing passage number. These results not only indicate that TGF-β and HPI are different molecules but also suggest that their inhibitory activity in these cells is mediated through different mechanisms. This finding is supported by previous studies which have demonstrated that HPI is a reversible inhibitor of proliferation of the RLE cells [1], while the inhibition of RLE cell proliferation produced by TGF-β appears to be irreversible and may in fact lead to a more differentiated phenotype [16]. A similar finding has been reported when human bronchial epithelial cells were treated with TGF-β [9]. Additional evidence indicating that HPI and TGF-β are different polypeptides is provided by the results of the experiments utilizing an anti-TGF-β antibody. Although the antibody was able markedly to reduce the inhibitory effects of TGF-β on the proliferation of RLE cells, it had no effect on the inhibition of growth induced by

HPI. The antibody (8.3 μg/ml) was able to abolish completely the inhibitory effect of the normal ID$_{50}$ concentration of TGF-β for these cells.

The mechanisms by which HPI and TGF-β mediate the growth arrest of normal cells are unknown. It has been clearly demonstrated that TGF-β does not compete with EGF for binding to the EGF-receptor [31,32], although it has been reported that TGF-β treatment produces a transient decrease in EGF-receptor affinity in NRK cells [33,34]. The binding of EGF to A431 cells was unaltered following pretreatment of these cells with HPI for 2 hr. A study on the effect of EGF binding to RLE cells was not possible as the level of specific binding of [^{125}I]-EGF was very low even in the absence of HPI. In addition it was not possible to examine the competition of HPI with [^{125}I]-EGF for specific binding to the EGF-receptor owing to the limited amounts of HPI available. Although these results suggest that HPI has no effect on EGF-receptor affinity, it is necessary to confirm this finding in cells known to be responsive to the growth-regulatory effects of HPI. The effect of HPI pretreatment on the binding of EGF to its receptor in hepatocytes is currently under investigation. Thus the present studies demonstrate that HPI is a growth inhibitor that is distinct from TGF-β. Work is currently in progress to determine the tissue specificity of HPI and its possible involvement in the neoplastic process.

ACKNOWLEDGMENTS

We wish to thank Dr. Chien-Hua Niu for his help with the EGF-binding experiments and Dr. Anita B. Roberts and Dr. James B. McMahon for helpful discussion. The gifts of pure human TGF-β and anti-TGF-β antibody from Dr. Michael B. Sporn are gratefully acknowledged.

REFERENCES

1. McMahon JB, Farrelly JG, Iype PT: Proc Natl Acad Sci USA 79:456–460, 1982.
2. Iype PT, McMahon JB: Mol Cell Biochem 59:57–80, 1984.
3. Krutzsch HC, Huggett AC, Richards WL, Konno R, McMahon JB, Thorgeirsson SS: (submitted).
4. Sporn MB, Roberts AB, Wakefield LM, Assoian RK: Science 233:532–534, 1986.
5. Anzano MA, Roberts AB, Sporn MB: J Cell Physiol 126:312–318, 1986.
6. Kehrl JH, Wakefield LM, Roberts AB, Jakowlew S, Alvarez-Mon M, Derynck R, Sporn MB, Fauci AS: J Exp Med 163:1037–1050, 1986.
7. Kehrl JH, Alvarez-Mon M, Fauci AS: Clin Res 33:610A, 1985.
8. Shipley GD, Pittelkow MR, Wille JJ, Scott RE, Moses HL: Cancer Res 46:2068–2071, 1986.
9. Masui T, Wakefield LM, Lechner JF, LaVeck MA, Sporn MB, Harris CC: Proc Natl Acad Sci USA 83:2438–2442, 1986.
10. Holley RW, Bohlen P, Fava R, Baldwin JH, Kleeman G, Armour R: Proc Natl Acad Sci USA 77:5989–5992, 1980.
11. Seyedin SM, Thomas TC, Thompson AY, Rosen DM, Piez KA: Proc Natl Acad Sci USA 82:2267–2271, 1985.
12. Florini JR, Roberts AB, Ewton DZ, Falen SL, Flanders KC, Sporn MB: J Biol Chem 261:16509–16513, 1986.
13. Ling N, Ying S-Y, Ueno N, Esch F, Denoroy L, Guillemin R: Proc Natl Acad Sci USA 82:7217–7221, 1985.
14. Cate RL, Mattaliano RJ, Hession C, Tizard R, Farber NM, Cheung A, Ninfa EG, Frey AZ, Gash DJ, Chow EP, Fisher RA, Bertonis JM, Torres G, Wallner BP, Ramachandran KL, Ragin RC, Manganaro TF, MacLaughlin DT, Donahoe PK: Cell 45:685–698, 1986.
15. Nakamura T, Tomita Y, Hirai R, Yamaoka K, Kaji K, Ichihara A: Biochem Biophys Res Commun 133:1042–1050, 1985.

16. McMahon JB, Richards WL, del Campo AA, Song M-K, Thorgeirsson SS: Cancer Res 46:4665–4671, 1986.
17. Hayashi I, Carr BI: J Cell Physiol 125:82–90, 1985.
18. Carr BI, Hayashi I, Branum EL, Moses HL: Cancer Res 46:2330–2334, 1986.
19. Evarts RP, Marsden E, Hanna P, Wirth PJ, Thorgeirsson SS: Cancer Res 44:5718–5724, 1984.
20. Assoian RK, Komoriya A, Meyers CA, Miller DM, Sporn MB: J Biol Chem 258:7155–7160, 1983.
21. Roberts AB, Sporn MB, Assoian RK, Smith JM, Roche NS, Wakefield LM, Heine UI, Liotta LA, Falanga V, Kehrl JH, Fauci AS: Proc Natl Acad Sci USA 83:4167–4171, 1986.
22. Richards WL, Song M-K, Krutzsch H, Evarts RP, Marsden E, Thorgeirsson SS: Exp Cell Res 159:235–246, 1985.
23. Laemmli UK: Nature 227:680–685, 1970.
24. Nakamura T, Nawa K, Ichihara A: Biochem Biophys Res Commun 122:1450–1459, 1984.
25. Bradford M: Anal Biochem 72:248–254, 1976.
26. Nestor JJ, Jr, Newman SR, Delustro B, Todaro GJ, Schreiber AB: Biochem Biophys Res Commun 129:226–232, 1985.
27. Tucker RF, Shipley GD, Moses HL, Holley RW: Science 226:705–707, 1984.
28. Roberts AB, Anzano MA, Wakefield LM, Roche NS, Stern DF, Sporn MB: Proc Natl Acad Sci USA 82:119–123, 1985.
29. Roberts AB, Anzano MA, Meyers CA, Wideman J, Blacher R, Pan Y-CE, Stein S, Lehrman R, Smith JM, Lamb LC, Sporn MB: Biochemistry 22:5692–5698, 1983.
30. Nakamura T, Teramoto H, Ichihara A: Proc Natl Acad Sci USA 83:6489–6493, 1986.
31. Roberts AB, Anzano MA, Lamb LC, Smith JM, Frolik CA, Marquardt H, Todaro G, Sporn MB: Nature 295:417–419, 1982.
32. Anzano MA, Roberts AB, Smith JM, Sporn MB, De Larco JE: Proc Natl Acad Sci USA 80:6264–6268, 1983.
33. Assoian RK: J Biol Chem 260:9613–9617, 1985.
34. Massague J: J Cell Biol 100:1508–1514, 1985.

Journal of Cellular Biochemistry 35:315–320 (1987)
Growth Regulation of Cancer 65–70

Interactions Between Growth Factor Receptors and Corresponding Monoclonal Antibodies in Human Tumors

Ulrich Rodeck, Meenhard Herlyn, and Hilary Koprowski

The Wistar Institute of Anatomy and Biology, Philadelphia, Pennsylvania 19104

Monoclonal antibodies (MAbs) to the human epidermal growth factor (EGF) receptor, the type I insulin-like growth factor (IGF) receptor, and the nerve growth factor (NGF) receptor were used to study the growth regulation of malignant cells. Anti-EGF receptor MAb 425 inhibited the growth of A 431 squamous carcinoma cells which express high numbers of EGF receptors on their surfaces. Growth inhibition induced by MAb 425 was accompanied by alterations of the cell-cycle distribution of these cells, indicating the ability of a monoclonal antibody to act as a biologically active ligand. Growth stimulation of melanoma cells by EGF was unrelated to EGF receptor expression on the cell surface. Insulin- and IGF-I-induced growth stimulation of melanoma cells was inhibited by MAb αIR-3 which reacts with the type I IGF receptor. This result indicates that the type I IGF receptor mediated growth stimulation not only by IGF-I but also by insulin. Normal melanocytes and cells of all stages of tumor progression expressed in tissue culture the receptor for NGF, but no effect on the growth of these cells has been observed.

Key words: cancer, growth regulation

Recent advances in the purification and the genetically engineered production of polypeptide growth factors have facilitated studies on the role of these factors in growth regulation of mammalian cells. For most of the known growth factors, receptors expressed on the cell surface of responding cells have been identified. Monoclonal antibodies (MAbs) binding to growth factor receptors provide valuable tools to study effects of growth factors in malignant cells and their normal counterparts. Here, we report on the utilization of MAbs to three growth factor receptors for studies on the growth regulation of malignant cells.

Abbreviations used: EGF, epidermal growth factor; FGF, fibroblast growth factor; IGF, insulin-like growth factor; PDGF, platelet-derived growth factor; NGF, nerve growth factor; MAb, monoclonal antibody; MHA, mixed hemadsorption assay; RIA, radioimmunoassay; SRBC, sheep red blood cells; TGF, transforming growth factor.

Received March 25, 1987; accepted June 19, 1987.

MATERIALS AND METHODS

MAb Binding Assay

Binding of MAbs to target cell surfaces in mixed hemadsorption assay (MHA) was determined using an indicator system consisting of sheep red blood cells (SRBC) precoated with mouse anti-SRBC antiserum and goat-antimouse immunoglobulin antiserum [1]. Positive cells were covered (>25% of perimeter) by rosettes of indicator cells. Binding of either ^{125}I-labeled MAb or ^{125}I-labeled growth factor to target cells was determined in radioimmunoassay (RIA) [2]. Nonspecific binding was defined as bound radioactivity in the presence of 50–100 M excess of unlabeled ligand [2].

Growth Assays

After time periods ranging from 1 to 12 days, cells grown in culture in the presence or absence of growth factors were trypsinized and cell numbers were determined using a Coulter cell counter [3].

RESULTS AND DISCUSSION

Table I identifies MAbs to the growth factor receptors for epidermal growth factor (EGF), insulin-like growth factor (IGF)-I, and nerve growth factor (NGF), all of which inhibit binding of the corresponding growth factor to the respective target cells. Six melanoma cell lines grown in a culture medium devoid of polypeptide growth factors (protein-free medium) were used in our studies. As shown in Figure 1 for melanoma cell line WM 239-A, insulin, EGF, and a combination of insulin, transferrin, and EGF significantly stimulated growth when compared to cultures deprived of growth factors. Growth stimulation by insulin could be demonstrated in cultures of all of five metastatic melanoma cell lines and by EGF in cultures of three out of five cell lines [3].

Epidermal Growth Factor Receptor

EGF-induced stimulation of growth of cells of four out of six melanoma cell lines occurred regardless of the expression of EGF receptors on the cell membrane of these cells (Table II). The lack of receptor expression may be explained by internalization of the receptor after ligand binding. There is no evidence that EGF is produced by melanoma cells in culture (unpublished data). However, transforming growth factor alpha (TGFα) is secreted by various melanoma cells [7–10]. TGFα competes with EGF for binding to the EGF receptor [7]. The hitherto undetermined amount of TGFα produced by our cells may contribute to the continuous downregulation of the EGF receptor on those cells.

TABLE I. Growth Factor Receptors Detected by Monoclonal Antibodies Used in Our Studies

Growth factor receptor	MAb	Isotype	Reference	Ligand binding inhibition	Growth modulation
IGF-I receptor	αIR-3	IgG1	[4]	Yes	ND[a]
EGF receptor	425	IgG2a	[2,5]	Yes	Yes
NGF receptor	ME 20.4	IgG1	[6]	Yes	No
	ME 82-11	IgG1	[6]	Yes	No

[a]ND = not determined.

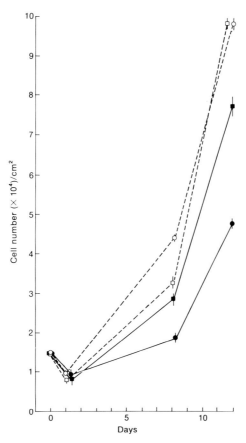

Fig. 1. Growth stimulation of metastatic melanoma cell line WM 239-A by EGF (1 nM) (■---■), insulin (1 μM) (□---□), and a combination of EGF, insulin, and transferrin (125 nM) (○---○). Cell numbers of cultures grown for 8 and 12 days in the presence of each growth factor were significantly (p < 0.05 in Student's t-test) higher than cell numbers of cultures grown in protein-free base medium (●---●). Results are given as mean cell counts ± SD of duplicate cultures.

The effect of anti-EGF receptor MAb 425 on EGF-receptor-expressing target cells was studied with human epidermoid carcinoma cell line A 431, which has $> 10^6$ EGF binding sites per cell [2]. Similar to growth inhibition induced by EGF, A 431 cells were growth inhibited by MAb 425 present in the culture medium at concentrations greater than 1 nM. As shown in Figure 2, growth inhibition of A 431 cells by MAb 425 was accompanied by a decrease in the number of cells in S-phase of the cell cycle, suggesting that the antibody induces specific alterations of the cell cycle.

Insulin and Insulin-Like Growth Factor Receptors

In order to study growth effects of insulin and IGF-I on melanoma cells, we used MAb αIR-3 (see Table I), which reacts with the human type I IGF receptor and blocks binding of insulin and IGF-I to the receptor. MAb αIR-3 partially inhibited growth stimulation of cells of three melanoma cell lines by both insulin and IGF-I (Fig. 3). These results strongly suggest that growth stimulation of melanoma cells induced by insulin is mediated via the type I IGF receptor.

TABLE II. Lack of Correlation Between EGF-
Receptor Expression and Growth Stimulation of
Melanoma Cells Induced by EGF*

Cell line	EGF-R expression[a]	Growth stimulation by EGF[b]
WM 266-4[c]	0	Yes
WM 239-A[c]	0	Yes
WM 373	0	No
WM 164	0	Yes
WM 115[c]	15	No
WM 852	45	Yes

*Melanoma cells used in these experiments have been
adapted to grow in serum-free (WM 115) or protein-
free medium.
[a]Expression assessed in mixed hemadsorption assays
with MAb 425; results expressed as % rosette-forming
cells. Similar results were obtained in radioimmunoassays using ^{125}I-labeled EGF and MAb 425.
[b]Stimulation of growth was determined in cell counting
assays; wells containing EGF (5 ng/ml) were scored
positive if they contained significantly (p < 0.05 in
Student's t-test) higher No. of cells than did wells with
medium devoid of exogenously added growth factors.
[c]Primary (WM 115) and metastatic (WM 239-A, WM
266-4) melanoma cell lines derived from the same
patient.

Nerve Growth Factor Receptor

Although normal melanocytes and cells of metastatic melanoma lines in culture
express the NGF receptor [11], none of the six cultured melanoma cells studied were
growth stimulated by NGF (not shown). This is not surprising since NGF-induced
effects of target tissues of neuroectodermal origin are rather related to survival and
differentiation [12,13]. Its effect on melanoma cells may thus be related to the
pathways of differentiation in situ and in vitro [11].

Other Growth Factor Receptors

Various other growth factors seem to be relevant in the growth regulation of
melanocytic cells. Halaban et al [14] have shown that basic fibroblast growth factor
(FGF) has mitogenic effects on normal melanocytes. Platelet-derived growth factor
(PDGF) [15], TGFα [7–10], and TGFβ [8] are the better characterized growth-
modulating activities produced by melanoma cells, but their effects on growth of the
cells still await detailed investigation. Equally, the corresponding receptor for melanoma growth-stimulating activity described by Richmond et al [10] remains to be
identified.

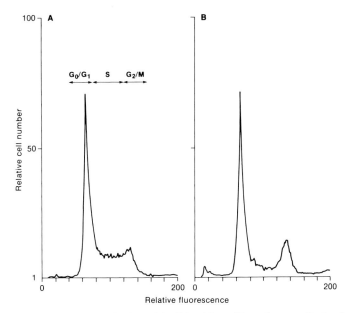

Fig. 2. Changes in cell cycle distribution of A 431 epidermoid carcinoma cells incubated with anti-EGF receptor MAb 425. **A** shows the cell cycle distribution of cells in untreated cultures; **B** demonstrates a clear decrease of the number of cells in S-phase in cultures treated with 32 nM MAb 425 after 4 days of culture. Decrease in S-phase cells in antibody treated cultures was statistically significant ($p < 0.05$) in Student's t-test when compared to control cultures.

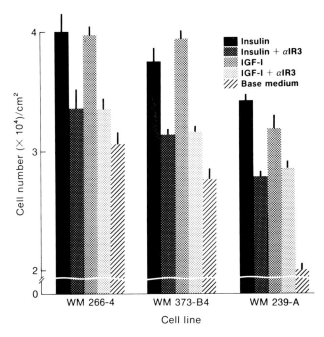

Fig. 3. Inhibition of insulin (1 μM)- and IGF-I (13 nM)-mediated growth stimulation in three malignant melanoma cell lines by MAb αIR3 (100 nM), which reacts with the type I IGF receptor. Results are given as mean cell counts $\pm$ SD of duplicate cultures.

ACKNOWLEDGMENTS

These studies were supported in part by grants CA-25874 and CA-2081 of the National Institutes of Health, and IM-402 of the American Cancer Society. We are grateful to Dr. S. Jacobs for providing MAb αIR3 and to Dr. R. Furlanetto for providing purified IGF-I. The excellent technical assistance of M. Coleman, G. Levengood, and M. Varello is greatly appreciated.

REFERENCES

1. Herlyn M, Guerry D, Koprowski H: J Immunol 134:4226, 1985.
2. Rodeck U, Herlyn M, Herlyn D, Molthoff C, Atkinson B, Varello M, Steplewski Z, Koprowski H: Cancer Res 47:3692, 1987.
3. Rodeck U, Herlyn M, Menssen HD, Furlanetto RW, Koprowski H: Int J Cancer (in press).
4. Jacobs S, Cook S, Svoboda ME, Van Wyk JJ: Endocrinology 118:223, 1986.
5. Murthy U, Basu A, Rodeck U, Herlyn M, Ross A, Das M: Arch Biochem Biophys 252:549, 1987.
6. Ross AH, Grob P, Bothwell M, Elder D, Ernst CS, Marano N, Ghrist BFD, Slemp CC, Herlyn M, Atkinson B, Koprowski H: Proc Natl Acad Sci USA 81:6681, 1984.
7. Marquard H, Todaro GJ: J Biol Chem 257:5220, 1982.
8. DeLarco JE, Pigott DA, Lazarus JA: Proc Natl Acad Sci USA 82:5015, 1985.
9. Kim MK, Warren TC, Kimball ES: J Biol Chem 258:6561, 1985.
10. Richmond A, Lawson DH, Nixon DW, Chawla, RK: Cancer Res 45:6390, 1985.
11. Herlyn M, Clark WH, Rodeck U, Mancianti ML, Jambrosic J, Koprowski H: Lab Invest 56:461, 1987.
12. Edgar D: J Cell Sci [Suppl] 3:107, 1985.
13. Dichter MA, Tischler AS, Greene LA: Nature 268:501, 1977.
14. Halaban R, Ghosh S, Baird A: In Vitro Cell Dev Biol 23:47, 1987.
15. Westermark B, Johnsson A, Paulsson Y, Betsholtz C, Heldin C-H, Herlyn M, Rodeck U, Koprowski H: Proc Natl Acad Sci USA 83:7197–7200, 1986.

Journal of Cellular Biochemistry 36:185–198 (1988)
Growth Regulation of Cancer 71–84

Melanoma Growth Stimulatory Activity: Isolation From Human Melanoma Tumors and Characterization of Tissue Distribution

Ann Richmond and H. Greg Thomas

V.A. Medical Center (Atlanta), Department of Medicine, Division of Endocrinology, Emory University School of Medicine, Atlanta, GA 30322

Melanoma growth stimulatory activity (MGSA) is an acid and heat stable, auto-stimulatory growth factor which was first isolated from culture medium conditioned by the Hs294T human melanoma cell line. In this report, we describe the purification of MGSA from acid ethanol extracts of Hs294T tumors grown in nude mice using a series of Bio-Gel P30, reverse phase-high performance liquid chromatography and heparin-sepharose steps. This modified procedure provides a 10-fold improved yield of MGSA over previously published procedures. Purified MGSA-stimulated melanoma cell growth in both ^{3}H-thymidine and cell number assays over a concentration range of 0.06 to 6 ng/ml. The MGSA bioactivity was primarily associated with fractions which exhibited molecular weights of 16 and 13–14 Kd based upon sodium dodecyl sulfate-polyacrylamide gel electrophoresis. Purified platelet-derived growth factor (PDGF), insulin-like growth factor (IGF-1), transforming growth factor-beta (TGF$_\beta$), and epidermal growth factor (EGF) in combination with TGF$_\beta$ did not stimulate ^{3}H-thymidine incorporation in Hs294T cells under the conditions used for MGSA bioassay. Monoclonal antibody to MGSA was used to screen melanoma and benign nevus cultures as well as fixed sectioned tissue for MGSA. The majority of the melanoma cultures were MGSA positive, while most nevus cultures were MGSA negative. However, when fixed sectioned tissue was screened for MGSA immunoreactivity, melanoma tissue was MGSA positive and three-fourths of the benign nevi were MGSA positive. In addition, epidermal keratinocytes and several tissues exhibiting proliferative disorders contained immunoreactive MGSA. These data suggest that MGSA may be a normal regulator of growth and that the microenvironment of the cell may regulate both production of MGSA and response to MGSA.

Key words: MGSA, growth factor, melanoma, autocrine

Human malignant melanoma cells have been reported to produce a variety of growth factors, including transforming growth factor-alpha (TGF$_\alpha$) [1], transforming

Address correspondence to: Ann Richmond, Ph.D., Research Service (151), V.A. Medical Center (Atlanta), 1670 Clairmont Road, Decatur, GA 30033.

Received March 5, 1987; revised and accepted July 16, 1987.

growth factor-beta (TGF$_\beta$), platelet-derived growth factor (PDGF) [3], fibroblast growth factor (FGF) [4], and melanoma growth stimulatory activity (MGSA) [5–7]. TGF$_\alpha$, TGF$_\beta$, PDGF, FGF, and MGSA have all been suggested as possible autocrine regulators of melanoma growth. These proposed autocrine mechanisms include both positive and negative signals for growth regulation. For example, TGF$_\beta$ is secreted by melanoma cells and in some instances inhibits the ability of melanoma cells to form colonies in soft agar, while other melanoma cultures have apparently lost their inhibitory response to TGF$_\beta$ [9]. TGF$_\alpha$ has been proposed to stimulate melanoma colony formation in soft agar, but EGF/TGF$_\alpha$ receptor availability is quite limited in most melanoma cultures [10]. It has been postulated that EGF receptors are unavailable for binding in radioreceptor assays because the receptor is already occupied by TGF$_\alpha$. Apparently, PDGF-A chain may be produced more frequently than PDGF-B chain in human melanoma, but investigators have been unable to demonstrate PDGF binding to these melanoma cells [3].

Recently, Halaban et al. have shown that antibodies to basic but not acidic FGF will inhibit the growth response of normal melanocytes to melanoma extracts [4]. We have previously demonstrated that pituitary-derived FGF produces a minimal, but significant, stimulation in melanoma cell growth [11]. However, secretion of basic FGF has not been demonstrated in melanoma cells.

An autocrine mechanism of growth stimulation has been previously demonstrated for MGSA in that: 1) MGSA released into the serum-free culture medium of the Hs294T melanoma cell line has been purified and demonstrated to stimulate the growth of Hs294T cells and exhibit specific, temperature-dependent, saturable binding to cultured Hs294T melanoma cells [8]; 2) monoclonal antibodies to MGSA inhibit the serum free growth of Hs294T melanoma cells [12].

The MGSA has been purified by gel exclusion chromatography, reverse phase high performance liquid chromatography (RP-HPLC), and preparative electrophoresis from melanoma serum-free conditioned medium. The activity resides in a family of proteins < 14 to 28 Kd. The most reproducibly active form of MGSA appears to be the 16-Kd polypeptide. Cultured melanoma cells respond to 0.3–30 pM concentrations of MGSA with increased growth. Amino acid analysis of MGSA preparations suggests that MGSA is different from other previously characterized growth factors [8]. Hs294T cells do not exhibit a growth response to EGF, insulin, transferrin, progesterone, or nerve growth factor as single agents or in combination with one another [11]. Monoclonal antibody FB2AH7 to MGSA will bind to the 16-Kd form of MGSA from tumor extracts after Western blot [12], but this antibody will not bind to other growth factors. We now report the purification of MGSA from Hs294T melanoma tumors with the use of a series of gel filtration and reverse phase high performance liquid chromatography steps. These experiments demonstrate that MGSA is present in melanoma tumor tissue in sufficient quantity to recover appreciable amounts of the growth factor and that the preparative electrophoresis step previously described for purification of MGSA from conditioned medium [8] can be replaced with chromatography on a Vydak Hi-Pore C$_{18}$ column and heparin-sepharose, with the end result of purification providing an approximately 10-fold increase in recovery of purified MGSA. We also report that though MGSA has been isolated from melanoma-conditioned medium and melanoma tumor extracts, immunoreactive MGSA is not restricted to melanoma tissue but is found in a number of proliferating tissues. Finally, in no instance did TGF$_\beta$, EGF in combination with TGF$_\beta$, PDGF, or IGF-I mimic the growth-stimulatory activity of MGSA on Hs294T cells under the conditions of MGSA bioassay. Altogether, these data suggest that MGSA is a novel growth factor which not only has the capacity to autostimulate the growth of human melanoma cells, but may also affect the growth of other types of cells.

MATERIALS AND METHODS

Tissue culture materials and media were supplied as described previously [2]. The Hs294T cells were obtained from the American Type Tissue Culture, and a population of cells was selected which would grow on serum-free culture medium without supplementation with hormones or growth factors. Athymic nude nu/nu mice (4–5-week-old females) were obtained from the NCI Frederick Cancer Research Facility, Frederick, MD.

Tumor Formation and Extraction

Tumor formation in athymic nude mice was induced by intra-scapular injection of 1×10^6 Hs294T human melanoma cells per mouse. Palpable tumor formation was observed approximately 7 days after injection. As the tumors reached maximal size (at 24–30 days, prior to the mice becoming moribund), they were removed, minced, homogenized, and extracted with ethanolic hydrochloric acid as previously described [5].

Purification of MGSA

Bio-Gel P-30 chromatography was performed on acid ethanol extracts of tumors as described previously [7]. Fractions eluting between the ribonuclease A and the insulin molecular weight markers were pooled, lyophilized, and applied to a Waters u-Bondapak C_{18} column, eluting with a 60-min linear gradient of acetonitrile:water:TFA (6:94:0.05 to 60:40:0.05) as previously described [8]. Absorbance was monitored at 206 nm. The sensitivity range was 2.0 AUFS. The flow rate was 1.0 ml per min, and 1.0-ml fractions were collected. Fractions were lyophilized and redissolved in 100-μl of 4 mM HCl and 1/10 aliquots were assayed for recognition by the FB2AH7 antibody for MGSA in the modified dot blot enzyme-linked immunoadsorbent assay (ELISA) [12]. An ELISA-positive peak was identified that eluted from the u-Bondapak column at ~39% acetonitrile. Fractions from this peak were then re-fractionated on the Vydak Hi-Pore C_{18} column by using a 60 min linear gradient of acetonitrile:water:heptafluorobutyric acid (25:75:0.05 to 45:55:0.05). Absorbance was monitored at 214 nm and a sensitivity of 1.0 AUFS. The flow rate was 1.0 ml per min, and fractions were manually collected as peaks appeared in the chromatogram. An aliquot of each fraction was examined by SDS-polyacrylamide gel electrophoresis. The fractions eluting at 37% and 38% acetonitrile contained the 16- and 13- to 14-Kd moieties previously shown to contain MGSA bioactivity in similar preparations from Hs294T conditioned medium. Fractions corresponding to major peaks were lyophilized and re-run separately under the same conditions as above.

Heparin-Sepharose Chromatography

The RP-HPLC-purified MGSA was lyophilized, redissolved in 10 mM Tris, pH 7.5, and subjected to heparin-sepharose chromatography. A 10×50 mm column of heparin-sepharose CL-6B was equilibrated in 10 mM tris hydroxymethylaminomethane (Tris), pH 7.5. After loading the partially purified MGSA onto the column, the material which did not bind to heparin-sepharose was removed by continued flow of 10 mM Tris, pH 7.5. A 200-ml linear gradient of 10 mM Tris, pH 7.5, to 10 mM Tris, 1M sodium chloride, pH 7.5, was followed by elution with 100 ml 10 mM Tris, 2M sodium chloride, pH 7.5, and finally eluted with 100 ml 6M guanidine hydrochloride. Absorbance was monitored at 280 nm, at a sensitivity of 0.1 AUFS. The flow rate was 0.5 ml/min, and 8-ml fractions were collected. Fractions were pooled based on the absorbance at 280 nm of material eluting from the heparin-sepharose, then pooled fractions were subjected to bioassay.

MGSA Bioassay and Immunoassay

The MGSA bioactivity was affirmed by using the ^{3}H-thymidine incorporation assay, with the Hs294T melanoma cells serving as the responding cell as described previously [8]. Briefly, 8,000 cells were plated in 28 × 61-mm glass scintillation vials (Wheaton #225288) in 2 ml of Ham's F-10 medium supplemented with 10% fetal bovine serum (FBS). Twenty-four hours later, cells were washed with 2 ml of phosphate-buffered saline (PBS: 8 g NaCl, 1.15 g Na_2HPO_4, 0.2 g KCl, 0.2 g KH_2PO_4, 0.1 g $MgCl_2:6H_2O$, 0.1 g $CaCl_2$ per liter of water, pH 7.4) and placed on serum-free F-10 medium containing HEPES (30 mM) and ovalbumin (10 μg/ml). Eight hours later ^{3}H-thymidine (5 μCi) was added to each vial and the incubation was continued for another 16 hours. The reaction was stopped by addition of methanol:ethanol (3:1). Unincorporated ^{3}H-thymidine was removed by a repeated wash with methanol, then 10 ml of counting fluid (Scintiverse II) was added to each vial, and radioactivity incorporated into DNA was counted in a Beckman liquid scintillation counter (LS-1800).

For cell number experiments, 72 hours after seeding 8 × 10^3 Hs294T cells into Wheaton scintillation vials in F-10 culture medium containing 10% fetal bovine serum, the medium was aspirated and the cells were placed on serum-free F-10 medium. Twenty-four hours later, the medium was aspirated, and dilutions of MGSA or fetal bovine serum in serum-free binding buffer (F-10 culture medium containing 30 mM HEPES and 75 μg/ml ovalbumin) were added. On the third day after growth factor additions, cells were released with trypsin, and cell number was determined from aliquots of suspended cells counted in a hemocytometer (n=4 for each point). For MGSA immunoassay, the FB2AH7 antibody was used in the modified dot blot ELISA described previously [12].

Sodium Dodecyl Sulfate-Polyacrylamide Gel Electrophoresis (SDS-PAGE)

Purified preparations of MGSA were analyzed by SDS-PAGE according to a modification of the methods of Laemmli [13]. Double strength sample buffer containing the growth factor preparation or molecular weight standards (14.4–94 Kd) was not boiled and did not contain reducing agent. The 12% polyacrylamide gels were pre-run for 1 hour prior to the addition of samples and standards. After fixing in methanol:acetic acid:H_2O (40:10:50), the gels were stained with Coomassie Blue R-250 (0.01%) and/or silver.

Newly Established Melanoma and Nevus Cultures

This study was approved by the Human Investigations Committee at Emory University. Primary cultures were established as previously described [13] from tissue samples obtained after informed consent from melanoma patients undergoing surgical resection (without prior antitumor therapy), or from patients having nevi biopsied for histologic examination.

Monoclonal Antibodies

Monoclonal antibody FB2AH7 to MGSA has been previously characterized [12]. This antibody inhibits the in vitro growth of Hs294T cells and recognizes the 16 Kd form of MGSA in Western blot analysis.

Immunocytochemistry

At the time of subculture of melanoma and nevus cultures, cells were split such that slide chambers could be made for immunocytochemical assay and the L-dopa tyrosinase assay [15]. Nevus or melanoma cells were cultured at a density of 2.5×10^4 cells per well in two chamber/slides (Lab-tek) with 2 ml of F-10 culture medium containing 10% fetal bovine serum. After a 24-hour incubation, the cells were washed twice with PBS and then incubated with serum free F-10. After another 24 hours, slide cultures were fixed with 10.7% formalin/0.2% gluteraldehyde/0.6% Tris-buffered saline (TBS) (pH 7.5). Endogenous peroxidase was quenched by addition of 0.3% H_2O_2 in methanol for 30 min. The slides were washed in TBS for 10 min, nonspecific binding was blocked with a 1:100 dilution of normal serum (Vector Laboratories), then the slides were incubated for 30 min at 37°C with a 1:10 dilution of FB2AH7 monoclonal antibody to MGSA. As a control, a nonspecific IgM_k monoclonal antibody to alpha-lipoteichoic acid was used in place of FB2AH7. Slide chambers were then processed by using the Vectastain ABC kit according to procedures described by Vector Laboratories. The color was developed by using the peroxidase substrate, amino-ethyl-carbazole. Slides were counterstained with Mayer's hemotoxylin, washed 5 min with deionized H_2O, treated for 1 min with ammonium hydroxide, washed 5 min with running deionized H_2O, and mounted in glycerol:PBS (1:1).

Immunohistochemistry

Fixed and sectioned tissues were deparaffinized by 5-min changes of xylene; tissues were hydrated through a graded alcohol series (3 min/dilution), rinsed for 5 min in distilled water, fixed, and processed as described for immunocytochemistry.

RESULTS
RP-HPLC Purification of MGSA

Acid-ethanol extracts of melanoma tumors have been previously demonstrated to contain MGSA bioactivity [5]. In this study, acid-ethanol extracts of Hs294T tumors developed in nude mice were subjected to gel exclusion chromatography in a Bio-Gel P-30 column as previously described [8]. The Bio-Gel P-30 fractions from Pool B (lower Mr) containing MGSA bioactivity were subsequently subjected to RP-HPLC with modification of the procedure described previously for isolation of MGSA from conditioned medium, only a combination of uBondapak C_{18} and Vydak Hi-Pore columns were used. The MGSA ELISA-positive fractions eluted at ~39% acetonitrile from RP-HPLC. These fractions were pooled, lyophilized, and subjected to a second RP-HPLC step on the Vydak column eluting with a 60 min linear gradient of acetonitrile:water:HFBA (25:75:0.05 to 45:55:0.05). Fractions eluting at 37%–38% acetonitrile (Fig. 1) contained the 16- and 13-Kd bands, respectively, previously identified as MGSA positive [9] (Fig. 2). Bioassay and ELISA assays for MGSA reconfirmed that the 16-Kd and 13- to 14-Kd containing fractions did contain the majority of MGSA. The 16 Kd moiety was found to be present primarily in those fractions eluting at 37% acetonitrile, while a 13- to 14-Kd moiety predominated in the fraction eluting at 38% acetonitrile. The 16-Kd material eluting at 37% acetonitrile and the 13- to 14-Kd material eluting at 38% acetonitrile were then separately reinjected on to the Vydak column and eluted as described earlier with the 25%– 45% acetonitrile gradient and HFBA in the mobile phase. The optical density profile at 214 nm revealed a sharp peak at 37% acetonitrile (Fig. 3), and analysis of the peak by SDS-polyacrylamide gel electrophoresis revealed a single 16-Kd band as was shown in Fig. 2, lane 4. Similar results were found with the 13–14 Kd material eluting at 38% acetonitrile. The fractions eluting at both 37% (16 Kd) and 38% (13–14 Kd) acetonitrile were active in the MGSA bioassay, producing a stimulation of ^{3}H-thymidine incorporation 166% to 200% of control at concentrations in the nanogram per milliliter range.

Amino acid sequence analysis revealed that there was a unique peptide in the 16-Kd preparation. However, there was also a contaminating protein with a high percentage homology with the protein histone 2A. Contaminating histone 2A has subsequently been removed by heparin-sepharose chromatography. The more basic H2A binds more strongly to heparin-sepharose than MGSA. The MGSA bioactivity elutes from tumor extract MGSA preparations and from similar MGSA preparations derived from Hs294T conditioned medium between 0.1 and 0.3M NaCl, while histone 2A (H2A) cannot be eluted with 2M NaCl but requires 6M guanidine-HCl for elution. There was no MGSA bioactivity associated with H2A. This combined

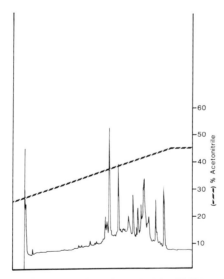

Fig. 1. RP-HPLC profile of MGSA on Vydak column. MGSA ELISA-positive fractions which eluted at ~39% acetonitrile from the u-Bondapak C_{18} column were rechromatographed on the Vydak Hi-Pore C_{18} column. A 60-min linear gradient of acetonitrile:water:HFBA (25:75:0.05 to 45:55:0.05) was employed as the mobile phase at a flow rate of 1.0 ml/min. The absorbance was monitored at 214 nm and a sensitivity of 1.0 AUFS.

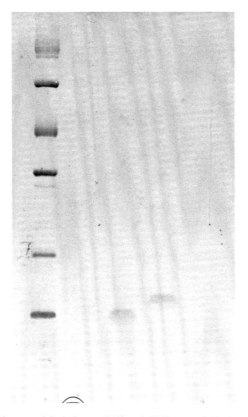

Fig. 2. SDS-PAGE of the material eluting at 37% and 38% acetonitrile from the Vydak column. A modification of the Laemmli method was employed by utilizing double strength sample buffer and omitting addition of the reducing agent to the samples or molecular weight standards. The 12% polyacrylamide gel was pre-run for 1 hour prior to the addition of samples and molecular weight standards. Lanes 1–4 consist of the following: **Lane 1**, Mr standards (phosphorylase b 94Kd, bovine serum albumin 67Kd, ovalbumin 43Kd, carbonic anhydrase 30Kd, soybean trypsin inhibitor 20.1Kd, and alpha lactalbumin 14.4Kd); **Lane 2**, blank; **Lane 3**, material eluting at 38% acetonitrile from the Vydak column; **Lane 4**, material eluting at 37% acetonitrile from the Vydak column.

RP-HPLC and heparin-sepharose chromatography procedure thus allows final purification of MGSA (Table I and Figure 4). The purified MGSA was active at concentrations of 6 to 0.06 ng/ml, producing a maximal stimulation in ^{3}H-thymidine incorporation of 171% of control and an approximately twofold increase in cell number (Fig. 5). The 5 μg of MGSA purified from 53 g of Hs294T tumor tissue contained 260,000 units, representing a recovery of 8% of the activity present in the Hs294T tumor extract. (One MGSA unit produces a stimulation in ^{3}H-thymidine incorporation into DNA half-maximal to that produced by unfractionated Hs294T-conditioned medium.)

Effects of Other Growth Factors on Hs294T Melanoma Cells

In order to determine whether other endogenous growth factors stimulate the growth of the Hs294T melanoma cells in serum-free culture medium, HPLC-purified PDGF (Collaborative Research), recombinant IGF-I (Am-Gen), and TGF$_\beta$ (the kind gift of Dr. Harold Moses) as a single agent and in combination with EGF (Collabo-

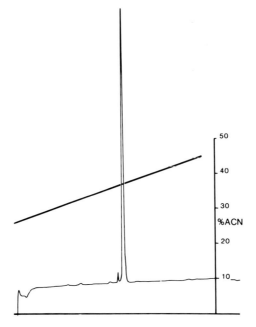

Fig. 3. RP-HPLC of 16Kd moiety. The 16 Kd material which eluted at 37% acetonitrile from the Vydak column was rechromatographed by using the 25:75:0.05 to 45:55:0.05% acetonitrile:water: HFBA 60-min linear gradient at a flow rate of 1.0 ml/min. The absorbance was monitored at 214 nm and a sensitivity of 0.5 AUFS.

TABLE I. Purification of MGSA From Hs294T Tumor Extract

Source of MGSA (Stage of Purity)	Protein content	Purification (n-fold)
Tumor tissue	53.0 g	
EtOH-HCL extraction of Hs294T tumors	289.0 mg	184
Bio-Gel P-30 Chrom. Pool B fr. 51-73	33.0 mg	1,600
RP-HPLC 6–60% ACN, 0.05% HFBA	560.0 μg	94,000
RP-HPLC Vydak C$_{18}$ 25–45% ACN, 0.05% HFBA	53.0 μg	1,000,000
Heparin-sepharose chromatography	5.0 μg	10,000,000

rative Research, receptor grade) were assayed for MGSA-like activity. These agents were tested over a concentration range similar to that required for MGSA bioactivity in low-density Hs294T cultures. Neither PDGF or IGF-I had growth stimulatory activity for Hs294T cells under the conditions of the bioassay developed for MGSA (Fig. 4). However, less pure preparations of both of these factors from Collaborative Research have exhibited ability to occasionally, but not reproducibly, stimulate Hs294T melanoma growth at high concentrations. Since the activity was not present in more purified preparations of these growth factors, it is possible that a contaminant in these impure growth factor preparations was responsible for the stimulation of growth of the melanoma culture. The EGF and TGF$_\beta$ had no significant effect on Hs294T cell growth, and combinations of these growth factors did not stimulate Hs294T cell growth (Fig. 4).

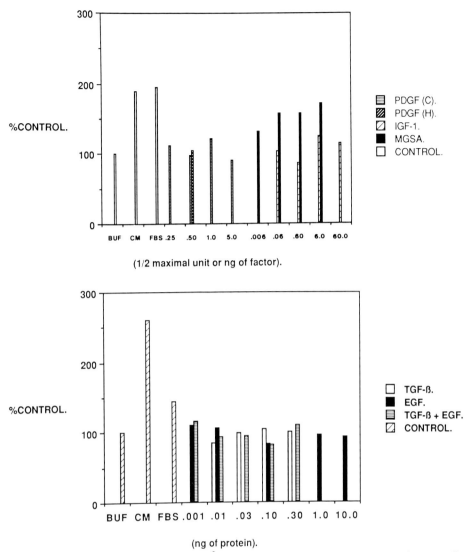

Fig. 4. Effects of other growth factors on ^{3}H-thymidine incorporation in Hs294T melanoma cells. Hs294T cells were plated into sterilized Wheaton scintillation vials in 2 ml of Ham's F-10 medium plus 10% fetal bovine serum at a density of 1×10^4 cells per vial. Cells were incubated overnight (16 hours) at 37°C, 95% air/5% CO_2, and the next day the media was aspirated, the cell layer was washed twice with serum free Ham's F-10 medium (SF-F10), and the cells were fed with 2 ml SF-F10 prior to incubation overnight. On day 3, the medium was aspirated and replaced with SF-F10 containing 20 μg/ml ovalbumin and EGF, TGF$_\beta$, PDGF, IGF-1, or purified MGSA at the concentrations indicated. Six hours later 5 μCi of ^{3}H-thymidine was added to each vial, and the cultures were incubated for an additional 18 hours. The cells were then fixed and processed for determination of radioactivity incorporated into DNA as described previously (8). Each bar represents the mean of three individual determinations except for the crude PDGF data, where each bar represents the mean of 5 separate experiments with a total of 15 individual determinations per bar. In the assays which included both TGF$_\beta$ and EGF, 1 ng of EGF was included per milliliter of binding buffer. Abbreviations: **BUF**, binding buffer-control, F-10 media plus 20 μg/ml ovalbumin and 30 mM HEPES; **CM**, conditioned medium from a confluent Hs294T culture processed by low spin centrifugation; **FBS**, Ham's F-10 medium containing 1% fetal bovine serum; **PDGF (C)**, units of culture grade PDGF from Collaborative Research; **PDGF (H)**, units of HPLC grade PDGF from Collaborative Research; **IGF**, 1 ng of purified recombinant IGF-1 from AmGen; **MGSA**, 1 ng of MGSA purified by RP-HPLC and heparin-sepharose. Bars in the upper figure from left to right illustrate effects of binding buffer; conditioned medium; **FBS**; **PDGF (C)** 0.25 max units; **PDGF (C)**, **PDGF (H)** 0.5 max units; **PDGF (C)** 1.0 max units; **PDGF (C)** 5.0 max units; **MGSA** 0.006 ng; **IGF-1**, **MGSA** 0.06 ng; **IGF-1**, **MGSA** 0.06 ng; **IGF-1**, **MGSA** 6.0 ng; **IGF-1** 60 ng.

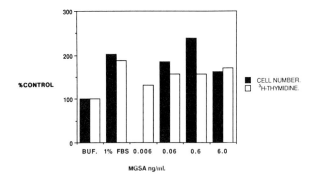

Fig. 5. Comparison of MGSA Effects on ^{3}H-Thymidine Incorporation and Cell Number. The ^{3}H-thymidine bioassay was performed on Hs294T cells as described in Figure 4. MGSA which had been purified by RP-HPLC and heparin-sepharose chromatography was assayed for growth-promoting activity on low-density Hs294T cultures at concentrations ranging from .006 ng/ml to 6 ng/ml. An *n* of four was used for each concentration and data are recorded as percent of the binding buffer control (BUF). The positive control was 1% fetal bovine serum (FBS). Cell number experiments were also performed on MGSA preparations. Briefly, 8×10^3 Hs294T cells were plated into Wheaton scintillation vials on Ham's F-10 medium containing 10% FBS. Three days later, the medium was aspirated and cells were placed on serum free F-10 medium. At 24 hours later, the medium was aspirated, and dilutions of MGSA or FBS in serum-free binding buffer (F-10 culture medium containing 30 mM HEPES and 75 μg/ml ovalbumin) were added. Controls received binding buffer alone. On the third day after growth factor additions, cells were released with trypsin, and cell number was determined from aliquots of suspended cells counted on a hemocytometer (n = 4 for each point).

Comparison of MGSA Effects on ^{3}H-Thymidine Incorporation and Cell Number

Purified MGSA is able to stimulate an increase in both ^{3}H-thymidine incorporation and cell number in low-density cultures of human Hs294T melanoma cells. Though there is some difference in the optimal concentration for maximal response between the two bioassays (optimal response with 6 ng/ml in H-thymidine bioassay versus optimal response with 0.6 ng/ml in the cell number bioassay), this difference can probably be accounted for by the differences in duration of the assays (Fig. 5).

Utilization of Monoclonal Antibody to MGSA to Evaluate the Prevalence of MGSA in Cultured Melanoma and Nevus Cells and in Fixed Tissue

Newly established cultures from human melanoma tumors and benign nevi have been examined by immunocytochemical assay for the presence of MGSA by using a monoclonal antibody to MGSA. Twenty five of 32 nevus cultures studied have been MGSA negative. In contrast, 19 of 27 melanoma cultures were positive for MGSA by immunocytochemistry (Table II, and Fig. 6). The MGSA-positive cultured nevus cells tended to be chromosomally abnormal [14]. Greater than 50% of the nevus cultures were melanin-positive and representative samples of melanin-negative nevus cultures were demonstrated to contain premelanosomes by electron microscopy.

In contrast, 10 of 15 fixed sectioned nevus tissues were MGSA positive by immunohistochemistry (Table II, and Fig. 6). These data suggest that MGSA may be involved in proliferation of nevocytes in vivo, but in vitro culture conditions are not compatible with expression of MGSA. In fixed sectioned tissue, keratinocytes and cells derived from the basal epithelium from normal skin were also MGSA positive by IHC (Table II, Fig. 6) as were three other tissues exhibiting proliferative disorders:

TABLE II. MGSA Reactivity

MGSA-negative Tissues	MGSA-positive Tissues
Metastatic adenocarcinoma (lung)	Sarcoidosis
Lymphoma	Mesangial proliferative
Testis (normal)	glomerulonephritis/tubulo interstitial nephritis
Vascular smooth muscle	Metastatic small cell
Fibroblasts	anaplastic carcinoma
Vascular endothelium	Basal cell carcinoma
Alveolar macrophages	Cirrhotic hepatic tissue
Lymphocytes	with bile ductule proliferation
Intestinal epithelium	Melanoma (4/4)
Benign nevi (7)	Benign nevi (10)
Cultures	**Cultures**
Melanoma cultures (8)	Melanoma cultures (19)
Benign nevi (25)	Benign nevi (7)[a]

[a]MGSA positive benign nevi exhibited a high incidence of chromosomal abnormality.

renal tissue exhibiting mesangial proliferative glomerulonephritis, small cell carcinoma metastatic to the liver, and sarcoidosis tissue (Table II). Associated connective tissues were MGSA negative including both cells (lymphocytes, fibroblasts, and macrophages) and fibers (collagen and elastin). In addition, alveolar macrophages, vascular endothelial cells, lung epithelium, intestinal epithelium, and testicular tissue were negative (Table II).

DISCUSSION

The substance MGSA was first described as an endogenous growth factor released into the culture medium of human malignant melanoma cells. In this study, we have determined that MGSA is not only released by cultured human melanoma tumors, but sufficient quantities of growth factor are stored in the tumor cells to enable isolation from acid-ethanol extracts of melanoma tumors. A combination of RP-HPLC and heparin-sepharose chromatography were utilized, bypassing the preparative electrophoresis step reported earlier for purification of MGSA from conditioned medium and providing a 10-fold increased yield for purified MGSA. The heparin-sepharose chromatography step enabled removal of very basic contaminants and demonstrated that MGSA differs from acidic and basic FGF as well as the endothelial growth factors which exhibit a high affinity for heparin-sepharose [16].

Studies with MGSA monoclonal antibody FB2AH7 demonstrate that approximately 70% of cultures established from human melanoma tumors are MGSA positive by immunocytochemistry while most cultures established from benign nevi were MGSA negative. Since 10 of 15 nevi were MGSA positive by immunohistochemistry when fixed sectioned tissue was studied, one might suspect that the nevocyte cultures were overgrown by fibroblasts. Several points argue against this possibility: 1) a selective low Ca^{2+} culture medium was used for the nevocyte cultures (MCDB-151), which enhances proliferation of epithelial cells and inhibits fibroblast proliferation;

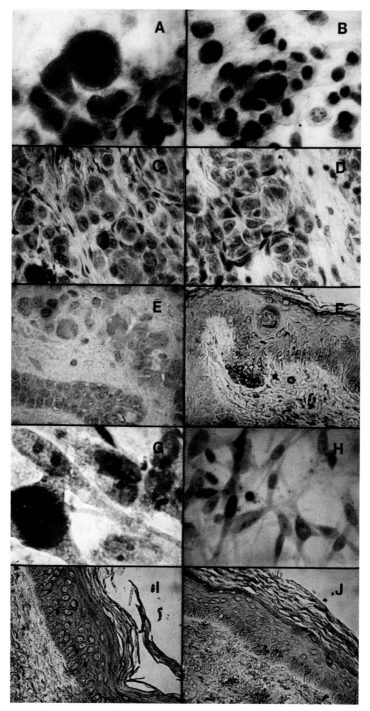

Fig. 6. Cellular localization of MGSA in cultured cells by immunocytochemistry and in fixed and sectioned tissue by immunohistochemistry. **A.** A melanoma cell culture treated with monoclonal antibody to MGSA, FB2AH7. 40× objective. **B.** A melanoma cell culture treated with non-specific monoclonal antibody. Note absence of red staining in cytoplasm. 40×. **C.** Section of a metastatic melanoma lesion treated with MGSA monoclonal antibody. 20×. **D.** Section of a metastatic melanoma lesion treated with control buffer. Note absence of red staining in cytoplasm of tumor cells. 20×. **E.** Section of a nevus lesion treated with MGSA monoclonal antibody. 20×. **F.** Section of a nevus lesion treated with control monoclonal antibody. Note absence of red staining in cytoplasm. 100×. **G.** Nevus cell culture N-48 treated with MGSA antibody. Note absence of red staining in cytoplasm. 100×. **H.** Nevus cell culture N-48 treated with control monoclonal antibody. 40×. **I.** Section of normal skin treated with MGSA antibody. 20×. **J.** Section of normal skin treated with control monoclonal antibody. Note absence of pink staining associated with epidermis. 20×.

2) electron microscopy of representative cultures of nevocytes revealed the presence of premelanosomes and/or melanosomes. Therefore, it is unlikely that the MGSA negativity in these cultures is due to failure to grow out the correct cells from the nevus tissue. Alternatively, the appropriate culture conditions (matrix molecules, growth factors, and/or nutrients) may not be present in the in vitro environment for optimal differentiation and growth. Since melanoma cells are known to produce fibronectin and specific proteoglycans in vitro which normal melanocytes do not produce in culture [17], it is possible that if the nevocytes were cultured on an appropriate substrate, then the nevocytes would be able to produce MGSA in vitro as the melanoma cultures do.

Localization of immunoreactive MGSA in the stratum spinosum of the epithelium of the skin was an unexpected finding. These data suggest that MGSA may affect the growth of a number of other cell types in addition to melanocytes. Several other tissues exhibiting proliferative disorders (small cell carcinoma of the lung metastatic to the liver, mesangial proliferative glomerulonephritis, and sarcoid tissue) also suggest that MGSA may play a role in regulation of growth of a number of tissue types, though it does appear to be most concentrated in the epithelium of the skin.

We have previously demonstrated that pituitary-derived FGF and FSH produce a minimal but significant stimulation in Hs294T cell growth. However, insulin, transferrin, progesterone, LHRH, NGF, and EGF had no effect on Hs294T cell growth as single agents or in combination [11]. We now can add IGF-1, TGF_β, EGF in combination with TGF_β, and PDGF to this list of growth factors which are not active in the MGSA ^{3}H-thymidine bioassay.

Failure of other growth factors such as PDGF, IGF-1, EGF, and TGF_β to mimic MGSA, along with amino acid analysis data suggesting that MGSA differs from these growth factors [8] lead us to conclude that MGSA is unlike other growth factors previously described. In addition the data shown here demonstrate that the heparin-sepharose binding capacity of MGSA differs from that of acidic or basic FGF. The MGSA appears to contribute to the relatively autonomous growth of malignant melanoma cells, and, based on localization of immunoreactive MGSA in other proliferating tissues, this growth factor may also serve as a mitogen for a number of other cell types.

ACKNOWLEDGMENTS

We are indebted to Dr. Bryan Noe for his consultation in the design of the protocol for final purification of MGSA; to Chris Engel, Robert G.B. Roy and Eddie Balentein for excellent technical assistance; to Dr. Robert Fine, Dr. Douglas Murray and Dr. V.A. Varma for the tissue samples used in this study; Dr. Harold Moses for the TGF_β; and Margaret Miles for the electron microscopy studies. Research was supported by NCI grant CA 34590 and V.A. Merit Award.

REFERENCES

1. Marquardt H, Todaro GJ: J Biol Chem 257:5220, 1982.
2. Richmond A, Lawson DH, Nixon DW, Chawla RK: Cancer Res 45:6390, 1985.
3. Westermark B, Johnson A, Paulson Y, Betsholtz C, Heldin CH, Herlyn M, Rodeck U, Koprowski H: Proc Natl Acad Sci USA 83:7197, 1986.

4. Halaban R, Ghosh S, Baird A: In Vitro 23:47, 1987.

5. Davoren PR. Biochim Biophys Acta 63:150, 1962.

6. Richmond A, Lawson DH, Nixon DW: Cold Spring Harbor Conf Cell Prolif 9:885, 1982.

7. Richmond A, Lawson DH, Nixon DW, Stevens JS, Chawla RK: Cancer Res 43:2106, 1983.

8. Richmond A, Thomas HG: J Cell Physiol 129:375, 1986.

9. Roberts AB, Anzano MA, Wakefield LM, Roche NS, Stern DG, Sporn MB: Proc Natl Acad Sci USA 82:119, 1985.

10. Todaro GJ, DeLarco JE, Marquardt H, Bryant ML, Sherwin SA, Sliski AH: Cold Spring Harbor Conf Cell Prolif 6:113, 1979.

11. Richmond A, Lawson DH, Nixon DW, Stevens JS, Chawla RK: Cancer Res 42:3175, 1982.

12. Lawson DH, Thomas HG, Roy RGB, Gordon D, Nixon DH, Chawla RK, Richmond A: J Cell Biochem 24:168, 1987.

13. Laemmli UK: Nature 227:680, 1972.

14. Richmond A, Fine R, Murray D, Lawson DH, Priest JH: J Invest Derm 86:295, 1986.

15. White R, Hu F, Roman NA: Stain Tech 58:13, 1983.

16. Lobb R, Sasse J, Sullivan R, Shing Y, D'Amore P, Jacobs J, and Klagsburn M: J Biol Chem 261:1924, 1986.

17. Rettig WJ, Real FX, Spengler BA, Biedler JL, Old LJ: Science 231:1281, 1986.

Journal of Cellular Biochemistry 36:237–248 (1988)
Growth Regulation of Cancer 85–96

Swiss 3T3 Mouse Embryo Fibroblasts Transfected With a Human Prepro-GRP Gene Synthesize and Secrete Pro-GRP Rather Than GRP

Anne-Marie Lebacq-Verheyden, Shoshana Segal, Frank Cuttitta, and James F. Battey

NCI-Navy Medical Oncology Branch, National Cancer Institute (A.-M.L.-V., S.S., F.C., J.F.B.), and Department of Medicine, Uniformed Services University of the Health Sciences, National Navy Medical Center (S.S., F.C.), Bethesda, Maryland 20814-20815

A prepro-gastrin-releasing peptide (GRP) gene was introduced into Swiss 3T3 mouse embryo fibroblasts by DNA transfection in an attempt to establish autocrine growth stimulation. Clonal transfectants expressed varying amounts of GRP encoding mRNA. They synthesized and secreted a ~15-kd pro-GRP hormone but not fully processed 2.8-kd GRP. Accordingly, no changes in growth properties were associated with GRP gene expression. We postulate that Swiss 3T3 fibroblasts lack the enzymes necessary to process significantly pro-GRP into biologically active peptides and that this deficiency may be responsible for the failure to establish autocrine growth stimulation in the transfected cells.

Key words: autocrine growth, transfection, prohormone processing, bombesin

The gastrin-releasing peptide (GRP) is a 27-amino-acid neuropeptide homologous to the amphibian tetradecapeptide bombesin [1,2]. Both peptides bind to cell-surface receptors through their identical carboxyl heptapeptide [3], which triggers a physiological response in various central and peripheral neurons, in smooth muscle cells, and in secretory cells [4]. In addition, bombesin and GRP are potent mitogens for a number of cultured cells including Swiss 3T3 mouse embryo fibroblasts [5], human bronchial epithelial cells [6], and small-cell lung cancer cells [7,8]. The latter cells both contain and secrete a bombesinlike immunoreactive peptide [9–12] that was shown by cDNA cloning to be the 27-amino-acid GRP [13]. When a monoclonal antibody reacting with the carboxyl heptapeptide of GRP prevented this ligand from binding to its cell-surface receptors, the growth of some small-cell lung cancer cell lines was significantly impaired, both in soft agar and in nude mice [14]. Taken together, these data suggested that GRP could stimulate the growth of the cells that

Received March 9, 1987; revised and accepted August 5, 1987.

synthesized and secreted it. Such autocrine growth stimulation is thought to contribute to the acquisition of a malignant phenotype [15], and indeed both autocrine growth stimulation and tumorigenicity were induced in a factor-dependent hemopoietic cell line given a constitutively expressed GM-CSF growth factor gene [16], as well as in rat fibroblasts transfected with a TGF-α gene [17]. We tried to reconstitute an autocrine growth stimulation system by giving Swiss 3T3 mouse embyro fibroblasts a constitutively expressed prepro-GRP gene. These cells have a well-characterized mitogenic response to GRP [18], mediated by high-affinity cell-surface receptors [19], but do not normally synthesize or secrete this hormone. For DNA transfection, we used a cDNA clone of the human prepro-GRP gene [13,20] that encodes a 23-amino-acid signal sequence, the 27-amino-acid GRP, and a novel 95-amino-acid GRP-gene-associated peptide hereafter called GGAP. The present work shows that prepro-GRP transfected Swiss 3T3 cell lines synthesize and secrete large amounts of 15-kd pro-GRP but fail to process significantly this prohormone into biologically active GRP (2.8 kd).

MATERIALS AND METHODS
Prepro-GRP Expression Vectors

Two 8.1-kb GRP expression constructs were assembled (Fig. 1). Each construct contained the prepro-GRP and neomycin coding regions transcribed from opposite strands, with both genes being driven by the SV40 early region promoter (0.3-kb PvuII-HindIII fragment) and followed by the SV40 t antigen splice and polyadenylation site. The two constructs differ in that one transcribes the GRP coding region in a sense orientation with respect to the promoter, while the other should transcribe antisense GRP. To build these vectors, the pJB327 plasmid [21] (pBR322, with

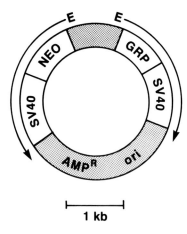

1 kb

Fig. 1. Prepro-GRP sense and antisense expression vectors. Arrows indicate that the GRP and the neomycin genes are driven on opposite strands by the SV40 early promoter and enhancer (E). The only difference between the sense and antisense vectors is that they transcribe the prepro-GRP coding sequences in either the sense (5′-3′) or antisense (3′-5′) orientation. GRP = 0.7-kb EcoRI-DraI fragment from prepro-GRP cDNA form I [13]. NEO = 1.4-kb BamHI fragment from pmyc-neo [23]. SV40 = SV40 sequences, including the splice (0.6 kb) and polyadenylation (0.22 kb) sites from pSV2-gpt [22]. Stippling = pJB327 sequences, including the ampicillin resistance gene (AMP^R) and the origin of replication (ori) [21].

nucleotides 1,427–2,516 deleted, and the EcoRI-HindIII fragment replaced by the mp11 EcoRI-HindIII polylinker region) was reduced in size by deleting 737 bp in the tetracycline gene, eliminating the unique HindIII and EcoRV sites. This plamid, pJBΔ, was digested with SmaI and EcoRI, and a 2.9-kb PvuII-EcoRI fragment from pSV2-gpt [22] (which contained the Ecogpt coding region under control of the SV40 early promoter, followed by SV40 t antigen splice and polyadenylation site) was ligated into these sites. This plasmid, pJBΔ-gpt, was digested with EcoRV, and a HindIII linker was added by ligation. Subsequent digestion with HindIII released a 0.6-kb fragment containing the 5′ portion of the gpt coding sequence. The prepro-GRP coding region was then substituted for the gpt coding region, by (1) preparing a 0.7-kb EcoRI-DraI fragment encoding the prepro-GRP cDNA form I [13], (2) filling in the ends with Klenow polymerase, (3) adding HindIII linkers by ligation, and (4) ligating this fragment into pJBΔ-gpt missing the 0.6-kb HindIII-EcoRV gpt encoding fragment. Plasmids were selected which contained the prepro-GRP in either sense (5′–3′) or antisense (3′–5′) orientation. These two plasmids were linearized with NruI, and a 2.6-kb BamHI fragment from pmyc-neo [23] encoding the neomycin gene was ligated into the NruI site after filling in the staggered termini with Klenow polymerase. Plasmids carrying the prepro-GRP gene and the neomycin gene in opposite orientations were grown in *E. coli* LE392 and purified by CsCl density centrifugation [24] for transfection.

GGAP and GRP/GGAP Expression Vectors

The human GGAPI and GGAPIII cDNA sequences [13] were cloned in frame into the pUR290 expression vector [25], in order to produce β-galactosidase/GGAP fusion proteins (Fig. 2). This was done (1) by digesting pUR290 with BamHI and filling in the ends with Klenow polymerase; (2) by digesting further the linearized pUR290 with HindIII; and (3) by cloning a 0.5-kb RsaI-HindIII cDNA fragment encoding all but the first 21 amino acids of human GGAPI and GGAPIII (95 and 85 amino acids, respectively) into the modified BamHI and HindIII sites of pUR290. A 0.8-kb SmaI-HindIII cDNA fragment encoding the last amino acids of the signal sequence, GRP_{1-27} and $GGAPI_{1-95}$, was cloned into the same vector. The DNA regions containing the β-galactosidase junctions were sequenced by the dideoxy method [24], which showed that the three fragments had been cloned in frame. *E. coli* RR1Δm15 cells were transformed with the pUR290, pUR290-GGAP, and pUR290-GRP-GGAP plasmids. For expression, 20-ml bacterial cultures were grown at 37°C to an OD_{600} of 0.3 and induced for 30 min at the same temperature with 40 μl of 0.1 M IPTG. The bacterial pellets were washed once in 50 mM Tris-HCl, pH 7.5, containing 150 mM NaCl and 5 mM EDTA, boiled for 5 min in SDS sample buffer (62.5 mM Tris-HCl pH 6.8, 2% SDS, 5% beta-mercaptoethanol, 10% glycerol), and cleared by centrifugation. The protein concentration of the lysates was determined by the Biorad colorimetric assay, using lysozyme as a standard. For Western blot analysis, 10 μg of total proteins were electrophoresed on a 7.5% SDS-polyacrylamide gel [26], transferred to nitrocellulose [27], and incubated with 1:200,000 anti-GGAPI antiserum or 1:5,000 anti-N-GRP antiserum followed by ^{125}I-protein A (380,000 cpm/ml), as described below.

Transfected Cell Lines

The Swiss 3T3 mouse embryo fibroblast cell line was obtained from the American Type Culture Collection (CCL 92) and grown in Dulbecco's Modified

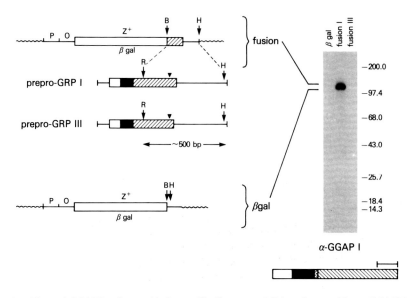

Fig. 2. The anti-GGAPI antiserum binds specifically to near full-length recombinant GGAPI in Western blot analysis. **Left:** prepro-GRP I and III: cDNA clones encoding the human prepro-GRP hormones I and III [13], ⊢—⊣ = untranslated sequences; nucleotides encoding the signal sequence (□), GRP$_{1-27}$ (■), and the GRP-gene-associated peptide GGAP (hatched bar); the arrowhead indicates the point from which the carboxyl-termini from GGAPI and GGAPIII differ; R = RsaI site; H = Hind III site; B = BamHI site. A 500-bp fragment encoding most of GGAPI or of GGAPIII was fused to the 3′ end of the β-galactosidase gene (Z$^+$) in pUR290 [25], thus generating two fusion protein expression vectors (fusion); the unmodified pUR290 vector expresses β-galactosidase (βgal); p = promotor; o = operon. **Right:** Western blot analysis (10 μg/lane) with the anti-GGAPI antiserum that was raised against the synthetic peptide identified by the horizontal bar above the prepro-GRP cartoon; βgal, fusion I, and fusion III: lysates from bacteria transformed with the βgal, GGAPI, and GGAPIII vectors, respectively; molecular weight markers, in kilodaltons, are shown on the right; the bars on the left indicate the positions of the ~ 130-kd fusion proteins and of the 115-kd unfused βgal.

Eagle's Medium with 10% fetal bovine serum at 37°C in a humidified atmosphere with 5% CO_2. One million cells in 100-mm tissue culture dishes were transfected with 25 μg of purified DNA in TE buffer (10 mM Tris–HCl, pH 8.0, 1 mM EDTA), using the calcium phosphate DNA transfection method [24]. Mock transfections were done with TE buffer alone. Twenty-four hours after transfection, cells were plated for neomycin selection in 24-well microtiter plates, using 10^4 cells/well and 400 μg/ml of the biologically active aminoglycoside G-418 (Geneticin, Gibco). Preliminary experiments had established that in these conditions, all parent Swiss 3T3 cells were killed within 10–14 days of selection. Accordingly, after 2 wk of selection, none of the 84 wells containing mock-transfected cells showed evidence of growth, whereas 33% of the wells with sense or antisense transfected cells (104/312) contained at least one clone of growing cells, thus indicating an approximate transfection efficiency of 1:30,000. The contents of 24 wells were cloned by limiting dilution, generating 15 independent sense and four independent antisense transfected cell lines.

Northern Blot Analysis

Methods were essentially as described [24]. Total cellular RNA was prepared by the guanidine-isothiocyanate method, electrophoresed through a formaldehyde-containing 1% agarose gel, and transferred to nitrocellulose. The filters were hybridized to DNA fragments purified by gel electrophoresis and nick-translated to a specific activity of 100–500 cpm/pg of DNA. The GRP probe was a 0.9-kb full-length prepro-GRP cDNA [13] that had been excised with HindIII from pBR322; the neomycin probe was a 1-kb HindIII-SmaI fragment of pSV2-neo [28] that contained exclusively neomycin coding sequences.

In Vitro Transcription and In Vitro Translation of the Human Prepro-GRP Gene

A 0.7-kb EcoRI-DraI fragment of the human prepro-GRP cDNA form I [13] was cloned into the EcoRI and SmaI sites of the expression vectors pSP64 and pSP65 (Promega). In these vectors, the bacterial SP6 promoter directs the transcription of RNA either identical (sense RNA) or complementary (antisense RNA) to the prepro-GRP mRNA. The plasmids were grown in *E. coli* HB101 and purified by CsCl density centrifugation; restriction mapping confirmed that they contained a single insert in the correct orientation; 5 μg of linearized and gel-purified plasmid DNA was capped and transcribed in vitro (Promega catalogue, 1987). Ten percent of the synthesized RNA (1 μl) was electrophoresed on a formaldehyde-containing 1% agarose gel. A single 0.7-kb band was visible after ethidium bromide staining and shown by Northern blot analysis to hybridize to the nick-translated GRP probe; 2 μl of prepro-GRP RNA was translated in an RNAase-treated rabbit reticulocyte lysate (Promega), using 75 μCi of ^{35}S-methionine (Amersham) and methionine-free amino acids in a total volume of 50 μl.

Antisera and Iodinated Protein A

The antisera used in this paper are described in detail elsewhere (F. Cuttitta et al., submitted for publication). Briefly, synthetic peptides corresponding to the 15 amino-terminal amino acids of human GRP (N-GRP$_{1-15}$) and to the 23 carboxyl-terminal amino acids of human GGAPI (GGAPI$_{73-95}$) were conjugated in equal weight ratios to keyhole limpet hemocyanin in the presence of 0.125% glutaraldehyde and injected subcutaneously into New Zealand White rabbits; the resulting antisera bound specifically to the immunizing peptides in a solid-phase radioimmunoassay; their specificity is being further characterized in this paper. Purified protein A (Pharmacia) was labeled with ^{125}I (Amersham) by the chloramine T method [29] to a specific activity of 25 μCi/μg (1 Ci = 3.7 $\times$ 10^{10} becquerels).

Cell Lysates and Western Blot Analysis

Monolayers of Swiss 3T3 transfected cell lines and cells from the GRP-producing human small-cell lung cancer cell line NCI-H209 [30] were lysed in SDS-sample buffer (62.5 mM Tris-HCl, pH 6.8, 2% SDS, 5% β-mercaptoethanol, 10% glycerol). The lysates were cleared by ultracentrifugation and their protein concentration was determined by the Biorad colorimetric assay. Equal amounts of proteins were electrophoresed on a 15% SDS-polyacrylamide gel [26] and transferred electrophoretically to nitrocellulose [27]. The filters were coated with 5% skimmed milk in Tris buffer (50 mM Tris-HCl pH 7.5, 5 mM EDTA, 150 mM NaCl, 0.02% NaN$_3$) for 1 hr at 40°C and further incubated at room temperature with rabbit antisera followed by iodinated protein A (380,000 cpm/ml) diluted in the same buffer. After extensive washes, including one final 10-min wash in 0.5% NP40, filters were processed for autoradiography.

Metabolic Labeling and Immune Precipitation

Half-confluent monolayers of Swiss 3T3 transfected cell lines in T150 culture flasks ($\pm$ 5 $\times$ 10^6 cells/flask) were labeled for 4 hr at 37°C with 500 μCi of ^{35}S-methionine (Amersham) in 10 ml of methionine-free medium containing 2% dialyzed fetal bovine serum. Culture supernatants were centrifuged, made 250 μM PMSF, and fractionated on Sep-Pak C18 cartridges (Waters Associates). A fraction was eluted with 50% acetonitrile in 0.1 N NH_4OH after equilibrating the column with 15% acetonitrile in water, and the eluted material was lyophilized and resuspended in 1 ml of precipitation buffer (10 mM Tris-HCl pH 7.5, 150 mM NaCl, 1% NP-40, 1% Na deoxycholate). This procedure concentrated proteins smaller than 20 kd and allowed recovery of more than 90% of the ^{125}I-porcine GRP_{1-27} (Amersham) added to Swiss 3T3 culture supernatant. For immune precipation, 90,000 cpm of ^{125}I-porcine GRP_{1-27}, 150,000 TCA-insoluble cpm of reticulocyte lysate, and 350,000 TCA-insoluble cpm of culture supernatant in 450 μl of precipitation buffer were precleared twice for 1 hr in the cold with 50 μl of normal rabbit serum followed by 50 μl of protein A–Sepharose 4B CL (Pharmacia). After centrifugation, the supernatants were immune precipitated with 1:10 anti-N-GRP antiserum, followed by protein A–Sepharose 4B CL. After extensive washes [31], the immunoadsorbents were boiled for 10 min in SDS-sample buffer; the supernatants were electrophoresed on a 15% SDS-polyacrylamide gel that was eventually processed for fluorography.

RESULTS

Transfected cell lines were first analyzed at the nucleic acid level. Total RNA from 19 independent Swiss 3T3 transfected cell lines and from the GRP-producing small-cell lung cancer line NCI-H209 was assayed by Northern blot analysis (Fig. 3). As previously described, a major 0.9-kb prepro-GRP transcript was observed in the NCI-H209 cell line [13]. In the transfected cell lines, the prepro-GRP transcripts were expected to include the SV40 early promoter (0.34 kb), the prepro-GRP cDNA fragment (0.7 kb), the 3' untranslated end of the gpt gene (0.5 kb), and the SV40 t antigen splice and polyadenylation signals (0.6 kb and 0.2 kb, respectively). Accordinly, $\pm$ 2.3-kb transcripts were detected in 13/15 sense and 4/4 antisense transfected cell lines. Minor 1.8-kb and 4.8-kb transcripts were also observed in these lines; they were possibly generated by the use of alternative SV40 polyadenylation sites. The levels of prepro-GRP mRNA varied from barely detectable to as high as those observed in a good GRP-producing small-cell lung cancer cell line. Hybridization of the same blot to the neomycin probe confirmed that all the transfected lines expressed the expected 2.6-kb neomycin transcript, as well as some other minor transcripts (not shown). Southern blot analysis of genomic DNA prepared from four of these lines showed that multiple copies of both unaltered and rearranged prepro-GRP genes had been integrated (not shown). Finally, the identity of the sense and of the antisense transfected lines was confirmed in an S1 nuclease protection assay, where total cellular RNA protected the appropriate single-stranded DNA probes [13] from S1 nuclease digestion (not shown).

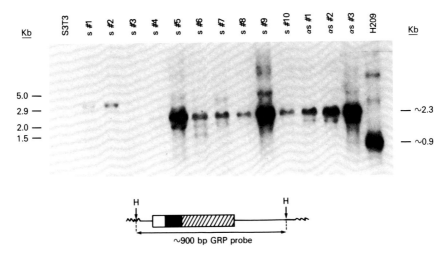

Fig. 3. Transfected Swiss 3T3 cell lines express varying amounts of prepro-GRP-encoding mRNA. Northern blot analysis of total cellular RNA (10 μg/lane) prepared from Swiss 3T3 mouse embryo fibroblast cell line (S3T3), from human small-cell lung cancer cell line NCI-H209 (H209), as well as from cloned Swiss 3T3 transfected cell lines; s# and αs# refer to cell lines transfected with sense and antisense prepro-GRP expression vectors, respectively. The probe is a 900-bp prepro-GRP cDNA, excised with HindIII (H) from pBR322 [13]. Molecular weight standards are indicated on the left; the approximate size of the transfected (2.3 kb) and endogenous (0.9 kb) GRP mRNAs are shown on the right.

Four transfected cell lines were further evaluated for protein expression. In a preliminary Western blot analysis, the anti-GGAPI antiserum bound specifically to the ± 130-kd β-galactosidase/GGAPI fusion protein, as well as to some minor degradation products of the latter (Fig. 2). It failed to react with bacterial lysates that contained either the unfused β-galactosidase (115 kd) or the β-galactosidase/GGAPIII fusion protein. This experiment confirmed that the anti-GGAPI antiserum bound specifically to near-full-length recombinant GGAPI. When the transfected cell lysates were analyzed in the same way, the anti-GGAPI antiserum bound specifically to a single 15-kd GRP precursor present in the NCI-H209 cell line, as well as in the two sense, but not in the two antisense, transfected cell lines (Fig. 4). Strikingly, the transfected cell lines contained at least ten times more GRP precursor than the NCI-H209 line. This precursor could formally be either prepro-GRP or pro-GRP. The former would have retained its signal sequence while the latter would have lost it (calculated molecular weights of 16 kd and 13.5 kd, respectively). Since in mammalian cells, the removal of signal sequences is usually a cotranslational procedure [32], it was assumed that the 15-kd GRP precursor was pro-GRP. In order to detect in cell lysates not only the 15-kd putative pro-GRP, but also processed GRP_{1-27} (calculated molecular weight of 2.8 kd), we used the anti-N-GRP antiserum in Western blot analysis. However, the latter antiserum failed to react with any of the cell lysates previously tested with the anti-GGAPI antiserum (not shown). This was probably due to the low affinity of this antiserum, since at high concentrations it failed to react in Western blot analysis with the ± 135-kd β-galactosidase/GRP-GGAPI fusion protein unless the latter was visible by Coomassie blue staining (at least 0.5 μg/lane).

Since cell-surface receptor-mediated autocrine growth requires the presence of processed GRP_{1-27} not only in the cells but also in the culture medium, the latter was

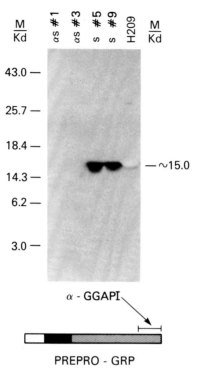

Fig. 4.   Cell lysates from Swiss 3T3 cells transfected with the sense (s#5, s#9) but not with the antisense (αs#1, αs#3) prepro-GRP expression vector contain at least ten times more pro-GRP than a small-cell lung cancer cell line lysate (H209). Western blot analysis (500 μg/lane) with the anti-GGAPI antiserum (see legend Fig. 2); the filter was exposed for 24 hr at −70°C to Kodak XAR film in the presence of an intensifying screen; molecular weight markers, in kilodaltons, are shown on the left; the apparent molecular weight of the pro-GRP hormone is shown on the right.

immune precipitated with the anti-N-GRP antiserum. In a preliminary experiment, we tested reticulocyte lysates that contained the in vitro labeled and in vitro translated products of the sense and of the antisense prepro-GRP mRNAs (Fig. 5). The anti-N-GRP antiserum immune precipitated a single 17.0 kd prepro-GRP hormone, which further suggested that the 15-kd GRP precursor (Fig. 3) was pro-GRP. In another experiment, 50 fM of iodinated porcine GRP_{1-27} was mixed with Swiss 3T3 culture medium and immune precipitated by the anti-N-GRP antiserum as a 2.8-kd molecular species (Fig. 5). However, when culture supernatants of two Swiss 3T3 transfected cell lines were immune precipitated with the anti-N-GRP antiserum, a single ± 15-kd pro-GRP hormone was recovered from the medium surrounding the sense but not the antisense transfected cell line (Fig. 5). When the same experiment was done on NCI-H209 culture supernatants, no GRP-containing peptides of any size were detected, which suggested that only very small amounts of such unbound and undegraded peptides were available for immune precipitation (not shown).

In accord with the immune precipitation data, none of the sense transfected cell lines displayed any obvious growth advantage over the antisense transfected lines. In medium with 10% fetal bovine serum, sense transfectants displayed a wide range of growth rates that could always be matched by an antisense counterpart; in medium with 2% or 0% fetal bovine serum, some of the sense as well as some of the antisense

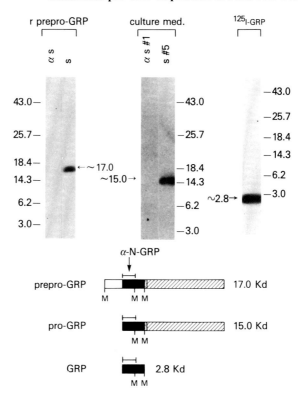

Fig. 5. **Left:** The anti-N-GRP antiserum immune precipitates a ~17.0 kd recombinant prepro-GRP hormone (r prepro-GRP); the synthetic peptide used to raise this antiserum is identified by the horizontal bar above the cartoons; s and α s: in vitro translation products of in vitro–transcribed sense and antisense prepro-GRP mRNA; fluorography exposed for 24 hr at −70°C to Kodak XRP film. **Right:** The anti-N-GRP antiserum does immune precipitate a ~2.8-kd iodinated GRP$_{1-27}$ (^{125}I-GRP) added to Swiss 3T3 culture medium; autoradiography exposed for 4 days at −70°C to Kodak XAR film. **Middle:** Swiss 3T3 cells transfected with the sense (s#5) but not with the antisense (αs#1) prepro-GRP expression vector synthesize and secrete the pro-GRP hormone rather than fully processed GRP$_{1-27}$; immune precipitation with anti-N-GRP antiserum of culture medium (culture med) from in vitro–labeled cells; fluorography exposed for 5 days at −70°C to Kodak XAR film; molecular weight markers are shown in kilodaltons; the apparent molecular weights of prepro-GRP, pro-GRP, and GRP$_{1-27}$ are indicated on the gels and on the corresponding cartoons; M = position of ^{35}S-methionine.

transfected cell lines managed to grow. However, none of these growth variations could be related to the expression of the prepro-GRP gene.

DISCUSSION

In this paper, we show that Swiss 3T3 mouse embryo fibroblasts express a transfected human prepro-GRP gene but that they secrete the 15-kd prohormone rather than processed GRP. Concomitantly, prepro-GRP transfected cell lines fail to show any obvious growth advantage over control transfected cell lines. We also provide the first data available on human GRP precursor proteins. Thus, the immune precipitation of recombinant human prepro-GRP establishes its apparent molecular weight as 17.0 kd. This strongly suggests that the 15-kd GRP precursor is the pro-GRP hormone, which was formally demonstrated in later experiments (A.M. Lebacq-

Verheyden et al., submitted for publication). However, nothing is known about the processing intermediates that separate the prohormone from the free hormones. The latter include at least GRP_{1-27} and GP_{18-27}, which were identified by radioimmunoassay in acid-boiled and size-fractionated extracts of human fetal lung [33,34], and of small-cell lung cancers [35]. Whether in all these tissues free peptides were being generated by a physiological process or by the experimental conditions remains unclear. Our inability to immune precipitate GRP_{1-27} from the supernatant of a small-cell lung cancer cell line that was shown in the past both to contain [10,30] and to secrete [36] bombesinlike immunoreactive material suggests that only very small amounts of free GRP are presently available in the culture medium. We are currently investigating the processing of prepro-GRP in several small-cell lung cancer cell lines in order to identify the GRP-related peptides that can be involved in autocrine growth stimulation [15].

In order to achieve autocrine growth stimulation, small-cell lung cancer cells and prepro-GRP transfected Swiss 3T3 cells need (1) to synthesize, process, and secrete biologically active GRP; (2) to bind this hormone to high-affinity cell-surface receptors [19]; and (3) to signal this binding through second messengers that include inositol 1,4,5-trisphosphate breakdown and calcium flux [18,37]. Failure at any of these three levels could account for the observed lack of autocrine growth stimulation. The data presented here suggest that Swiss 3T3 fibroblasts lack the enzymes required for processing pro-GRP into biologically active peptides. In common with many other peptide hormones [38], GRP needs to be α-carboxyl-amidated in order to bind to its receptor and exert its biological activities [39]. From processing data published about other prohormones [32,40,41], it can be inferred that the processing of pro-GRP should at least include (1) the trypsinlike cleavage of the 15-kd prohormone at a dibasic lys-lys in the sequence Met-Gly-Lys-Lys-Ser, where Met is the carboxyl-terminal amino acid of GRP_{1-27} [20]; (2) the removal of the two basic residues; and (3) the cleavage of the glycine—that is, the amide donor—with amidation of the methionine. For pro-insulin, proparathyroid hormone and pro-opiomelanocortin, it has been demonstrated that most if not all of the processing occurred in secretory granules [reviewed in 40]. Hence, it may not be surprising that Swiss 3T3 fibroblasts, devoid of secretory granules, do not process efficiently some prohormones. Indeed, monkey-fibroblastlike cell lines (namely, AGMK, CV1, and COS) transfected with the rat or with the human prepro-insulin gene synthesize and presumably secrete pro-insulin rather than insulin [42,43]. Similarly, COS cells transfected with the porcine pro-opiomelanocortin gene synthesize and secrete authentic POMC, which is subsequently degraded into smaller immunoreactive peptides, distinct from the biologically active peptides, by nonspecific proteases present in the culture medium [44]. In contrast, some mature somatostatin-14 was secreted by COS cells transfected with angler fish preprosomatostatin, thus showing that at least some simple processing, involving only a trypsinlike cleavage of a single pair of basic amino acids, could occur in fibroblastlike cells [45].

In conclusion, the immune precipitation data and the absence of autocrine growth stimulation support the view that Swiss 3T3 cells transfected with the human GRP gene synthesize and secrete readily detectable amounts of the 15-kd prohormone but fail to process significantly this precursor into GRP_{1-27}. From these experiments, it is clear that GRP may function as an autocrine growth factor only in certain specific cell types which possess the necessary enzymatic activities to process biologically active GRP from its prohormone precursor.

ACKNOWLEDGMENTS

We wish to thank Joe Fedorko for the generous gift of iodinated protein A, Phil Kasprzyk for his valuable advice on peptide concentration, and Gena Parris for the expert typing of this manuscript. In addition, we thank E. Rozengurt for his generous gift of GRP-sensitive Swiss 3T3 fibroblasts, which were used in comparative transfection studies. A.M.L.-V. is a permanent research associate from the Fonds National de la Recherche Scientifique (Belgium) and was partially supported by an EORTC fellowship.

REFERENCES

1. Anastasi A, Erspamer V, Bucci M: Experientia 27:166, 1971.
2. McDonald TJ, Jörnvall H, Nilsson G, Vagne M, Ghatei M, Bloom SR, Mutt V: Biochem Biophys Res Commun 90:227, 1979.
3. Westendorf JM, Shonbrunn A: J Biol Chem 258:7527, 1983.
4. O'Donohue TL, Massari VJ, Pazoles CJ, Chronwall BM, Shultz CW, Quirion R, Chase TN, Moody TW: J Neurosci 4:2956, 1984.
5. Rozengurt E, Sinnett-Smith J: Proc Natl Acad Sci USA 80:2936, 1983.
6. Willey JC, Lechner JF, Harris CC: Exp Cell Res 153:245, 1984.
7. Weber S, Zuckerman JE, Bostwick DG, Bensch KG, Sikic BI, Raffin TA: J Clin Invest 75:306, 1985.
8. Carney DN, Cuttitta F, Moody TW, Minna JD: Cancer Res 47:821, 1987.
9. Wood SM, Wood JR, Ghatei MA, Lee YC, O'Shaughnessy D, Bloom SR: J Clin Endocrinol Metab 53:1310, 1981.
10. Moody TW, Pert CB, Gazdar AF, Carney DN, Minna JD: Science 214:1246, 1981.
11. Sorenson GD, Bloom SR, Ghatei MA, Del Prete SA, Cate CC, Pettengill OS: Regul Pept 4:59, 1982.
12. Erisman MD, Linnoila RI, Hernandez O, Di Augustine RP, Lazarus LH: Proc Natl Acad Sci USA 79:2379, 1982.
13. Sausville EA, Lebacq-Verheyden AM, Spindel ER, Cuttitta F, Gazdar AF, Battey JF: J Biol Chem 261:2451, 1986.
14. Cuttitta F, Carney DN, Mulshine J, Moody TW, Fedorko J, Fischler A, Minna JD: Nature 316:823, 1985.
15. Sporn MB, Roberts AB: Nature 313:745, 1985.
16. Lang RA, Metcalf D, Gough NM, Dunn AR, Gonda TJ: Cell 43:531, 1985.
17. Rosenthal A, Lindquist PB, Bringman TS, Goeddel DV, Derynck R: Cell 46:301, 1986.
18. Rozengurt E: Science 234:161, 1986.
19. Zachary I, Rozengurt E: Proc Natl Acad Sci USA 82:7616, 1985.
20. Spindel ER, Chin WW, Price J, Rees LH, Besser GM, Habener JF: Proc Natl Acad Sci USA 81:5699, 1984.
21. Sausville E, Carney D, Battey J: J Biol Chem 260:10236, 1985.
22. Mulligan RC, Berg P: Mol Cell Biol 1:449, 1981.
23. Johnson BE, Battey J, Linnoila I, Becker KL, Makuch RW, Snider RH, Carney DN, Minna JD: J Clin Invest 78:525, 1986.
24. Davis LG, Dibner MD, Battey JF: "Basic Methods in Molecular Biology." New York: Elsevier, 1986.
25. Rüther U, Müller-Hill B: EMBO J 2:1791, 1983.
26. Laemmli UK: Nature 227:680, 1970.
27. Towbin H, Gordon J: J Immunol Methods 72:313, 1984.
28. Southern PJ, Berg P: J Mol Appl Genet 1:327, 1982.
29. Hunter WM, Greenwood FC: Nature 194:495, 1962.
30. Carney DN, Gazdar AF, Bepler G, Guccion JG, Marangos PJ, Moody TW, Zweig MH, Minna JD: Cancer Res 45:2913, 1985.
31. Curran T, Teich NM: J Virol 42:114, 1982.
32. Docherty K, Steiner DF: Annu Rev Physiol 44:625, 1982.

33. Yoshizaki K, de Bock V, Solomon S: Life Sci 34:835, 1984.
34. Price J, Penman E, Bourne GL, Rees LH: Regul Pept 7:315, 1983.
35. Yamaguchi K, Abe K, Kameya T, Adachi I, Taguchi S, Otsubo K, Yanaihara N: Cancer Res 43:3932, 1983.
36. Moody TW, Russel EK, O'Donohue TL, Linden CD, Gazdar AF: Life Sci 32:487, 1983.
37. Takuwa N, Takuwa Y, Bollag WE, Rasmussen H: J Biol Chem 262:182, 1987.
38. Tatemoto K, Mutt V: Proc Natl Acad Sci USA 78:6603, 1981.
39. Moody TW, Pert CB, Rivier J, Brown MR: Proc Natl Acad Sci USA 75:5372, 1978.
40. Lazure C, Seidah NG, Pelaprat D, Chretien M: Can J Biochem Cell Biol 61:501, 1983.
41. Hilsted L, Rehfeld JF: Anal Biochem 152:119, 1986.
42. Gruss P, Khoury G: Proc Natl Acad Sci USA 78:133, 1981.
43. Laub O, Rutter WJ: J Biol Chem 258:6043, 1983.
44. Noel G, Zollinger L, Lariviere N, Nault C, Crine P, Boileau G: J Biol Chem 262:1876, 1987.
45. Warren TG, Shields D: Cell 39:547, 1984.

Journal of Cellular Biochemistry 36:249–260 (1988)
Growth Regulation of Cancer 97–108

Effect of Mutations Affecting Na$^+$:H$^+$ Antiport Activity on Tumorigenic Potential of Hamster Lung Fibroblasts

Alain E. Lagarde, Arlette J. Franchi, Sonia Paris, and Jacques M. Pouysségur

Mount Sinai Hospital Research Institute, Division of Cancer and Cell Biology, and Department of Medical Genetics, University of Toronto, 600 University Avenue, Toronto, Ontario, M5G 1X5, Canada (A.E.L.); Centre de Biochimie, CNRS, Université de Nice, Parc Valrose, 06034 Nice, France (A.J.F., S.P., J.M.P.)

Mutants unable to regulate intracellular pH through the Na$^+$:H$^+$ antiport system were found to evolve tumors less frequently than wild-type CCL39 hamster lung fibroblasts, after transplantation in athymic nude mice. When rare tumors arose, they comprised cells which were transformed in vitro, but which upon retransplantation grew at a lower rate than tumor cells originating from CCL39 cells. Both parental and mutant cells became transformed after transfection of the activated Harvey *ras* oncogene, but transfectants derived from the mutants had a weaker tumorigenic potential. These results suggest that transformed characteristics can be acquired independently from the Na$^+$:H$^+$ antiporter. However, the presence of this system provides a selective growth advantage when cells are confronted with natural environments, as it occurs during the expansion of tumors in a host.

Key words: Na$^+$:H$^+$ antiport, pH regulation, cell proliferation, neoplastic transformation

It is well established that an amiloride-sensitive Na$^+$:H$^+$ antiport system catalyzes the reversible and electroneutral exchange of Na$^+$ and H$^+$ ions across the plasma membrane of mammalian cells [1]. This system allows intracellular pH (pHin) to be maintained within narrow values compatible with cell viability and optimal proliferation [2]. It also becomes activated shortly after quiescent cells are stimulated to divide in response to growth factors or tumor-promoting phorbol esters [3–7]. The

Abbreviations used: pHin, intracellular pH; pHo, extracellular pH; THR, α-thrombin; EGF, Epidermal growth factor; INS, insulin; DME/F12, Dulbecco's modified minimal essential medium/Ham's F12 medium; FCS, fetal calf serum; Hepes, N-2-hydroxyethylpiperazine-N'-2-ethane sulfonic acid; Mes, 2-N-morpholino ethane sulfonic acid; Mops, 3-N-morpholino propane sulfonic acid; DMA, 5-N,N'-dimethylamiloride; DIDS, 4,4'-diisothiocyanostilbene-2,2'disulfonic acid.

Received February 19, 1987; revised and accepted August 18, 1987.

modest but persistent pHin alkalinization which results from this activation is believed to trigger rate-limiting reactions implicated in the conversion of growth factor signals into a proliferative response [8]. However, in bicarbonate-buffered medium, pHin may also be adjusted through the coordinate action of carbonic anhydrase and of a Na^+-dependent $HCO_3^-:Cl^-$ exchange system [9,10]. It has therefore been argued that a functional $Na^+:H^+$ antiport is not an essential component of the signal transducing pathways conducting the mitosis [11–13].

Methods were recently developed to isolate $Na^+:H^+$ antiport-defective mutants from Chinese hamster lung fibroblasts (CCL39) [14], mouse L cells [15], and pig kidney epithelial cells [16]. The division of mutants of the CCL39 cell line was found to obey the same dependence on extracellular pH (pHo) as their parent, in regular HCO_3^-/CO_2-buffered medium [2]. However, in the absence of bicarbonate, these mutants needed to be exposed to pHo values above 7.2, instead of 6.8, before they could be recruited to proliferate in response to factors such as α-thrombin (THR) and insulin (INS) [2,14]. In addition, they could not compensate for acute intracellular acidifying conditions with enough efficiency to prevent the process from becoming lethal [12].

In this study we examined the consequences that the loss of a functional $Na^+:H^+$ antiport activity might have on the acquisition of malignant attributes and on the development of tumors. We found that mutants unable to catalyze $Na^+:H^+$ exchange implanted less successfully in nude mice or grew at a slower rate than cells whose transport activity was intact. This trend was observed regardless of whether or not the cells had inherited an elevated anchorage-independent growth potential, a reduced requirement for growth factors, or were transformed with an activated *ras* oncogene. We conclude that if the $Na^+:H^+$ antiporter plays no crucial role in the transformation process, it does confer a selective advantage to malignant tumor cells proliferating in situ.

MATERIALS AND METHODS
Cell Lines

The growth factor dependence and malignant evolution of the Chinese hamster lung fibroblast CCL39 cell line (ATCC) were described in previous reports [17–19]. 39T10 is a malignant cell line which was isolated from a tumor growing at the site of subcutaneous (sc) inoculation, after transplanting CCL39 cells into athymic nude mice [17]. PS33, PS200, and PS120 are three mutants which were obtained after mutagenic treatment of CCL39 fibroblasts, followed by selection under conditions which specificially eliminate cells mediating $Na^+:H^+$ exchange [14]. The pHO6T1 plasmid was transfected into CCL39 and PS120 cells by Ca^{++}-phosphate precipitation, followed by selection in G418 (400 μg/ml)-containing medium, and 39ras5, 120ras1, and 120ras5 colonies were isolated. This vector contains the 6.6-kilobase (kb) Harvey *ras* oncogene of the human EJ bladder carcinoma, flanked by two potent viral enhancers, as well as the *neo*-resistance marker [20]. Expression of the human Ha-*ras* gene in the transfectants was verified by immunoprecipitation of the p21 protein with a specific antibody (Triton Biosciences Inc., Alameda, CA). Karyotype analysis indicated that all cell lines retained the same modal chromosomal number (2n = 22) as diploid CCL39 cells.

Tissue Culture Conditions

Cells were routinely propagated in DME/F12 medium (GIBCO, Grand Island, NY) supplemented with 2 mM L-glutamine, 2 g/liter sodium bicarbonate, 5 μg/ml human transferrin, and 10% FCS, without antibiotics. In experiments designed to test individual growth factors, FCS was either omitted (serum-free medium, SFM) or substituted with bovine insulin (INS 10 μg/ml), mouse EGF (10 ng/ml), or human α-thrombin (THR, 1 U/ml) from Sigma Chemical Co. (St. Louis, MO). Cells were plated in FCS-containing medium to allow attachment, and were subsequently rinsed twice with SFM before being exposed to purified factors on day 0. Cell counts were determined after a 6-day incubation period at 37°C in a humidified 5% CO$_2$–95% air atmosphere. The mean number of cell population doublings occurring between day 0 and 6 was calculated from duplicate cultures.

Cell growth in HCO$_3^-$/CO$_2$-free medium was followed at daily intervals by substituting sodium bicarbonate with 30 mM Hepes buffer adjusted to pH 7.0, 7.4, and 7.8. These media also included hypoxanthine (50 μM), uridine (50 μM), and dialyzed FCS (10%) and were replaced every 2 days, as described previously (14).

Colony Formation in Agarose

Eight thousand cells resuspended in SFM were mixed with 0.3% agarose (Type I, Sigma) and the appropriate concentrations of FCS (0 to 10%) and layered on a 0.5% agarose basal layer in 35-mm Petri dishes. Duplicate dishes were incubated for 8 days at 37°C in a humidified atmosphere of 5% CO$_2$–95% air. Colonies were scored under a microscope using a calibrated grid. Results were expressed as a percentage of colonies formed per seeded cell.

Measurement of DNA Synthesis

Cells inoculated in 24-well tissue culture plates were starved for 24 hr before being exposed to bicarbonate-free medium supplemented with dialyzed FCS (10%) and [methyl-^{3}H] thymidine (Amersham Corp., Oakville, ON, Canada; 1 μCi/ml, 2 μM). The amount of radioactivity incorporated into trichloroacetic acid-precipitable material during the next 24 hr in a CO$_2$-free incubator was determined by liquid scintillation counting. In this assay, which measures the re-initiation of DNA synthesis following G$_0$-arrest, the pH of the medium was initially adjusted with 30 mM of either Mes (pH = 6.25 to 6.7) or Mops (pH = 7.0 to 8.2), as described earlier [2,14].

Tumorigenicity Assays

Inocula comprising 1, 5, or 10 $\times$ 10^5 viable cells suspended in 0.2 ml phosphate-buffered saline were injected subcutaneously (sc) into the flank of 1-month-old BALB/c (*nu/nu*) mice. The presence of a progressively growing and localized tumor was assessed twice a week by palpation. Its size was measured with a ruler at weekly intervals thereafter. When tumors reached a size equivalent to 10 cm^3, the animals were sacrificed and inspected for the presence of macroscopic metastases in the lungs.

Measurement of Na$^+$ Uptake and Intracellular pH

The rate of ^{22}Na$^+$ uptake driven by an outwardly directed proton efflux, was estimated exactly as described previously [12,14]. Conditions for measuring pHin variations in response to NH_4^+-induced cytoplasmic acidification were also reported earlier [10].

RESULTS

Tumorigenic Potential of CCL39 Variants Exhibiting Altered Na^+:H^+ Antiport Activity

Earlier observations demonstrated that CCL39 fibroblasts were not tumorigenic at the onset since their injection in the peritoneal cavity or the tail vein of athymic nude mice resulted in no tumor formation [18]. However, inoculation of CCL39 cells at a sc site allows the outgrowth of rare variants which have inherited a complete transformed phenotype [17–19]. Accordingly, a relatively long latency period (~1 month) precedes the emergence of tumors in CCL39-injected animals, as shown in Figure 1. To address the question of whether the loss of a functional Na^+:H^+ antiport activity would affect this clonal evolution process, three independent mutants were characterized.

PS33, PS200, and PS120 mutants were isolated using a procedure which counterselects cells undergoing an acute and persistent intracellular acidification through the Na^+:H^+ antiport system [14]. Unlike PS200 and PS120 cells, PS33 cells retained some 30–40% normal antiport activity presumably because only one instead of two alleles of the responsible gene had been inactivated in this mutant [14]. As illustrated in Figure 1, sc injection of these mutants into nude mice led to the formation of tumors in 80% (PS33), 25% (PS120), and 0% (PS200) of the animals, respectively. Increasing the size of the inocula by a factor of ten did not enhance the incidence of tumors, and did not shorten their time of appearance. These findings suggest that unlike cells which are fully (CCL39) or partially (PS33) competent for mediating Na^+:H^+ exchange, mutants completely devoid of activity are not (PS200) or less frequently (PS120) converted into malignant variants once they are confronted with in vivo environments prevailing in nude mice.

As summarized in Table I, the growth characteristics of mutant and parental cells in tissue culture did not differ appreciably. In defined medium containing bicarbonate (pHo = 7.4) they arrested easily in G_0 upon removal of growth factors, and the same relative numbers of cell population doublings were induced in response to either serum, THR or THR and INS. EGF, with or without INS, appeared to be

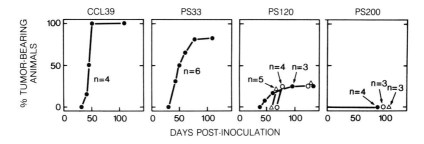

Fig. 1. Tumorigenicity of antiport-defective CCL39 mutants. Single cells suspensions containing $1\times$ (●), $5\times$ (○), and 10×10^5 cells (△) were injected subcutaneously into the flank of 4–6-week-old Balb/c athymic nude mice. The animals were followed on a weekly basis for the emergence of tumors growing progressively at the site of inoculation. n = number of animals inoculated per group.

TABLE I. Growth Properties of Wild-Type and Mutant Cell Lines*

Medium composition	CCL39	PS33	PS120	PS200	39T10	PS120-T1
No. of cell population doublings						
SFM	−0.5	−0.9	0.5	−0.8	2.9	1.8
INS (10 μg/ml)	1.1	−0.3	1.3	0.2	3.0	3.8
EGF (10 ng/ml)	2.2	0.2	0.6	−0.2	5.4	3.0
THR (1 U/ml)	3.9	3.4	3.2	2.3	5.5	4.3
INS + EGF	4.8	1.4	2.0	1.6	5.8	5.2
INS + THR	4.5	4.9	3.5	3.7	5.8	5.1
Serum: (0.1%)	0.9	0.2	2.1	0.1	5.2	3.2
(5%)	5.2	4.3	4.5	5.3	5.9	5.7
% colonies in agarose						
Serum: (0%)	0	0	0	0	0.5	0.1
(1%)	0	0	0	0	8.0	3.5
(10%)	2.0	1.5	0.5	1.4	27.0	32.0

*In normally bicarbonate buffered medium (pHo = 7.4) as described in Materials and Methods.

less efficient in promoting the division of PS120 and PS200 cells, but this was also observed for PS33 mutants. The mutants had the same limited capacity to grow as spheroids in semisolid agarose as parental cells. The slightly lower plating efficiencies manifested by the mutants are within the range of clonal variability observed in CCL39 cell populations. The only discernible difference between PS200, PS120, and PS33 and CCL39 cells resides in the inability of the former two mutants to re-initiate DNA synthesis in response to growth factor stimulation when the extracellular pH is below 7.2 [2,14]. As illustrated in Figure 2, at this pHo value CCL39 cells replicated DNA at 30% of its optimal level, whereas PS120 cells had to be exposed to pHo = 7.6 in order to reach a comparable rate of division. Thus, we presume that the nature of the environments prevailing in nude animals is such that antiport-defective mutants do not survive or proliferate as well as competent cells. Consequently, the spontaneous emergence of transformed variants from these mutants might be handicapped, thus explaining the rarity with which tumors arose and progressed. When tumors arise occasionally, as is the case in some PS120-injected animals (Fig. 1) they should comprise cells having selectively overcome conditions that restrict the process of malignant transformation. To examine this question we establish cell lines from PS120 and CCL39 tumors and we compared their characteristics.

Malignant Properties of Tumor Cell Lines Derived From Na$^+$:H$^+$ Antiport-Competent Versus -Deficient Cells

As shown in Figure 3, when PS120 tumor-derived cells (PS120-T1) were re-implanted into nude mice, tumors formed in 100% of the animals. These tumors arose not only systematically but also earlier than those induced in PS120- or CCL39-injected mice (Fig. 1). They progressed steadily to reach a median size of ~3 cm^3 after 50 days. Likewise, CCL39 tumor-derived cells (39T10) produced tumors which expanded rapidly but which eventually attained a tenfold larger size (Fig. 3). This significant difference in the rate at which 39T10 and PS120-T1 tumors progressed might reflect the intrinsically weaker growth potential of PS120-T1 tumor cells which cannot regulate pHin through the Na$^+$:H$^+$ antiport system.

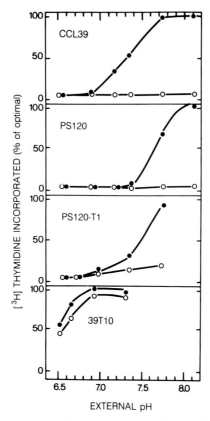

Fig. 2. pH dependence of the rate of DNA synthesis in CCL39, PS120, PS120-T1, and 39T10 cell lines. Cells were exposed to SFM for 24 hr in HCO_3^-/CO_2^- buffered medium, pHo = 7.4. They were then exposed to bicarbonate-free medium buffered with Mes or Mops, containing [^{3}H]thymidine, with (●) or without (○) 10% dialyzed serum. The amount of radioactivity incorporated 24 hr later was determined.

Results listed in Table I indicate that both 39T10 and PS120-T1 cells inherited features commonly associated with the transformed phenotype. They escaped G_0-arrest controls and therefore divided at a substantial rate in serum-free medium; they responded better to INS, EGF, or THR than CCL39 and PS120 parental cells; and they formed colonies in agarose at a ~20-fold higher frequency. However, PS120-T1 differed from 39T10 cells in that their rate of DNA replication (Fig. 2) and proliferation (Fig. 4A) were submitted to the same pHo controls as their PS120 progenitors. Under the same conditions (i.e. in bicarbonate-free medium), 39T10 tumor cells replicated DNA between pHo 6.5 and 7.5, regardless of whether or not they were stimulated by growth factors (Fig. 2). Therefore external pH had a much greater restrictive influence on the division of PS120-T1 cells than on that of 39T10 cells.

Additional experiments depicted in Figure 4B and 4C confirm the absence of a functional $Na^+{:}H^+$ antiport system in PS120-T1 cells. Firstly these cells were unable to rapidly re-establish an initial pHin value following NH_4^+-induced acid load (Fig. 4B). CCL39 cells were shown previously to readjust acidification [12]. In both PS120 and PS120-T1 cells, protection against a persistent cytoplasmic acidification was

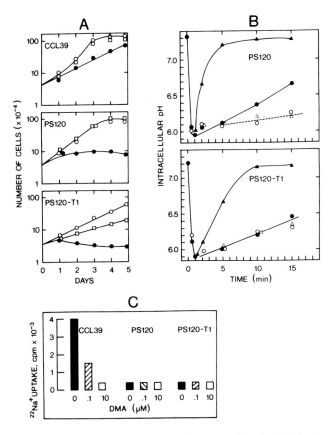

Fig. 3.   Properties of PS120 and PS120-T1 cell lines. **A:** Cell proliferation in bicarbonate/CO$_2$-free medium buffered at pHo 7.0 (●), 7.4 (□), and 7.8 (○). Medium supplemented with 10% dialyzed fetal calf serum, hypoxanthine, uridine, and appropriate buffer solutions was changed on day 0, 2, and 4, as described previously [14]. **B:** Kinetics of pHi recovery following NH$_4^+$-induced intracellular acidification in the absence (●) and presence of 1 mM DIDS (○), 5 mM NaHCO$_3$ (▲), 5 mM NaHCO$_3$ and 1 mM DIDS (△). Cells were pre-incubated with 20 mM NH$_4$Cl for 45 min. At time 0, extracellular NH$_4^+$ was removed and radiolabelled benzoic acid intracellular content was measured at time intervals to determine pHi as described previously [10]. **C:** Rate of ^{22}Na$^+$ influx in CCL39, PS120, and PS120-T1 cells in the absence and presence of 5-N, N$^{'}$-dimethylamiloride (DMA). Conditions for measuring ^{22}Na$^+$ uptake driven by H$^+$ efflux were described previously [14].

afforded through the Na$^+$-dependent HCO$_3^-$ exchange system [10], as indicated by experiments involving addition of bicarbonate ions (Fig. 4B). This protection was abolished when the specific inhibitor of the anionic exchange system, DIDS, was added in conjunction with bicarbonate (Fig. 4B). Secondly, no amiloride-sensitive ^{22}Na$^+$ uptake could be detected in PS120 or PS120-T1 cells (Fig. 4C). These findings indicate that the oncogenic events which were at the origin of the PS120-T1 tumor did not involve the partial recovery of a functional Na$^+$:H$^+$ antiport activity, or the expression of another transport system possessing an equivalent pH-regulating function. Instead, in the course of their first passage into the animal, PS120 cells acquired an enhanced proliferative potential whose expression remains restricted by adverse environmental conditions requesting appropriate pHin regulation.

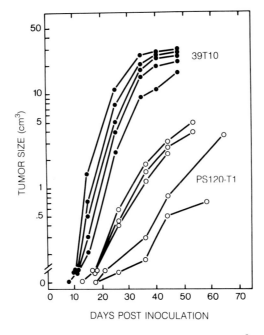

Fig. 4. Tumorigenicity of 39T10 and PS120-T1 tumor-derived cells. 1×10^5 cells were injected sc into groups of six Balb/c nude mice, and tumor size was measured at regular intervals.

Properties of CCL39 and PS120 Harvey ras Transfectants

The possibility that the differential tumorigenic potential of 39T10 and PS120-T1 cells resulted from the deregulation of unrelated oncogenes rather than from their distinct ability to respond to pH variations could not be excluded. We therefore investigated whether the deliberate introduction of a potent oncogene into CCL39 and PS120 cells would confer upon them similar transformed characteristics. A plasmiol vector encoding the activated form (VAL^{12} mutation) of the human Ha-*ras* oncogene was transfected into CCL39 and PS120 fibroblasts, and three neomycin-resistant colonies—39ras5, 120ras1, and 120ras5—were characterized. Immunoprecipitation experiments of p21 proteins indicated that 120ras5 cells express ~5-fold less *ras* products than 39ras5 and 120ras5 (not shown). This level was nevertheless tenfold higher than in CCL39 or PS120 cells because of the strong viral promoters driving the *ras* gene [20]. All three transfectants were transformed according to conventional criteria (Fig. 5): they were highly refractile and displayed altered morphological features; they cloned in semisolid agarose with an elevated frequency; and they divided in the absence of growth factor stimulation. However, whereas sc inoculation of 39ras5 cells into nude mice led to the systematic formation of tumors growing at a rate of ~5 cm^3 per month, tumors formed in only 75% and 50% of the cases in 120ras5 and 120ras1-injected animals, respectively (Fig. 5). Furthermore, some of the latter tumors grew for approximately a month and subsequently regressed so that the overall incidence of persisting tumors was respectively 100% (39ras5), 50% (120ras1), and 25% (120ras5). Another noticeable difference between the two classes of *ras*-transfectants was that 39ras5 tumors were invasive and disseminated to the lungs, whereas only one animal among those injected with 120ras1 and 120ras5 cells showed pulmonary metastases, after 60 days. Histological sections of 120ras1 and

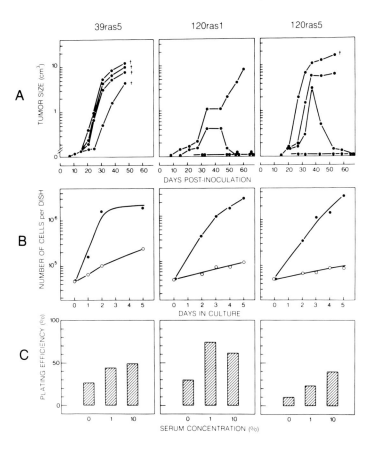

Fig. 5. Properties of 39ras5, 120ras1, and 120ras5 transfected cell lines. **A:** Tumorigenic potential. 1×10^5 cells were injected sc into groups of four nude mice, and tumor size was measured at regular intervals. Pulmonary metastases were detected in all 39ras5-injected animals at day 50, but in only one 120ras5-injected mouse (†). **B:** Proliferation in serum-free (○) and serum-containing medium (●) buffered at pHo $= 7.4$ with bicarbonate-CO_2. Serum was removed at day 1, and on day 0 monolayers were fed with either SFM or 5% serum. Cultures were trypsinized at daily intervals and cell numbers were determined. Mean of duplicated determinations is shown. **C:** Percentage colonies forming in semisolid agarose supplemented with 0%, 1% and 10% serum.

120ras5 tumors at day 50 revealed extensive zones of necrosis extending from the center to the periphery. Therefore, despite the fact that transfection of the *ras* oncogene induced similar transformed characteristics in parental and mutant cells the tumor-forming ability of cells unable to mediate Na⁺:H⁺ exchange was comparatively lower.

DISCUSSION

The mechanisms by which the Na⁺:H⁺ antiporter regulates the intracellular pH of mammalian cells are receiving considerable attention [1]. In this study we attempted to confirm the role previously attributed to this system in the pH control of cell proliferation [2,21]. To this end we took advantage of the recent isolation of fibroblast mutants unable to catalyze $Na^+:H^+$ exchange [14] to examine whether such a defect would affect the extent of cell division, as determined in an in vivo context. We compared preneoplastic, malignant, and *ras*-transformed CCL39-cell lines, lacking or not $Na^+:H^+$ antiport activity, for their ability to evolve tumors after implantation into nude mice.

We first showed that two mutants (PS200, PS120) induced tumors less frequently than their CCL39 parent. We believe the significantly lower tumor incidence is directly accountable for the complete lack of transport activity since another mutant (PS33) which had retained residual activity was nearly as tumorigenic as CCL39 cells (Fig. 1). However, we ignore the reasons that PS200 did not form tumors at all, whereas PS120 cells did so occasionally. We found no discernible difference between these two mutants concerning their rate of proliferation in response to growth factors or in semisolid media (Table I). They similarly failed to take up $^{22}Na^+$ ions in an amiloride-sensitive manner, and did not replicate at external pHs below 7.2, two properties associated with the loss of a functional $Na^+:H^+$ antiport activity [2,14]. We noticed that PS200 and PS120 mutants were characteristically less responsive to EGF at concentrations which are weakly mitogenic to normal CCL39 cells. This observation is unlikely to explain the modest tumorigenic potential of these mutants, since PS33 cells were also less responsive to EGF, but were nevertheless able to form tumors. Fewer EGF binding sites (50% less than normal) were detected on the membrane of PS120 cells, but it was demonstrated that the process of ligand internalization was not impaired in such a mutant [22]. The tumorigenic potential of CCL39 fibroblasts was previously shown to reside in the propensity of these cells to generate authentic malignant variants at low frequency when implanted at a sc site in nude mice [17,18]. We speculate that conditions prevailing in this particular environment are poorly permissive to mutant cells which require either high concentrations of Na^+ and bicarbonate ions, or a slightly alkaline medium (pHo $>$, 7.2) [2,14] in order to undergo a minimum number of divisions before malignant variants arise.

The lack of antiport activity did not preclude cells from acquiring a completely transformed phenotype. Not only did rare PS120-derived tumors such as PS120-T1 comprise cells which manifested transformed features in vitro (Table I), but mutant cells could also become transformed after transfection of the Ha-*ras* oncogene (Fig. 5). However, despite the fact that PS120-T1, 120 ras1, and 120ras5 cells inherited an increased capacity to grow without anchorage and partially escaped growth factor requirements, their tumorigenic potential was comparatively weaker than that of 39T10 and 39ras 5 cells. If PS120-T1 cells initiated tumors much earlier and more frequently than PS120 cells, these tumors expanded less rapidly than 39T10 cells which were not impaired in the ability to exchange Na^+ and H^+ ions (Fig. 2). Likewise, tumors arose less frequently and did not always persist in animals challenged with *ras*-transformed antiport-less mutants, whereas they were extremely aggressive in mice receiving implants of *ras*-transformed competent cells (Fig. 5). We believe these differences reflect the distinct fate of cell populations that can or cannot overcome exposure to low pH values. It is well documented that hypoxia and acidosis develop in rapidly growing tumors, and that these factors are in part responsible for necrosis [23,24]. Direct measurements using microelectrodes [25] and telemetry capsules [26] have revealed that the intratumoral pH of some tumors may be as low as 6.3 $\pm$ 0.1. Such values are clearly below the threshold (pHo = 6.8) at which fibroblasts can divide [2,27]. Antiport-deficient cells whose threshold pH is even more alkaline (pHo $= 7.2$) would conceivably be vulnerable even under less severe conditions. The excessive production of lactic acid by tumor cells is recognized to be responsible in part for the marked acidification of their immediate environment [28]. This process has clearly been shown to be one of the metabolic consequences of activation of the *ras* oncogene [29]. Levels of lactate production would have to be compared among the cell lines that we characterized to determine whether there is any correlation between the stage of transformation, the extent of acidification due to lactic acid release, and the kinetics of tumor expansion in vivo.

The present report strongly suggests that the Na$^+$:H$^+$ antiporter is a limiting factor in cell proliferation by virtue of its ability to maintain a steady pHin under conditions when other pHin-regulating systems operate less efficiently. Its controls apply to normal as well as to neoplastically transformed cells. The recent suggestion that this exchange system contributes to the development of the malignant phenotype [27] is contradicted by our observation showing that CCL39 fibroblasts can acquire this phenotype even when this function is deleted by mutations. We also obtained evidence that CCL39 mutants which overexpress the Na$^+$:H$^+$ antiport activity [30] do not inherit a selective advantage to grow as tumors in comparison to CCL39 parental cells (unpublished results).

The conclusions drawn from this study regarding the role of the Na$^+$:H$^+$ antiporter in the development of tumors assume that mutations abrogating the exchange activity are indeed affecting the gene encoding the transporter molecule. The possibility that they affect a distinct protein which would regulate the antiporter as well as other cellular processes cannot be formally excluded. However, recent transfection experiments point to the contrary [15], and the molecular characterization of the human gene which can restore a wild-type phenotype in Hamster mutants should resolve this ambiguity.

ACKNOWLEDGMENTS

This work was supported by grants from the National Cancer Institute of Canada (N.C.I.C.), the Centre National de la Recherche Scientifique, and the Institut National de la Recherche Médicale. A.E.L. is the recipient of an N.C.I.C. Research Scholarship award, and of a short-term I.C.R.E.T.T. fellowship. We gratefully acknowledge the technical assistance of J. Dixon and the secretarial help of Astrid Eberhart.

REFERENCES

1. Moolenar WH: Annu Rev Physiol 48:363, 1986.
2. Pouysségur JA, Franchi A, L'Allemain G, Paris S: FEBS Lett 190:115, 1985.
3. Besterman JM, Cuatrecasas P: J Cell Biol 99:340, 1984.
4. Burns CP, Rozengurt E: Biochem Biophys Res Commun 116:931, 1983.
5. Cassel D, Rothenberg P, Zhyang Y, Deuel TF, Glaser L: Proc Natl Acad Sci USA 80:6224, 1983.
6. Grinstein S, Cohen S, Goetz D, Rothstein A, Gelfand EW: Proc Natl Acad Sci USA 82:1429, 1985.
7. Moolenar WH, Tertoolen LGJ, de Laat SW: J Biol Chem 259:7563, 1984.
8. Rozengurt E: Science 234:161, 1986.
9. Jentsch TJ, Stahlknecht TR, Hollwede H, Fisher DG, Keller SK, Wiederholt: J Biol Chem 260:795, 1985.
10. L'Allemain G, Paris S, Pouysségur J: J Biol Chem 260:4877, 1985.
11. L'Allemain G, Franchi A, Cragoe E, Pouysségur J: J Biol Chem 259:4313, 1984.
12. L'Allemain G, Paris S, Pouysségur J: J Biol Chem 259:5809, 1984.

13. Besterman JM, Tyrey SJ, Cragoe EJ, Cuatrecasas P: Proc Natl Acad Sci USA 81:6762, 1984.
14. Pouysségur J, Sardet C, Franchi A, L'Allemain G, Paris S: Proc Natl Acad Sci USA 81:4833, 1984.
15. Franchi A, Perucca-Lostanlen D, Pouyssegur J: Proc Natl Acad Sci USA 83:9388, 1986.
16. Agarwal NH, Haggerty E, Adelberg E, Slayman C: Am J Physiol 251:C825, 1986.
17. Perez-Rodriquez R, Chambard JC, Van Obberghen-Schilling E, Franchi A, Pouysségur J: J Cell Physiol 109:387, 1981.
18. Renwick D, Franchi A, Pouysségur J, Lagarde A: J Natl Cancer Inst 77:105, 1986.
19. Van Obberghen-Schilling E, Perez-Rodriquez R, Franchi A, Chambard JC, Pouysségur J: J Cell Physiol 115:123, 1983.
20. Spandidos DA, Wilkie NM: Nature 310:469, 1984.
21. Busa WB, Nuccitelli R: Am J Physiol 246:R409, 1984.
22. Hwang J, Pouysségur J, Willingham MC, Pastan I: J Cell Physiol 128:18, 1986.
23. Rotin D, Robinson B, Tannock IF: Cancer Res 46:2821, 1986.
24. Rotin D, Wan P, Grinstein S, Tannock IF: Cancer Res 47:1497, 1987.
25. Jain RK, Shah SA, Finney PL: J Natl Cancer Inst 73:429, 1984.
26. Hinsull SM, Colson RH, Franklin A, Watson BW, Bellamy D: J Natl Cancer Inst 73:463, 1984.
27. Ober SS, Pardee AB: Proc Natl Acad Sci USA 84:2766, 1987.
28. Sauer LA, Douchy RT: J Biol Chem 260:7496, 1985.
29. Racker E, Resnick RJ, Feldman R: Proc Natl Acad Sci USA 82:3535, 1985.
30. Franchi A, Cragoe E, Pouysségur J: J Biol Chem 261:14614, 1986.

Journal of Cellular Biochemistry 36:341–352 (1988)
Growth Regulation of Cancer 109–120

Assessment of Biological Activity of Synthetic Fragments of Transforming Growth Factor-Alpha

Krzysztof Darlak, Glen Franklin, Philip Woost, Elaine Sonnenfeld, Daniel Twardzik, Arno Spatola, and Gregory Schultz

Departments of Biochemistry (G.F., P.W., E.S., G.S.) and Chemistry (K.D., A.S.), University of Louisville, Louisville, Kentucky 40292, and Oncogen (D.T.) Seattle, Washington 98121

Transforming growth factor-alpha (TGF-α) is a single chain polypeptide hormone of 50 amino acids that stimulates growth of some human cancer cells via an autocrine mechanism. The domain(s) of TGF-α that bind and activate its receptor have not been reported. Hydrophilicity plots of TGF-α indicate three discrete sequences that are theoretically exposed on the hormone's surface and thus potentially able to interact with the TGF-α receptor. Fragments of TGF-α encompassing these hydrophilic domains were prepared by using solid-phase peptide synthesis (SPPS) techniques and purified by use of high performance liquid chromotography (HPLC). Assessment of biological activity of the TGF-α fragments indicated that none of the fragments significantly inhibited binding of EGF to the receptor, stimulated DNA synthesis of cells, inhibited EGF-induced DNA synthesis of cells, stimualted growth of cells in soft agar, or induced phosphorylation of the receptor or p35 protein. These results indicate that the receptor binding domain of TGF-α is not totally encompassed by any of the separate fragments tested and probably is formed by multiple separate regions of TGF-α.

Key words: **peptides, mitogens, solid-phase peptide synthesis**

TGF-α is a mitogenic hormone that is thought to play important roles in normal fetal development and in tumor growth. Northern analysis of RNA isolated from rat embryos indicated that TGF-α transcripts were expressed at high levels during early development (8–10 days) then declined to undetectable levels at birth [1]. Analysis of normal adult human tissues for TGF-α transcripts found no mRNA for TGF-α but approximately half of 39 human tumor specimens contained mRNA for TGF-α [2]. Also, TGF-α was detected in urine of patients with various malignancies [3] and was secreted in vitro by a variety of malignant human cells [2]. Recently, TGF-α was shown to be the agent responsible for growth of MCF-7 human breast cancer cells in vivo by an autocrine mechanism [4]. Estrogen appears to stimulate growth of MCF-7 cells indirectly by inducing synthesis and secretion of TGF-α.

Received February 23, 1987; revised and accepted September 10, 1987.

TGF-α is synthesized as a large, single chain, transmembrane glycoprotein of 160 amino acids from which the smaller 50 amino acid polypeptide hormone of is cleaved by the action of an uncharacterized protease that cleaves between Ala-Val residues at both the N- and C-terminals [5]. TGF-α has 30% sequence homology with epidermal growth factor (EGF) and vaccinia virus growth factor (VGF) [6]. All three growth factors share similar placement of three intrachain disulfide loops and all three bind and activate the tyrosine kinase activity of a common membrane receptor. The domain(s) of TGF-α that bind and activate its receptor have not been reported. Hydrophilicity plots of TGF-α indicate three discrete sequences that are theoretically exposed on the hormone's surface and thus potentially able to interact with the TGF-α receptor. We synthesized and purified fragments of TGF-α encompassing these hydrophilic domains using solid-phase peptide synthesis (SPPS) techniques and high performance liquid chromatography (HPLC) and analyzed the fragments for biological activity in several assays. In some cases where disulfide bridging overlapped, selected cysteine residues were replaced by alanine to conserve structural and hydrophobic parameters.

MATERIALS AND METHODS
Synthesis of TGF-α Fragments

The primary amino acid sequence of rat TGF-α (1–50) is shown in Figure 1. Fragments of TGF-α are listed in Table I and peptides 1–7 were prepared by SPPS using the standard Merrifield method [7] with a Peptides International Synthor 2000 automated synthesizer (Louisville, KY) and peptides 8–13 were prepared by Peninsula Laboratories (San Carlos, CA). Alpha-amino groups were protected with t-butyloxy-carbonyl (Boc) group and the following side chain protecting groups were used: Arg(Tos), Asp(Cxl), Cys(Acm) or Cys(Meb), Glu(Cxl), His(Bom), Lys(Cl-Z), Ser(Bzl), and Tyr(Dcb). Each synthetic cycle consisted of 1) 5-min and 25-min deprotection with 40% trifluoroacetic acid (TFA)/10% anisole/50% dichloromethane, 2) 5-min neutralization with 10% triethylamine/dichloromethane, and 3) double couplings (3-hr and 16-hr) with Boc-amino acid in the presence of N-hydroxybenzotriazole (HOBt) and dicyclohexylcarbodiimide (DCC), all at 2.5-fold mole excess over amino acid on resin. Asn and Gln were coupled with their preformed p-nitrophenyl esters in the presence of HOBt, and Arg(Tos) and Gly were coupled with DCC omitting HOBt. All couplings were monitored with the Kaiser test. Triethylamine was distilled from ninhydrin; dichloromethane was distilled from potassium carbonate; dimethylformamide was distilled under reduced pressure. Other solvents and reagents were of analytical grade.

Peptides were deprotected and cleaved from resin with anhydrous HF (1 hr at 0°C) in the presence of 5% p-cresol (v/v) and 5% dimethyl sulfide (v/v). After evaporation of HF and scavengers, solid residues were washed with diethyl ether, extracted with 10% acetic acid and lyophilized. Residues were dissolved in 30% acetic acid and desalted on a Sephadex G-25 column eluted with 30% acetic acid. The major peak of each peptide was pooled, lyophilized, and purified by reversed phase preparative high performance liquid chromatography (HPLC) using a Vydac C-18 column (250 × 10 mm, 300-angstrom pore size, Separations Science, Hesperia, CA) with a gradient of 15% to 30% acetonitrile/water containing 0.05% TFA. HPLC columns had not been used previously to purify any growth factors.

Peptides containing cystine disulfide bonds were produced by washing the residues obtained after HF cleavage with diethyl ether containing 1% 2-mercaptoethanol, then extracted with 10% acetic acid under nitrogen. After lyophilization, residues were dissolved in 0.2% acetic acid saturated with nitrogen, and 2 N aqueous ammonia was added gradually to give a final pH of 7.0 to 7.5. Solutions of the peptides were treated with 20 μM $K_3Fe(CN)_6$ until a permanent yellow color was generated and then stirred for an additional 20 min. The pH was adjusted to 4–5 with acetic acid, and then the solutions were stirred with anion exchange resin (AG 3 $\times$ 4, acetate form) to remove excess ferri- and ferrocyanide ions and then lyophilized. Residues were desalted by chromatography on a Sephadex G-15 column eluted with 30% acetic acid and then purified by HPLC as described above.

Competition of EGF Binding

Peptides were tested for their ability to compete for ^{125}I-EGF binding using two receptor sources: placental cell membranes and A-431 cells. Normal term human placenta was homogenized at 4°C with a Brinkman Polytron in a solution of 250 mM sucrose, 1 mM calcium chloride buffered to pH 7 with 10 mM Tris, then filtered through four layers of cheese cloth [8]. Aliquots of placental membrane (50 μg) were incubated with a constant amount of ^{125}I-EGF and increasing amounts of unlabeled EGF or peptides for 2 hr at 37°C. Four milliliters of cold buffer was then added and reaction tubes were centrifuged at 7,000g for 20 min at 4°C and pellets counted with a Beckman gamma scintillation counter. Values represent the mean of triplicate determinations. Competition binding assays using A-431 cells were conducted as described and the values reported represent the mean of duplicate determinations [9].

Induction of DNA Synthesis

Peptides were tested for their ability to stimulate DNA synthesis using diploid human foreskin fibroblasts (HFF) or mouse 3T3 fibroblasts. Confluent, quiescent cultures of HFF, which had been seeded into 96-well plates and held in 0.2% calf serum for 2 days, received 10 ng/ml of TGF-α or 100 ng/ml of peptides. After 8 hr, cultures were labeled with 5-^{125}I]iodo-2-deoxyuridine (Amersham, 10 μCi/μg) and the amount of isotope incorporated into TCA-insoluble material measured in triplicate wells [9]. Assays using mouse 3T3 fibroblasts were conducted as described below.

Inhibition of EGF-Induced DNA Synthesis

Confluent cultures of the J-2 clone of mouse 3T3 fibroblasts (H. Green, Harvard University) were washed with PBS and held in chemically defined medium (CDM) (equal parts of Dulbecco's modified Eagle medium, Medium 199, Ham's F-10, and buffered with 25 mM HEPES to pH 7.4) containing 0.5% calf serum for 24 hr and then harvested with trypsin. Twenty-four-well plates were seeded with 30,000 cells in 500 μl of CDM containing 0.5% calf serum and tritiated thymidine (1 μCi/ml, Amersham, [methyl,1',2'-^{3}H]thymidine, final specific activity 100 μCi/mmol). Five hundred microliters of CDM containing 0.5% calf serum and the indicated levels of serum EGF or peptides was added and incubated for 72 hr. Culture wells were washed twice with PBS, 5% TCA, methanol, then dissolved in 1 N sodium hydroxide and radioactivity measured with a beta scintillation counter. Quadruplicate wells were measured and averaged.

Stimulation of Anchorage-Independent Cell Growth

Soft agar growth assay was performed using normal rat kidney cells (NRK) [9]. The number of colonies represents those colonies containing a minimun of 20 NRK cells per 6 random low power fields 10 days after seeding plates with TGF-α or peptides. Plates contained 2 ng/ml of TGF-β purified from human platelets [10] and the designated amounts of TGF-α or peptides. Plates of NRK cells treated with TGF-β alone did not form colonies.

Growth Factor-Induced Phosphorylation

Placental membranes (50 μg) were added to a reaction mixture at 4°C containing TGF-α or peptides at the designated amounts and ^{32}P-ATP and AMP-PNP to reduce phosphatase activity. After 5 min reactions were stopped by addition of SDS and processed by polyacrylamide gel electrophoresis and autoradiography [8].

RESULTS
Chemical Characterization of TGF-α Fragments

The primary amino acid sequence of rat TGF-α [11] is shown in Figure 1. The hydrophilicity plot [12] of TGF-α is shown in Figure 2. Three regions contain high indexes of hydrophilicity and encompass amino acids 8–13, 25–31, and 42–47. These sequences are located essentially within the three disulfide loops. Table I lists the fragments of TGF-α synthesized and Table II lists expected and measured amino acid compositions of the TGF-α fragments (1–6). Values for all the peptides are within experimental error of predicted values. Table III lists the physiochemical properties of the TGF-α fragments (1–6), and all the peptides were greater than 95% pure by HPLC analysis and gave a single spot in two TLC systems.

Competition of EGF Binding

As shown in Figure 3, EGF effectively competes for ^{125}I-EGF binding to human placental membranes with 50% displacement at approximately 2 nM and 90% of the

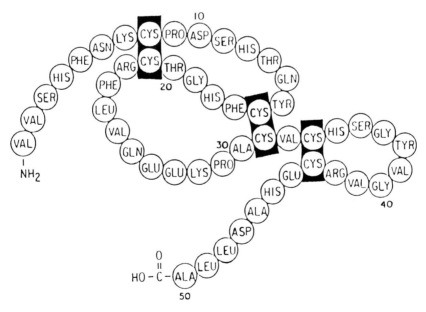

Fig. 1.   Primary amino acid sequence of rat TGF-α. TGF-α has substantial sequence homology with EGF and VGF including the alignment of the three disulfide bonds.

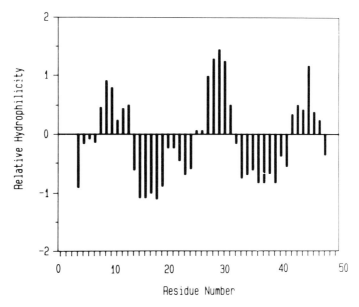

Fig. 2.   Hydrophilicity plot of rat TGF-α. TGF-α contains three separate regions of hydrophilicity.

TABLE I. TGF-α Fragments*

Sequence	Peptide number
TGF-α (34–50)	1
Ac-TGF-α (34–43)-NH$_2$	2
[S-AcmCys^{21,32}]TGF-α (21–33)	3
[Ala^{32}]TGF-α (22–43)-NH$_2$	4
[Ala^{16}]TGF-α (1–21)-NH$_2$	5
[S-AcmCys^{16,32}Ala^{21}]TGF-α (15–33)	6
[Ala^{21}]TGF-α (16–33)	7
TGF-α (1–15)	8
[Tyr^{32}]TGF-α (22–32)	9
TGF-α (34–50)	10
TGF-α (34–43)	11
TGF-α (41–50)	12
TGF-α (26–36)	13

*Peptides 1 through 7 were prepared by Merrifield method of solid phase peptide synthesis, and peptides 8 through 13 were prepared by Peninsula Laboratories.

total binding displaced by 10 μM unlabeled EGF. In contrast, none of the TGF-α fragments (1–7) effectively competed for ^{125}I-EGF binding even at 100 μM concentrations. By the use of A-431 cells as the receptor source the same results were obtained: EGF (10 nM) displaced 92% of ^{125}I-EGF binding while none of the TGF-α fragments (1–5, 7) competed for ^{125}I-EGF binding even at 100 μM (Fig. 4).

Induction of DNA Synthesis

TGF-α (10 ng/ml) stimulated incorporation ^{125}IdU sevenfold over control cultures of human foreskin fibroblasts (Table IV). Fragments of TGF-α (1–5, 7) tested

TABLE II. Amino Acid Composition of Synthetic TGF-α Peptides*

Amino acid	Peptide 1	Peptide 2	Peptide 3	Peptide 4	Peptide 5	Peptide 6	Peptide 7
Ala	2.06 (2)	—	0.87 (1)	0.87 (1)	1.01 (1)	2.03 (2)	1.99 (2)
Asp	0.98 (1)	—	—	—	1.79 (2)	—	—
Arg	0.97 (1)	1.17 (1)	0.93 (1)	0.93 (1)	—	1.04 (1)	0.97 (1)
(Cys)$_2$	1.08 (1)	0.89 (1)	—	—	0.60 (1)	—	ND
Glu	1.05 (1)	—	3.01 (3)	3.02 (3)	1.00 (1)	3.07 (3)	3.23 (3)
Gly	2.00 (2)	2.07 (2)	—	—	1.00 (1)	1.00 (1)	1.00 (1)
His	1.92 (2)	1.08 (1)	—	—	3.06 (3)	1.01 (1)	0.86 (1)
Leu	2.09 (2)	—	1.00 (1)	1.00 (1)	—	0.98 (1)	1.01 (1)
Lys	—	—	0.98 (1)	0.97 (1)	0.89 (1)	1.06 (1)	1.00 (1)
Phe	—	—	0.98 (1)	0.98 (1)	1.98 (2)	1.96 (2)	1.89 (2)
Pro	—	—	1.22 (1)	1.42 (1)	1.25 (1)	1.46 (1)	1.29 (1)
Ser	0.87 (1)	0.83 (1)	—	—	1.59 (2)	—	—
Thr	—	—	—	—	1.76 (2)	0.89 (1)	0.91 (1)
Tyr	1.03 (1)	1.14 (1)	—	—	0.98 (1)	0.96 (1)	—
Val	2.10 (2)	2.00 (2)	1.95 (2)	1.95 (2)	1.52 (2)	1.82 (2)	2.11 (2)

*Peptides (0.5 mg) were hydrolyzed with constant boiling hydrochloric acid (0.4 ml) containing phenol (20 μl) in evacuated and sealed ampules for 24 hours at 110°C. Analyses were performed on a Dionex analyzer. Values in parentheses are predicted molar ratios. ND, not determined.

TABLE III. Physiocochemical Properties of TGF-α Fragments*

Peptide number	R_f		K'
	BAW	BAWP	HPLC
1	0.08	0.77	2.90
2	0.05	0.76	3.96
3	0.09	0.78	4.40
4	0.02	0.70	3.39
5	0.15	0.74	4.55
6	0.05	0.78	3.18
7	0.16	0.77	3.92

*Purified peptides shown in Table II gave the indicated relative migration in thin layer chromatography systems: BAW, 1-butanol-acetic acid-water (4:1:5, v/v, upper phase); BAWP, 1-butanol-acetic acid-water-pyridine (15:12:10:3, v/v). Analytical C-18 reversed phase HPLC was performed using 20-min linear gradient (flow rate 1 ml/min) from 15–40% acetonitrile/water v/v containing 0.05% trifluoroacetic acid.

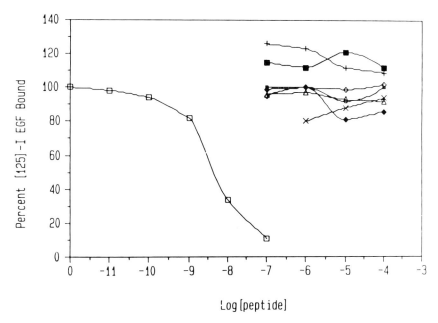

Fig. 3. Competition of EGF binding to human placental membranes. Aliquots of placental membranes (50 μg) were incubated with a constant amount of ^{125}I-EGF (100 pM) and unlabeled EGF or peptides at the indicated levels. After 2 hr at 37°C, tubes were centrifuged and pellets counted. Values are the mean of triplicate samples. Peptides are EGF (⊡), peptide 1 (◇), peptide 2 (△), peptide 3 (◆), peptide 4 (×), peptide 5 (■), peptide 6 (□), and peptide 7 (+).

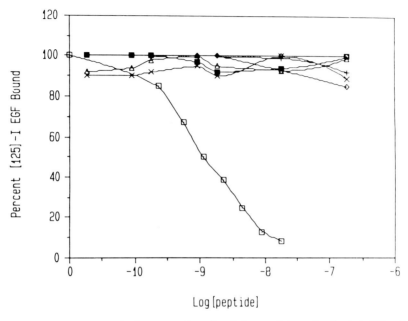

Fig. 4. Competition of EGF binding to A-431 cells. Cultures of formalin fixed A-431 cells were incubated with ^{125}I-EGF (300 pM) and increasing amounts of unlabeled peptides. After 1 hr at 37°C, wells (16 mm) were washed and radioactivity measured. Values are the mean of triplicate samples. Peptides are EGF (□), peptide 1 (◊), peptide 2 (△), peptide 3 (◆), peptide 4 (×), peptide 5 (■), and peptide 7 (+).

TABLE IV. Induction of DNA Synthesis*

Peptide	[125I]IdU incorporated (cpm/dish)
TGF-α	7,824
1	856
2	1,012
3	956
4	979
5	1,005
7	804
No addition	1,075

*Quiescent cultures of diploid human foreskin fibroblasts were seeded into 96-well plates and cultured in medium containing 0.2% calf serum. After 2 days TGF-α (10 ng/ml) or peptides (100 ng/ml) were added and 8 hr later labeled with [125I]IdU for 8 hr and TCA insoluble radioactivity measured. Values are mean of triplicate samples.

at 100 ng/ml all failed to stimulate DNA synthesis above control levels. When 3T3 fibroblasts were used for mitogenesis assay, EGF (1 nM) stimulated thymidine incorporation twofold over control cultures and peptides 1 to 4 (100 μM) again failed to stimulate DNA synthesis.

Inhibition of EGF-Induced DNA Synthesis

As shown in Figure 5, 3T3 cells incubated in CDM containing 0.5% calf serum incorporated small amounts of tritiated thymidine. Addition of 10% calf serum increased thymidine incorporation fivefold and addition of 1 nM EGF increased thymidine incorporation twofold over incorporation in the presence of 0.5% calf serum. Simultaneous addition of 1 nM EGF with each of TGF-α fragments 1 through 4 at 100 μM failed to reduce thymidine incorporation below the level of stimulation measured with EGF alone.

Stimulation of Anchorage-Independent Cell Growth

TGF-α stimulated extensive numbers of colonies of NRK cells in soft agar. In contrast, peptides 1–5 and 7 failed to stimulate colony formation even at tenfold higher concentration (50 ng/ml) (Table V).

Growth Factor-Induced Phosphorylation

Autoradiography of SDS polyacrylamide gels of placental membranes incubated with EGF or TGF-α (2 μM) and ^{32}P-ATP showed enhanced phosphorylation of the EGF/TGF-α receptor (170,000 daltons) and p35 (35,000 daltons) relative to membranes incubated without the growth factors (Fig. 6). Placental membranes incubated

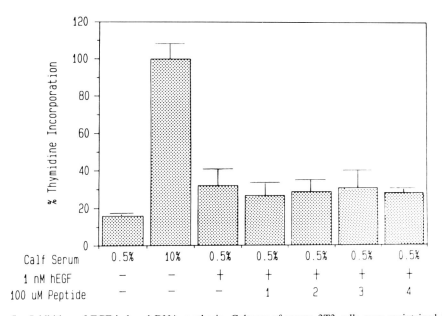

Fig. 5.   Inhibition of EGF-induced DNA synthesis. Cultures of mouse 3T3 cells were maintained in low serum (0.5%) containing tritiated thymidine (1 μCi/ ml) and EGF alone or with the indicated peptides. After 72 hr, cultures were washed and radioactivity measured. Values are the mean and standard error of quadruplicate samples.

TABLE V. Stimulation of Anchorage-Independent Cell Growth*

Peptide	Concentration (ng/ml)	Soft agar colonies
TGF-α	5	253
1	5	<20
	50	<20
2	5	<20
	50	<20
3	5	<20
	50	<20
4	5	<20
	50	<20
5	5	<20
	50	<20
7	5	<20
	50	<20

*Normal rat kidney (NRK) cells were seeded in soft agar containing 2 ng/ml TGF-β purified from human platelets and TGF-α or peptides at the designated concentrations. The number of soft agar colonies represents the number of colonies containing a minimum of 20 NRK cells per 6 random low power fields 10 days after seeding (1.4×10^4 cells/ml) with TGF-α or peptides. Plates treated with TGF-β alone did not form colonies.

with TGF-α fragments (1–5, 7) at 200 μM showed no increased phosphorylation of the EGF/TGF-α receptor or p35 above control.

DISCUSSION

Hydrophilicity plots of TGF-α indicate three discrete sequences with high indexes of hydrophilicity separated by stretches of hydrophobic amino acids. Each of the three hydrophilic sequences is located nearly entirely within one of the three internal disulfide loops. It is highly probable that the hydrophilic sequences are located on the surface of TGF-α and, therefore, bind to the receptor. The three-dimensional structures of TGF-α or EGF have not been reported. We synthesized seven peptides encompassing the hydrophilic sequences of TGF-α using SPPS techniques and purified them to homogeneity by HPLC. Amino acid analysis confirmed the correct composition of the fragments.

Analysis of the peptides for activities characteristic of TGF-α gave uniformly negative results in five different assays. The peptides did not compete for ^{125}I-EGF binding to receptors of intact A-431 cells or human placental membranes even at 1,000 times the concentration of EGF that completely displaced the labeled EGF. Concentrations of the peptides up to 10 μM did not stimulate DNA synthesis of human foreskin fibroblasts or 3T3 cells nor did they stimulate anchorage-independent growth of NRK cells. Also, the peptides did not inhibit EGF-induced stimulation of DNA synthesis or stimulate phosphorylation of the EGF/TGF-α receptor or p35 even when added at 10 μM.

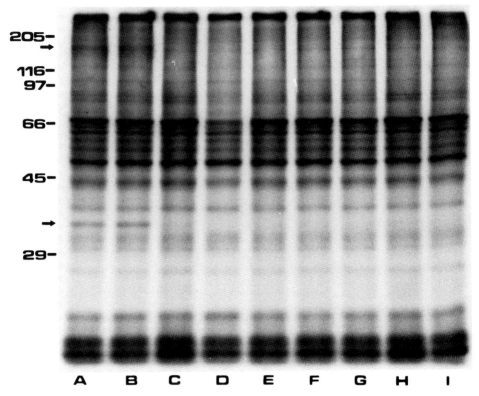

Fig. 6. Growth factor induced phosphorylation. Placental membranes (50 μg) were incubated with
^{32}P-ATP and AMP-PNP and peptides. After 5 min of reaction at 0°C, samples were chromatographed
on SDS PAGE and autoradiography performed. Lanes contained 2 μM EGF (**A**), 2 μM TGF-α (**B**),
buffer (**C**), or TGF-α peptide 5 (**D**), peptide 7 (**E**), peptide 2 (**F**), peptide 4 (**G**), peptide 3 (**H**), peptide
1 (**I**) all at 200 μM.

In addition to the seven peptides we synthesized, six peptides with sequences
overlapping our peptides were synthesized and purified by Peninsula Laboratories.
These peptides (8–13) also uniformly failed to produce any response characteristic of
TGF-α in the five assays. Thus, results of assays testing the 13 peptides consistently
indicate that the receptor binding domain of TGF-α is not contained within any of the
individual sequences tested.

Since EGF, VGF, and TGF-α all compete for specific binding of ^{125}I-EGF to
membrane receptors, it is likely that similar regions of the growth factors interact
with the receptor. The region with the highest conservation of amino acid residues common to all three growth factors encompasses the third disulfide loop of the TGF-α.
Nestor et al. [13] reported that a fragment of TGF-α comprising the third disulfide
loop (residues 34–43) had low affinity ($IC_{50} = 80$ μM) for EGF receptors of human
cells and that the affinity increased 10- to 100-fold when the N-terminal was blocked
by acylation and the C-terminal was blocked by methylation or amidation. These
decapeptides were antagonists of the mitogenic effect of EGF and TGF-α on fibroblasts. Also, Ac-TGF-α (34–43)-NHEt was reported to inhibit vaccinia virus infection
purportedly by occupying the EGF receptor of target cells [14].

We also synthesized and evaluated the peptides encompassing the third disulfide loop including fragments with nonblocked N- and C-termini (peptides 1 and 10) and with acylated N-termini and/or amidated C-termini (peptides 2, 4, 10, and 11). All of these peptides failed to show inhibition of EGF-induced DNA synthesis in our assay systems. The reason(s) for the different results is not known.

Synthetic fragments of EGF have been reported to contain a major receptor binding domain. Komoriya et al. [15] reported that the cyclic second disulfide loop [Ala^{23}]EGF-(14–31) and the linear [S-AcmCys^{21,31}]-EGF-(20–31) peptide induced all of the biological responses associated with intact EGF but were 10,000-fold less potent than intact EGF. Heath and Merrifield [16] reported that a fragment containing the cyclic third disulfide loop of EGF (residues 32–53) was 100,000-fold less potent than EGF in receptor binding and did not stimulate DNA synthesis. A fragment comprising 70% of EGF starting from the C-terminal (residues 15–53) was 10,000 times less potent than EGF in binding to the EGF receptor and stimulating DNA synthesis.

Based upon the failure of our 13 fragments of TGF-α to mimic or inhibit actions of intact TGF-α, we conclude the major receptor-binding domain is not contained entirely within any of the single peptide sequences reported here. This is supported by the reports that linear TGF-α and polymeric EGF molecules have 100- to 1,000-fold lower potency than the correctly folded hormones [16,17]. When the three dimensional structures of TGF-α or EGF become available, it may be possible to predict more accurately those sequences that form the receptor-binding domain. It is likely that the receptor binding domain is composed of separate regions of the TGF-α sequence that fold into the correct alignment when the hormone assumes its native conformation.

REFERENCES

1. Lee DC, Rochford R, Todaro GJ, Villarreal LP: Mol Cell Biol 5:3644–3646, 1985.
2. Derynck R, Goeddel DV, Ullrich A, Gutterman JU, Williams RD, Bringman TS, Berger WH: Cancer Res 47:707–712, 1987.
3. Sherwin SA, Twardzik DR, Bohn WH, Cockley KD, Todaro GJ: Cancer Res 43:403–407, 1983.
4. Lippman ME, Dickson RB, Bates S, Knabbe C, Huff K, Swain S, McManaway M, Bronzert D, Kasid A, Gelmann EP: Breast Cancer Res Treat 7:59–70, 1986.
5. Derynck R, Roberts AB, Winkler ME, Chen EY, Goeddel DV: Cell 38:287–297, 1984.
6. Reisner AH: Nature 313:801–803, 1985.
7. Barany G, Merrifield RB: In Gross E, Meienhofer J (eds): "The Peptides" Vol II. New York: Academic Press, 1980, pp 3–284.
8. Rao CV, Ramani N, Chegini N, Stadig BK, Carman FR, Woost PG, Schultz GS, Cook CL: J Biol Chem 260:1705–1710, 1985.
9. Twardzik DR, Brown JP, Ranchalis JE, Todaro GJ: Proc Natl Acad Sci USA 82:5300–5304, 1985.
10. Assoian RK, Komomya A, Meyers C, Komoriya A, Lamb L, Smith J, Sporn M: Cancer Res 42:4776–4778, 1982.
11. Lee DC, Rose TM, Webb NR, Todaro GJ: Nature 313:489–491, 1985.
12. Hopp TP,, Woods KR: Proc Natl Acad Sci USA 78:3824–3828, 1981.
13. Nestor JJ, Newman SR, DeLustro B, Todaro GJ, Schreiber AB: Biochem Biophys Res Commun 129:226–232, 1985.
14. Eppstein DA, Marsh YV, Schreiber AB, Newman SR, Todaro GJ, Nestor JJ: Nature 318:663–665, 1985.
15. Komoriya A, Hortsch M, Meyers C, Smith M, Kanety H, Schlessinger J: Proc Natl Acad Sci USA 81:1351–1355, 1984.
16. Heath WF, Merrifield RB: Proc Natl Acad Sci USA 83:6367–6371, 1986.
17. Hanauske AR, Buchok JB, Pardue RL, Muggia VA, Von Huff DD: Cancer Res 46:5567–5570, 1986.

Journal of Cellular Biochemistry 36:353–367 (1988)
Growth Regulation of Cancer 121–135

Human Cytokines, Tumor Necrosis Factor, and Interferons: Gene Cloning, Animal Studies, and Clinical Trials

Arthur P. Bollon, Susan L. Berent, Richard M. Torczynski, Norwood O. Hill, Yuri Lemeshev, Joseph M. Hill, Feng Lan Jia, Anwar Joher, Sathit Pichyangkul, and Amanullah Khan

Wadley Institutes of Molecular Medicine, Dallas, Texas 75235

Presented is a comprehensive program designed to isolate human cytokine genes and investigate their relative induction, and to analyze cytokine activities in cell culture, animal tumor models, and human clinical trials. Human cytokine cDNAs have been isolated from a cDNA library made from normal human peripheral blood leukocytes (PBLs) treated with Sendai virus and the relative induction of tumor necrosis factor (TNF), alpha and gamma interferons (IFN-α, IFN-γ), and interleukin-1 beta IL-1β) genes has been analyzed. In the Sendai virus-induced PBL system, IL-1β mRNA was shown to be approximately twofold higher than TNF or IFN-α mRNA whereas IFN-γ mRNA was 50–100-fold lower than TNF or IFN-α mRNA. The cytotoxic activity of TNF was analyzed on several cell lines and IFN-α and IFN-γ were shown to potentiate TNF cytotoxicity about 2–200-fold depending on cell lines. The LD_{50} for recombinant TNF in BALB/c mice was determined to be 6×10^7 U/kg and the therapeutic dose of recombinant TNF in sarcoma 180 bearing BALB/c mice was 3×10^5 U/kg, indicating a wide therapeutic index. Phase I clinical trials of recombinant TNF given I.V. indicated a tolerated dose of 150,000 U/kg with biphasic half-life (T-1/2) of 2 and 31 min following TNF injection. Phase II trials of TNF and trials of TNF combined with IFN-α are in progress. These studies indicate that cytokines such as TNF and IFN-α are subject to similar induction systems, potentiate each other's activities, and can be tolerated at specific doses for potential therapeutic use.

Key words: TNF, IFN, genes, clinical use

Cytokines are proteins involved in the modulation of the immune system [1] and are the targets of intense investigation due to their potential use for increasing our understanding of the immune system and for help in the development of new

Address correspondence to Arthur P. Bollon, Wadley Institutes of Molecular Medicine, 9000 Harry Hines Boulevard, Dallas, TX 75235.

Received April 12, 1987; revised and accepted October 7, 1987.

drugs. Some cytokines permit the activation of key immune cells such as T-lymphocyte activation by interleukin-1 (IL-1) and B-lymphocyte activation by B-cell differentiation factor (BCDF) [1]. Other cytokines function as growth factors, such as interleukine-2 (IL-2), which is the growth factor for T-lymphocyte helper and killer cells, or B-cell growth factor (BCGF), which is involved in the proliferation of B-lymphocytes [1]. Several cytokines have cytotoxic activities, such as tumor necrosis factor (TNF), which is produced by activated macrophages and has been shown to be cytotoxic for various tumor cell lines [2]. Cytokines such as alpha interferon (IFN-α) are produced by peripheral blood leukocytes (PBLs) and induced by Sendai virus, as well as by a large array of other inducers [3]. IFN-αs have potent antiviral activity and antiproliferative activities against a variety of tumor cell lines [3] and have recently been licensed as the treatment of choice for hairy cell leukemia.

Due to the occurrence of low levels of natural cytokines either circulating in patients with various diseases or in human cell culture systems, alternative methods have been required to produce cytokines cost-effectively. Recombinant DNA technology [4] has permitted the isolation of human cytokine genes and large-scale production of the respective proteins. Human IFN-α genes have been isolated by a number of investigators from cDNA libraries [5,6] and human genomic libraries [7,8]. We have isolated a novel human IFN-α gene, designated IFN-αWA, from a human genomic library by using 17-base oligonucleotide probes [8–10]. IFN-αWA contains differences at five amino acid positions which are conserved for all other IFN-α genes. The IFN-αWA gene appears to be a natural hybrid between IFN-αF at the 5′-end and IFN-αH at the 3′-end [10]. Human TNF cDNA was isolated from tumor cell lines HL-60 [11,12] and U-937 [13], and the human TNF gene was initially isolated from a human genome library by using rabbit TNF cDNA as a probe [14]. We have isolated TNF cDNA from normal human peripheral blood leukocytes (PBLs) induced with Sendai virus [15–17].

Since the immune system involves a network of different cytokines, we have been interested in the availability of all the known cytokines as well as new ones. Such availability of various cytokines is critical for our studies since we believe that although some cytokines may have therapeutic use when delivered alone, many cytokines will function best in combination. Our approach has been to establish human cDNA libraries which are screened for known cytokines and stored on filters for future screening. We have created a cDNA library from human PBLs induced with Sendai virus. From this cDNA library we have isolated several cytokine cDNAs such as TNF [15–17], IFN-α, IFN-β, and IL-1β cDNAs. In addition, we are screening the cytokine-enriched cDNA libraries with cytokine cDNA probes as well as oligonucleotide probes by using various hybridization strategies so as to isolate related but new cytokines.

To facilitate cytokine cDNA isolation and analysis of cytokine activities, we have had the advantage of a comprehensive cancer research center which includes several critical capabilities. The blood bank at Wadley has been a source of PBLs which have been resource material for the molecular genetics department, which has isolated cytokine cDNAs. The departments of molecular genetics and immunology have collaborated to study cytokine expression and activities in tumor cell cultures and animals. The fermentation facility has permitted large-scale production of cytokines from genetically engineered bacteria and yeast. Wadley's Granville C. Morton Cancer and Research Hospital has permitted the clinical trials of the respective cytokines.

This paper describes the isolation of the cytokine cDNAs, the analysis of their induction by Sendai virus, and the testing of the TNF on cells, animals, and human clinical trials, alone and in combination with IFN-α. Hence, these studies relate to the analysis of the cytokine network and their potential therapeutic use.

METHODS AND RESULTS

Human Peripheral Blood Leukocyte cDNA Library

We have established a human peripheral blood leukocyte (PBL) cDNA library which has been utilized for the isolation of various human cytokine cDNAs. The human PBLs were cultured according to the method of Cantell et al. [18] and induced with Sendai virus. As indicated in Figure 1, PBL cultures containing approximately 10^7 cells/ml were primed with 100 U/ml of IFN-α at -2 hr. Sendai virus was added at 0 hr to a concentration of 200 hemagglutination U/ml. The PBL cultures were incubated at 37°C. Either cells were centrifuged at specified times and processed for RNA isolation, or supernatants were assayed for cytokine activities. Poly(A)$^+$ RNA was isolated from PBL cultures induced for 4 hr and cDNA was synthesized. In addition, poly(A)$^+$ RNA was stored at -70°C. The cDNA was transformed into *E. coli* and approximately 30,000 colonies were generated on filters [17].

Transformed colonies were screened on filters for IFN-α genes by using the IFN-αWA gene [8] as a probe. At least 15 colonies hybridized with the IFN-α probe and more than half of these clones appeared to contain IFN-αD based on hybridization and restriction analysis. One clone which was fully characterized was shown to contain IFN-αD by DNA sequence analysis and was used in experiments shown in

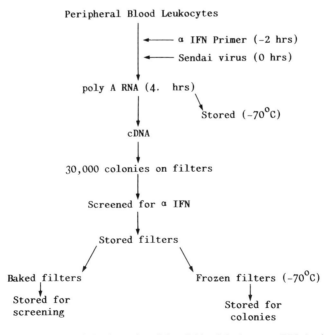

Fig. 1. The preparation and induction of peripheral blood leukocytes (PBLs), the synthesis and screening of cDNA, and the storage of filters were done as previously reported [17].

Figure 3. Duplicate filters, one containing transformed bacterial colonies and the other containing replica colonies baked at 80°C for screening the IFN-α genes, were stored at −70°C [17].

PBL poly(A)$^+$ RNA, isolated 4 hr after induction by Sendai virus, was subsequently removed after more than 12 mo of storage at −70°C and tested for hybridization by oligonucleotide probes complementary to the mRNA for several cytokines, including TNF cloned from leukemia cell line HL-60 [11,12]. No meaningful signals were observed for IFN-γ, IL-2, and lymphotoxin, whereas strong hybridization with the TNF probe was observed. Subsequently, the filters stored at −70°C which contained the cDNA library made with the 4-hr poly(A)$^+$ RNA were screened for TNF cDNA. Five positive clones were obtained after screening approximately 30,000 clones with the 17-base TNF probe [15–17]. The largest cDNA insert, pBR322-TNF1, was identical in sequence to the mature TNF obtained from leukemia cell lines HL-60 [11,12] and U-937 [13] which were induced with phorbol esters and endotoxin [17]. Screening of this same cDNA library with corresponding olignucleotide probes also yielded IFN-β cDNA and IL-1β cDNA clones.

The TNF cDNA was ligated with an expression vector containing a P_L promoter, a gene for the heat-sensitive repressor, and a consensus ribosomal binding site as indicated in Figure 2. The resulting expression vector pUC9-PL1-TNF1 was transformed into *E. coli* and the 17,300-dalton TNF was induced after a shift in temperature from 30°C to 42°C. Up to 3×10^6 U/ml of cytotoxic activity was obtained when cultures were grown for 3 hr after the shift from 30°C to 42°C at

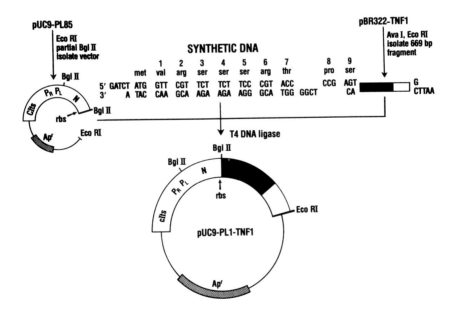

Fig. 2. Construction of a human TNF cDNA plasmid for expression in *E. coli*. An AvaI-EcoRI fragment containing the TNF cDNA was linked to an expression vector containing the bacteriophage P_L promoter, a gene for a temperature-sensitive repressor (cIts), and a consensus ribosome-binding site (rbs) by two complementary synthetic oligonucleotides. Black and white bars of the pBR322-TNF1 fragment represent portions of the structural gene and 3′-untranslated region, respectively. Regions surrounding the junction points were confirmed to be correct by nucleotide sequencing.

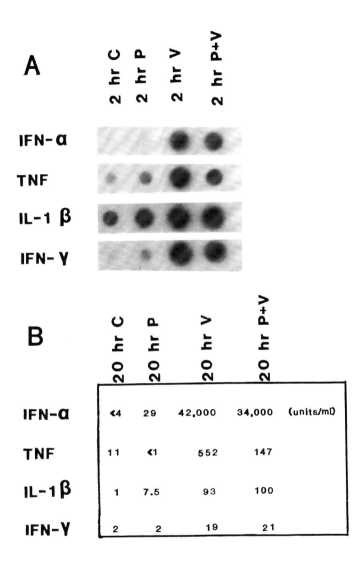

Fig. 3. Lymphokine activity in cultured PBLs under various induction conditions. PBLs were collected from 40 healthy individuals and then processed and cultured as previously described [17]. At −2 hr, some cell cultures were primed (P) with 100 U/ml of leukocyte IFN (10^6 U/mg), and at 0 hr, cultures were either not treated (C) or were induced with 200 hemagglutination U/ml of Sendai virus (V). **A:** Dot blots of total RNA isolated at 2 hr were hybridized with ^{32}P-RNA probes (2×10^8 cpm/μg) synthesized from cDNAs of IFN-αD, TNF, IL-1β, or IFN-γ by using SP6 RNA polymerase or T7 RNA polymerase as described [17]. Exposure times (−80°C, two screens) were 1 hr (IL-1β, TNF, and IFN-α) and 64 hr (IFN-γ). **B:** Assays of lymphokine activities. Twenty hours after virus infection, cell cultures were centrifuged and supernatants were stored at −70°C and then assayed for lymphokine activity. IFN-α, IL-1β, and IFN-γ activities were determined from radioimmune assay kits obtained from Bethesda Research Laboratories, Cistron, and Centocor, respectively. TNF activity was measured (triplicate assays) in cytotoxic units by using L_{929} cells and standardized against an internal purified TNF [17].

OD_{600} = 2.5 [17]. One unit is the amount required to give 50% cytotoxicity in the standard assay utilizing L_{929} cells [19].

Induction of IFN-α, IFN-γ, TNF, and IL-1β.

We examined the induction of various cytokines in populations of mixed human PBLs in response to Sendai virus infection. We compared the levels of their expression to that of IFN-α, whose induction is well characterized in this system [3]. All lymphokines we have examined (IFN-α, TNF, IL-1β, and IFN-γ) are induced to varying levels in virus-infected PBLs, as determined by RNA blot hybridizations and measurements of the proteins present in culture supernatants (Fig. 3). Since the RNA hybridization probes for the four genes were of equal specific activities and approximately equal lengths, the hybridization signals obtained for the RNA samples under the indicated culture conditions could be compared directly. As shown in Figure 3A for the virus-infected cultures, IL-1β mRNA is approximately twofold higher than TNF or IFN-α mRNA, whereas IFN-γ mRNA is 50–100-fold lower. Previously, we established that TNF and IFN-α mRNAs typically represent about 0.11% of the total virus-induced PBL mRNA [17]. In a cDNA library prepared from PBLs harvested 4 hr after Sendai virus infection, we identified TNF clones as 0.05% and IL-1β clones as 0.3% of the total. These results indicate that IL-1β is transcribed at high levels in PBL cultures, although the activity present in the culture supernatants is relatively low. IL-1β apparently lacks a leader peptide, as determined by cDNA sequence analysis, and recent studies indicate that IL-1β may be primarily a membrane-bound protein [20].

Although IFN-γ induction by PBLs treated with Sendai virus is low, previous work claimed IFN-γ expression was attributed solely to the mitogenic or antigenic stimulation of select T-cell populationsd. IFN-γ mRNA in phytohemagglutinin-stimulated lymphocytes was detected at low levels 3 hr post induction and peaked at 15 hr [21] as compared to IFN-α and TNF mRNA levels, which peaked 4 and 2 hr postinfection, respectively, in PBLs [17]. We have also observed low but reproducible levels of IFN-α mRNA in induced PBLs (Fig. 3A) that peaked 3–4 hr after virus infection and was barely detectable at 20 hr (unpublished results). IFN-γ induction in a similar system has been previously reported but this response was attributed to a mixed leukocyte reaction and presumably was not virus mediated [22]. However, we detected IFN-γ mRNA at only extremely low levels in uninfected PBLs as compared to virus-induced PBLs (Fig. 3A), with the concomitant levels of secreted IFN-γ appearing in culture supernatants. PBL cultures treated with lipopolysaccharide (LPS) (10 μg/ml) also produced low levels four-fold lower than virus-induced PBLs) of IFN-γ mRNA and secreted protein (unpublished results). IFN-γ mRNA was also detected from PBLs cultured in the presence of IFN-α alone (Fig. 3A).

We addressed the effect of pretreating mixed PBLs with human IFN-α (i.e., priming) prior to the addition of Sendai virus. An enhancement of IFN production has been observed by other investigators in certain primed, induced cells or cell lines as compared to unprimed, induced cells (see ref. 3 for a review). No enhancement of IFN-α mRNA or IFN-α production was observed in primed vs. unprimed virus-induced PBLs (Fig. 3, unpublished results). This observation holds for both PBLs primed with crude IFN (10^6 U/mg) or highly purified IFN (2×10^8 U/mg). No general pattern of either increased or decreased induction was observed for primed and induced PBLs, as compared to only induced PBLs, for the levels of mRNA, and secreted proteins of TNF, IFN-γ, or IL-1β.

Potentiation of TNF Cytotoxicity by IFN-α and IFN-γ

Recombinant human TNF produced at the fermentation facility at Wadley Institutes was purified to a specific activity of 1×10^7 U/mg and tested for cytotoxic properties. Recombinant TNF was added in different concentrations and incubated for 48 hr with different tumor cell lines, and the amount of TNF required to cause 50% cytotoxicity was determined by a dye uptake test (neutral red) using a Titertek multiscan reader [19]. As indicated in Table I, there was a range of TNF concentrations required to effect 50% cell kill depending on the cell lines tested. For example, the human breast tumor cell line BT-20 required 250 U/ml TNF for 50% kill whereas the human colon tumor cell line SK-CO-1 required 75,000 U/ml TNF for 50% kill. In fact, tumor cell lines of similar origin required different levels of TNF for 50% kill such as human breast tumor cell line SK-BR-3, which required 62,500 U/ml TNF in contrast to the 250 U/ml of TNF required for the BT-20 breast cell line.

Also indicated in Table I is the reduction in the amount of TNF required for 50% cell kill when IFN-α and IFN-γ were present. Pretreatment with IFN-α and IFN-γ for 24 hr prior to the addition of TNF resulted in 2–200-fold potentiation for various cell lines. Treatment of the cell lines in Table I with either IFN-α or IFN-γ at the concentrations used in the potentiation studies described above resulted in no apparent cytotoxic effects. The degree of potentiation varied with different cell lines. Although melanoma cell line G-361 was not potentiated by IFN-α, melanoma cell

TABLE I. Potentiation of TNF Cytotoxicity by IFN-(α, γ)

Human cell line[b,c,d]	TNF (U/ml) required to kill 50% of cells		
	TNF	TNF + IFN-α	TNF + IFN-γ
BT-20 (breast)	250	180 (1.3)[a]	30 (8.3)
HT-144 (melanoma)	312	40 (7.8)	12 (26.0)
ME-180 (cervix)	1,000	90 (48.6)	5 (200.0)
A-549 (lung)	30,000	30,000 (0)	6,700 (4.5)
SK-OV-3 (ovary)	50,000	8,750 (5.8)	4,350 (11.3)
BRO (melanoma)	19,000	1,500 (12.7)	1,200 (15.8)
SK-CO-1 (colon)	75,000	50,000 (1.5)	9,000 (8.0)
MLCL$_1$ (melanoma)	9,000	2,400 (3.8)	1,200 (7.5)
SK-BR-3 (breast)	62,500	1,875 (33.0)	13,000 (5.0)
734B (breast)	45,000	600 (75.0)	10,000 (4.5)
G-361 (melanoma)	20,000	20,000 (0)	7,700 (2.6)
Colon 205 (colon)	15,000	2,500 (6.0)	10,000 (1.5)

[a]Potentiation index $= \dfrac{\text{TNF (U/ml) causing 50\% cytotoxicity in the untreated cells}}{\text{TNF (U/ml) causing 50\% cytotoxicity in the treated cells}}$.

[b]Cells were grown in RPMI-1640 medium (Gibco, Grand Island, NY) supplemented with 10% fetal bovine serum (Gibco) and 50 g/ml of gentamycin (Shering Corp, Kennelworth, NJ).
[c]1–2×10^4 cells were seeded per well in a 96-well plate (Costar, Cambridge, MA) and incubated 24 hr at 37°C. For potentiation studies, 5,000 U/ml of IFN-α (natural IFN-α isolated from human PBLs induced with Sendai virus; 1–5×10^6 U/mg specific activity) or 500 U/ml IFN-γ (Cellular Products, Buffalo, NY; 5×10^6 U/mg specific activity) were present during the 24-hr incubation. After 24 hr, TNF was added for 48 hr and cell cytotoxicity was determined by dye uptake test (neutral red) by using a Titertek reader [19].
[d]Cell lines were obtained from American Type Culture Collection (Rockville, MD).

lines MLCL$_1$ and BRO were potentiated 3.8- and 12.7-fold respectively as indicated in Table I. Although it is difficult to conclude whether tumor cell lines of a specific tumor origin are resistant to TNF cytotoxicity or potentiation by IFN, it is possible to conclude that TNF cytotoxicity is potentiated by IFN-α and -γ with various degrees of efficiency depending on the cell lines employed. What in vivo significance these results represent in terms of tumor origin remains to be established since the cell lines have probably been altered since the cell lines were established. Nevertheless, potentiation of TNF cytotoxic activity by IFN-α and IFN-γ which has been observed by other investigators [23] could have significance in vivo and in combination therapy involving TNF and IFN.

Animal Testing of Recombinant TNF

Purified recombinant TNF (1 $\times$ 10^7 U/mg) was tested for cytotoxic activity against sarcoma 180 tumors in BALB/c mice as indicated in Figure 4. In BALB/c nu/ + mice, both doses of recombinant TNF (2.4 $\times$ 10^4 and 6 $\times$ 10^3 U/mouse) caused

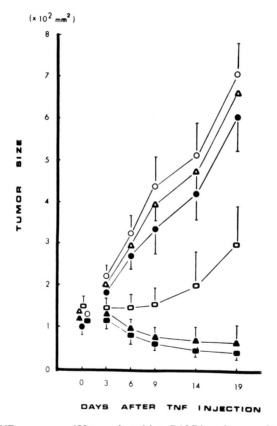

Fig. 4. Effect of TNF on sarcoma-180 transplanted into BALB/c nu/nu or nu/+ mice. Sarcoma-180 (1 $\times$ 10^7 cells) were inoculated s.c. 7 days prior to the administration of TNF. TNF (6 $\times$ 10^3 U/mouse ▲ nu/+, △ nu/nu, or 2.4 $\times$ 10^4 U/mouse ■ nu/+, □ nu/nu) was given as a single i.v. injection on day 0. Control mice received saline (● nu/+, ○ nu/nu). The results represent the mean value of six to eight animals and standard error. The tumor size of TNF treated nu/+ mice differs significantly after day 6 from nu/+ controls ($P < .001$). The tumor size of TNF-treated (24,000 U/mouse) nu/nu mice differs significantly after day 6 from TNF-treated (6,000 U/mouse) and control nu/nu mice ($P < .02$).

regression of sarcoma 180. However, in nu/nu mice, the lower dose of recombinant TNF (6×10^3 U/mouse) showed no effect. These data suggested that the T-cell-mediated immune response may be implicated in the antitumor effect of TNF. To test the acute toxicity of recombinant TNF, BALB/c mice were given purified recombinant TNF (1×10^7 U/mg specific activity) intravenously at different doses in 0.1-ml sterile phosphate-buffered saline containing human serum albumin (1 mg/ml). The control mice were injected with only phosphate-buffered saline and human albumin. The LD_{50} for recombinant TNF was determined to be 6×10^7 units of TNF/kg. The results of autopsies performed on BALB/c mice containing different concentrations of recombinant TNF are indicated in Table II. The cause of death at the LD_{50} appeared to be respiratory failure, which is consistent with interstitial lymphohistiocytic infiltrate presence in the lung at low TNF concentrations and pneumonitis at high concentrations, as indicated in Table II. Doses of 6×10^7 and 3×10^7 U/kg depressed the value of glucose and alkaline phosphatase and elevated blood urea nitrogen (BUN) and serum glutamate pyruvate transaminase (SGPT) as indicated in Table III. All values returned to normal after 72 hr for surviving animals. The therapeutic dose of TNF in sarcoma 180 bearing BALB/c mice was determined to be 3×10^5 U/kg [24]. These results indicate that TNF has a wide therapeutic index.

Clinical Trials of Recombinant TNF

Phase I clinical trials of purified recombinant TNF (1×10^7 U/mg) produced at the Wadley Institutes were initiated on September 25, 1985. Phase I clinical trials are primarily concerned with determining the side effects and tolerated dose of a drug. TNF was administered intravenous (I.V.) at escalated doses on alternate days by a modified Fibonacci scheme as indicated in Table IV. Eighteen patients having the malignancies indicated in Table V participated in the phase I studies. The highest doses received ranged from 3,000 U/kg to 250,000 U/kg. Also presented in Table V is the total dose received by patients having various forms of cancer.

The side effects for recombinant TNF are indicated in Table VI. Several of the side effects, such as chills, fever, and malaise, have been found for other cytokines, such as IFN-α [4]. At high doses of 250,000 U/kg, chills, fever, severe weakness, nausea, vomiting, diarrhea, and temporary neutropenia caused the dose to be lowered to more tolerable levels. The phase I clinical trials indicate that purified recombinant TNF can be administered I.V. three times per week up to 150,000 U/kg with tolerable side effects [25]. Patients had chills and fever within 10–15 min of injection with the fever ranging from 37.3 to 39.4°C. At least four patients who had been treated for over 4 wk showed a rise in triglycerides from 88.5 to 168.5 mg/dl. The half-life (T-1/2) of recombinant TNF was biphasic at 150,000 U/kg. The first phase T-1/2 was approximately 2 min and the second phase was 31 min following TNF injection.

Phase II clinical trials of recombinant TNF are in progress. Phase II trials are primarily concerned with determining drug effectiveness. The phase II trials of TNF involve a dose of 150,000 U/kg delivered I.V. three times per week. Twenty-three patients have participated in the phase II trials since its initiation. In addition to the clinical trials of recombinant TNF alone, clinical trials involving 90,000 U/kg of TNF delivered I.V. three times per week in combination with IFN-α are in progress.

DISCUSSION

Described is an organized effort employing gene cloning techniques and a comprehensive cancer center to analyze the immune network and develop immune

TABLE II. Autopsy Examination of BALB/c Mice 24 Hr After Single I.V. TNF Injection

Dose (U/kg)	Heart	Lungs	Liver	Spleen	Thymus	Lymph node	Kidney	G.I. tract
LD_{50} dead animal	Massive congestion	Focal pneumonitis	Subcapsular necrosis	Follicular hyperplasia	Lymphoid hyperplasia	Not identified	Severe congestion & proteinaceous material in tubules	Lymphoid aggregates in stomach
6×10^7 (LD_{50})	None	Focal pneumonitis	Vacuolization of hepatocytes	Follicular hyperplasia	Lymphoid hyperplasia	Follicular hyperplasia	Lymphohistiocytic infiltrate	Lymphoid hyperplasia of small intestine
3×10^7	None	Interstitial lymphohistiocytic infiltrate	Peripheral lymphohistiocytic infiltrate	Follicular hyperplasia	Lymphoid hyperplasia	None	Minimal interstitial lymphohistiocytic infiltrate	None
1.8×10^7	None	Interstitial lymphohistiocytic infiltrate	Peripheral lymphohistiocytic infiltrate	Follicular hyperplasia	Lymphoid hyperplasia	Follicular hyperplasia	Minimal interstitial lymphohistiocytic infiltrate	None
9×10^6	None	Interstitial lymphohistiocytic infiltrate	Peripheral lymphohistiocytic infiltrate	Follicular hyperplasia	Lymphoid hyperplasia	Follicular hyperplasia	Minimal interstitial lymphohistiocytic infiltrate	None
3×10^6	None	None	None	None	None	None	None	None

TABLE III. Acute Toxicity Study of TNF*

Dose (U/kg)	BUN (mg/dl)	Glucose (mg/dl)	Alk. Phos. (I.U./liter)	SGPT (I.U./liter)
6×10^7	110.0 ± 12.9	46.5 ± 1.7	42.0 ± 8.5	252.0 ± 53.4
3×10^7	80.7 ± 18.0	87.4 ± 21.5	54.2 ± 9.3	166.2 ± 69.1
1.8×10^7	25.5 ± 2.0	133.6 ± 7.4	59.4 ± 17.7	119.0 ± 4.0
9×10^6	32.7 ± 3.2	130.0 ± 5.4	77.2 ± 17.3	163.0 ± 24.9
3×10^6	30.4 ± 6.2	114.0 ± 9.7	64.2 ± 13.3	112.0 ± 30.3
Control	32.0 ± 5.6	98.6 ± 1.1	88.5 ± 27.4	86.0 ± 38.6

*Animals were injected intravenously with different TNF doses in 0.1 ml sterile phosphate saline containing human serum albumin (1 mg/ml). Each dose of TNF represents results of three BALB/c female mice. Determinations were made on animals 24 hr after TNF injection. Blood urea nitrogen (BUN), glucose, alkaline phosphatase (Alk. Phos.), and serum glutamate pyruvate transaminase (SGPT) levels were determined on an Abbott VP analyzer by the clinical chemistry laboratory of Granville C. Morton Hospital at Wadley Institutes.

TABLE IV. TNF Dose Escalation Regimen

Day	TNF (U/kg)[a]
1	1,000
3	2,000
5	3,000
7	5,000
9	8,000
11	13,000
13	21,000
15	34,000
17	55,000
19	89,000
21	144,000
23	234,000

[a]Based on a 70-kg human.

factors for therapeutic utility. Since several cytokines such as tumor necrosis factor, lymphotoxin [11], IFN-α, and IFN-β contain regions of homology in their gene and protein structures, the construction of cDNA libraries for proven cytokine genes may also permit the isolation of new but related cytokine cDNAs by using known cDNAs or related oligonucleotide probes for cDNA screening. As indicated above, we isolated TNF cDNA from a human PBL cDNA library, in contrast to tumor cell lines employed by others [11–13]. These results are significant because the PBL cDNA library was constructed primarily for IFN-α cDNA isolation, but the bacterial colonies were stored for future screening opportunities. At the time there was no reason to expect TNF cDNA to be present in this library, but the availability, 1 yr after the establishment of the PBL cDNA library, of the induced PBL RNA- and cDNA-containing colonies permitted rapid testing for the presence of TNF mRNA and eventually the isolation of a TNF cDNA clone [15–17]. We were able to isolate and engineer for expression in E. coli the recombinant TNF in only 5 wk. As indicated, we have also isolated several IFN-α clones including IFN-αD, which is consistent with previous studies [6] as well as IFN-β and IL-1β. Several potentially related but not identical cytokine cDNA clones from this cDNA library are under investigation.

Analysis of the induction of the various cytokine mRNAs indicated that the various cytokines tested, TNF, IFN-α, IL-1β, and IFN-γ, all respond to induction by

TABLE V. TNF Phase I Clinical Trial

Case no.	Diagnosis	Highest U/kg	Highest dose	Total dose
01	Chondrosarcoma	90,000	5,040,000	37,572,000
02	Ca. prostate	90,000	20,000,000	257,530,000
03	Melanoma	90,000	6,390,000	382,350,000
04	Ca. lung	3,000	210,000	420,000
05	Ca. lung	90,000	5,400,000	49,940,000
06	Ca. rectum	250,000	17,500,000	106,460,000
07	Ca. lung	55,000	3,850,000	9,960,000
08	A.G.L.	150,000	13,500,000	222,815,000
09	Ca. breast	55,000	3,410,000	12,215,000
10	Ca. breast	175,000	8,400,000	66,046,000
11	Osteosarcoma	175,000	9,950,000	100,500,000
12	Astrocytoma	200,000	10,000,000	94,075,000
13	Ca. colon	200,000	18,000,000	128,082,000
14	Ca. colon	5,000	363,000	363,000
15	Ca. breast	175,000	8,100,000	67,716,000
16	Ca. lung	175,000	12,775,000	255,500,000
17	A.M.L.	150,000	6,450,000	11,906,000
18	Ca. colon	175,000	7,390,000	123,959,000

TABLE VI. TNF Phase I — Side Effects

Effect	No. of patients	Beginning at TNF dose (units/kg)
Chills	17	1,000
Fever	18	1,000
Malaise	14	1,000
Fatigue	12	1,000
Anorexia	11	1,000
Nausea	10	1,000
Vomiting	9	1,000
Headache	7	3,000
Joint pain	3	8,000
Lower back pain	3	2,000
Diaphoresis	2	3,000
Shaking without chills	2	150,000
Flushing	1	21,000
Anxiety	1	90,000
Itching, no rash	2	34,000
Pallor	2	175,000
Shortness of breath	1 1	3,000
Dry mouth	1	1,000
Diarrhea	1	250,000

Sendai virus and that TNF and IFN-α mRNA are both induced at high levels (0.11% of total virus-induced PBL mRNA) [17]. These results contrast with TNF mRNA levels estimated from previous work for HL-60 cells of 0.0035% [11] and 0.002% [12] and for U-937 cells of 0.01% [13]. In addition, the inducers utilized in the previous studies were phorbol esters and endotoxin, not Sendai virus. Hence the availability and screening of the PBL cDNA library not only resulted in the isolation of useful cytokine cDNAs but also resulted in new insights into TNF induction and its relationship to other cytokines.

As indicated above and in previous studies [17] the level of TNF activity in induced PBL culture supernatants was about 200-fold lower than IFN-α activity. These results are in contrast to high levels of TNF and IFN-α mRNA levels. Previously we proposed that TNF mRNA may be less efficiently translated than IFN-α mRNA based on mixing studies [17]. Possibly related to these results is the potentiation of TNF activity by low levels of IFN-α and IFN-γ as indicated in Table II and by other investigators [23]. Perhaps low levels of TNF are sufficient for in vivo utility if IFN-α or -γ is present. The coexistence of TNF and IFN-α can be effected by induction by viruses such as Sendai virus. Whether TNF mRNA is subjected to translational regulation by factors such as other cytokines remains to be delineated.

Further evaluation of the in vivo function of TNF is necessary. TNF has been shown to contain a plethora of activities, such as cytotoxicity [2]; modulation of HLA-A, B antigens [26]; induction of IFN-β_2 [27]; activation of phagocytosis [28]; and induction of cachexia-related symptoms [29]. Delineation of cytokine function has involved analysis of cytokines on cells in culture, injection into animals, and human clinical trials as described in these studies and cited references. Some studies have involved the surveillance of cytokine mRNA and activities in response to other cytokines or inducers [17,30]. Clearly, exogenous delivery of cytokines has questionable relevance to the natural in vivo function of these proteins although such studies permit the evaluation of their therapeutic uses. One approach which has not been employed and which could be fruitful in generating insight into cytokine in vivo function would be to establish transgenic animals containing cytokine genes which are inducible to high levels. Such a system could permit the modulation of cytokine levels under controlled conditions and the evaluation of their effects under more natural conditions.

Since the animal studies indicated that recombinant TNF had a high therapeutic index it was with considerable interest that the clinical trials were initiated. As indicated in Table V, a range of doses were given 18 patients in the phase 1 clinical trials. Based on these studies 150,000 U/kg was determined to be the tolerated dose. These studies also indicated that the half-life of TNF was short and biphasic (2 min and 31 min T-1/2). The short half-life certainly may bear on its clinical effectiveness. Phase II clinical trials utilizing 150,000 U/kg are in progress. Preliminary phase II studies do not appear encouraging for TNF delivered I.V., but there is considerable interest in our trials involving intralesional TNF injections and TNF plus IFN-α.

The major issues for TNF utility appear to be high-dose toxicity and short half-life. During the clinical trials, a rapid reduction of circulating granulocytes was consistently observed in patients after TNF injection. Further study in vitro indicated that TNF rapidly binds to high-affinity receptors on granulocytes and induces cell adherence [31]. A parallel relationship was observed between TNF-induced granulocyte adherence and TNF-increased expression of surface adhesive proteins (Mac-1, p150,95) (unpublished data). The data suggested that TNF induced granulocyte adhesion by enhancing the expression of surface adhesive proteins. Enhanced granulocyte activities including phagocytic, antibody-dependent cell cytotoxicity and killing activity to parasites have also been reported [28,32]. The finding that TNF regulates granulocyte function is of particular interest, since this action may represent the role of TNF against infectious disease.

One of the limiting factors in the use of TNF as an antitumor drug is its toxicity at high doses. It has been shown that cyclooxygenase inhibitors, indomethacin or ibuprofen, can prevent the toxic effects of TNF in animals [33]. Combined administration of TNF with cyclooxygenase inhibitors may allow safer administration of high doses of TNF to cancer patients.

Further approaches to improving TNF delivery involve intralesional delivery of TNF; clinical trials involving the combination of TNF plus IFN-α which relate to the potentiation data described above; generation of TNF analogs which are presently under analysis; and combination of TNF with other cytokines. Further analysis of the immune network and testing of immune factors as described in these studies should result in an improved understanding of the immune system and development of new agents which may be useful for antiviral and anticancer therapies.

ACKNOWLEDGMENTS

We thank Sal Camparini, Bradley Hepner and Jerry Sanders for human leukocyte preparation; Dr. Karen Pennington for cytotoxicity assays; Saundra Davis, Paul John, and KaNan Vickroy for technical assistance; Dr. Steven J. Sandler, Dr. Rajinder Sidhu, and Cheryl Hendrix for development of pUC9-PL85; and Dr. S.J. Ahmed for assistance with clinical trial data. We thank Ms. Mickie Cox for the preparation of this manuscript. Some of this work was performed in the Oree Meadows Perryman Laboratory. This work was supported by the Meadows Foundation, the Samuel Roberts Noble Foundation, the Mary Kay Foundation, the Haggarty Foundation, and by a National Institutes of Health grant to A.P.B.

REFERENCES

1. Farrar JJ, Hiljiker ML: Fed Proc 41:263–268, 1982.
2. Old LJ: Science 230:630–632, 1985.
3. Stewart WE II: "The Interferon System." New York: Springer-Verlag, 1979.
4. Bollon AP: "Recombinant DNA Products: Insulin, Interferon and Growth Hormone." Florida: CRC Press, 1984.
5. Nagata S, Taira H, Hall A, Johnsrud L, Streuli M, Escodi J, Boll W, Cantell K, Weissmann C: Nature 284:316–320, 1980.
6. Goeddel DV, Yelverton E, Ullrich A, Heyneker HL, Miozzari G, Holmes W, Seeburg PH, Dull T, May L, Stebbing N, Crea R, Maeda S, McCandliss R, Sloma A, Tabor JM, Gross M, Familletti PC, Pestka S: Nature 287:411–416, 1980.
7. Goeddel DV, Leung DW, Dull TJ, Gross M, Lawn RM, McCandliss R, Seeburg PH, Ullrich A, Yelverton E, Gray PW: Nature 290:209–215, 1981.
8. Torczynski RM, Fuke M, Bollon AP: Proc Natl Acad Sci USA 81:6451–6455, 1984.
9. Bollon AP, Fuke M, Torczynski RM: Methods Enzymol 119:678–679, 1986.
10. Bollon AP, Torczynski RM, Sidhu RS, Hendrix LC: In Calendar R, Gold L (eds): "Sequence Specificity in Transcription and Translation." New York: Alan R. Liss, Inc., 363–376, 1985.
11. Pennica D, Nedwin GE, Hayflick JS, Seeburg PH, Derynck R, Palladino MA, Kohr WJ, Aggarwal BB, Goeddel DV: Nature (Lond) 312:724–729, 1984.
12. Wang AM, Creasey AA, Ladner MB, Lin LS, Stricker J, Van Arsdell JN, Yamamoto R, Mark DF: Science 228:149–154, 1985.
13. Marmenout A, Fransen L, Tavernier J, Van der Heyden J, Tizard R, Kawashima E, Shaw A, Johnson M-J, Semon D, Muller R, Ruysschaert M-R, Van Vliet A, Fiers W: Eur J Biochem 152:512–522, 1985.
14. Shirai T, Yamaguchi H, Ito H, Todd CW, Wallace RB: Nature 313:803–806, 1985.

15. Bollon AP, Torczynski RM, Hendrix LC, Sidhu RS, Berent SL: "The Biology of the Interferon System." Amsterdam: Elsevier Science Publishers B.V., 41–44, 1986.
16. Berent SL, Torczynski RM, Hill NO, Pichyangkul S, Jia F, Hill JM, Khan A, Bollon AP: "Advances in Gene Technology: Molecular Biology of the Endocrine System." New York: Cambridge University Press, 100–101, 1986.
17. Berent SL, Torczynski RM, Bollon AP: Nucleic Acids Res 14:8997–9015, 1986.
18. Cantell K, Hirvonen S, Kauppinen H-L, Myllyla G: Methods Enzymol 78:29–38, 1981.
19. Khan A, Weldon D, Duvall J, Pitchyangkul S, Hill NO: "Human Lymphokines." New York: Academic Press, 1982.
20. Matsushima K, Taguchi M, Kovacs EJ, Young HA, Oppenheim JJ: J Immunol 136:2883–2891, 1986.
21. Vaquero C, Sanceau J, Sondermeyer P, Falcoff R: Nucleic Acids Res 12:2629–2640, 1984.
22. Hiscott J, Cantell K, Weissmann C: Nucleic Acids Res 12:3737–3746, 1984.
23. Sugarman BJ, Aggarwal BB, Hass PE, Figari IS, Palladino MA, Jr, Shepard HM: Science 230:943–945, 1985.
24. Khan A, Joher A, Arfan M, Jia F, Pichyangkul S, Berent S, Hill NO, Bollon A: Proc Am Soc Cancer Res 27:320, 1986.
25. Khan A, Pardue A, Aleman C, Dickson J, Pichyangkul S, Hill JM, Hilario R, Hill NO: Proc Am Soc Clin Oncol 5:226, 1986.
26. Collins T, Lapierre LA, Fiers W, Strominger JL, Pober JS: Proc Natl Acad Sci USA 83:446–450, 1986.
27. Kohase M, Henriksen-DeStefano D, May LT, Vilcek J, Sehgal PB: Cell 45:659–666, 1986.
28. Shalaby MR, Aggarwal BB, Rinderknecht E, Svedersky LP, Finkle BS, Palladino MA, Jr: J Immunol 135:2069–2073, 1985.
29. Tracey KJ, Beutler B, Lowry SF, Merryweather J, Wolpe S, Milsark IW, Hariri RJ, Fahey TJ III, Zentella A, Albert JD, Hires GT, Cerami A: Science 234:470–473, 1986.
30. Tsujimoto M, Vilcek J: J Biol Chem 261:5384–5388, 1986.
31. Pichyangkul S, Schick D, Jia FL, Berent SL, Bollon AP, Khan A: Exp Hematol 15:1055–1059, 1987.
32. Silkerstein DS, David JR: Proc Natl Acad Sci USA 83:1055–1059, 1986.
33. Kettelhut IC, Fiers W, Goldberg AL: Proc Natl Acad Sci USA 84:4273–4277, 1987.

Journal of Cellular Biochemistry 36:369–376 (1988)
Growth Regulation of Cancer 137–144

Invasive Activity and Chemotactic Response to Growth Factors by Kaposi's Sarcoma Cells

Adriana Albini, Charles D. Mitchell, Erik W. Thompson, Ruth Seeman, George R. Martin, Alec E. Wittek, and Gerald V. Quinnan

Laboratory for Developmental Biology and Anomalies, National Institute of Dental Research, National Institutes of Health, Bethesda, MD 20892 (A.A., E.W.T., G.R.M.), Division of Virology, Office of Biologics Research and Review, Center for Drugs and Biologics, Food and Drug Administration, Bethesda, MD 20892 (C.D.M., R.S., A.E.W., G.V.Q.)

Kaposi's sarcoma (KS) is a relatively low grade neoplasm, classically occurring in the skin of elderly men. A more virulent and invasive form of Kaposi's sarcoma has been described in patients with acquired immune deficiency syndrome (AIDS). The origin and identification of the tumor cells in these lesions is controversial. Here we have studied the behavior of cells derived from KS lesions in an in vitro assay which measures the ability of cells to invade through a reconstituted basement membrane. In agreement with previous work, KS cells obtained under selective culture conditions were invasive showing activity comparable to that of malignant tumor cells. Normal fibroblasts, smooth muscle cells, and endothelial cells did not demonstrate invasive behavior under the same experimental conditions. To characterize further the nature of the KS cells we tested the chemotactic response of cells from the most invasive line to a variety of growth factors and compared their response to those of fibroblasts, smooth muscle, and endothelial cells. These studies suggest that normal cells respond to a unique repertoire of chemotactic factors. The chemotactic response of the KS cells most closely resembled that of smooth muscle cells and was quite distinct from endothelial cells. These results indicate that the KS-derived cultures contain invasive cells with a smooth muscle cell-like phenotype.

Key words: Kaposi's sarcoma, chemotaxis, invasion, growth factors

Kaposi's sarcoma (KS) presents as a progressive mesenchymal tumor involving the skin, mucosa, and digestive tract of up to 30% of patients with AIDS [1–4]. Kaposi's sarcoma differs from typical neoplasms in several characteristic ways. These

Adriana Albini's present address is Laboratory for Retinal Cell and Molecular Biology, NEI/NIH, Building 6, Room 224, Bethesda, MD 20892.

Received April 15, 1987; accepted October 23, 1987.

include the frequent regression of the lesion, the lack of aneuploidy in the cells, and the occurrence of multiple lesions of apparent multicentric origin [5–12]. Histological studies show that the lesions are principally composed of endothelial cells and spindle-shaped cells, although inflammatory cells are present in early lesions [13–18]. Consequently, some authors define KS as being an invasive granulation tissue, but KS has also been described as a hemangiosarcoma or highly vascularized fibrosarcoma. Thus, whether KS is indeed a neoplasm is still controversial [5,12].

Recently we have developed a method for establishing cell cultures from KS lesions using low serum to favor the growth of transformed cells over normal cells [17]. The cells selected in this fashion demonstrate anchorage-independent growth and exhibit invasive behavior when added to cultured skeletal muscle fragments. However, cells isolated from the KS lesions in this manner did not produce tumors when injected into nude mice.

The cultured cells morphologically resemble smooth muscle cells and possess myofibrils, which stained specifically by the Masson trichrome method. They show dense bodies by electron microscopy and do not differentiate to form capillaries in vitro or possess Weibel-Palade body or factor VIII-related antigen. Thus, these cultured cells are distinct from endothelial cells and resemble smooth muscle cells [17].

The aim of the present work was to investigate further the nature of the cultured KS cell populations by evaluating their invasive potential in vitro and their chemotactic response to specific growth factors. Our results confirm the previous suggestion that KS cells from patients with AIDS are invasive and show smooth muscle-like characteristics [17].

MATERIALS AND METHODS
Biopsies and Explant Culture

Skin specimens from four AIDS patients with Kaposi's sarcoma were obtained from the Clinical Center, National Institutes of Health. Tumor tissue was separated from normal dermis and epidermis, minced, and placed in culture in flasks with Medium 199 supplemented with 20% fetal bovine serum (FBS), antibiotics, 300 μg/ml of a crude preparation of endothelial cell growth factor (Meloy Labs., Springfield, VA), and 50 μg/ml of heparin (Hynson, Wescott & Dunning, MD). After a sufficient outgrowth of cells had appeared, they were removed with trypsin and replated. After one to five passages, cells derived from each biopsy were passaged in Medium 199 containing 2.5% serum, antibiotics, and 150 μg/ml of endothelial cell growth factor (ECGF), plus 50 μg/ml heparin. The majority of the cells in the flask failed to survive under these conditions, while the surviving cells proliferated and formed a confluent sheet after about 3 weeks. These cells were subsequently cultured in media containing 20% serum, 150 μg/ml of ECGF, and 50 μg/ml of heparin.

Other Cells

Normal skin fibroblasts were derived from skin biopsies. Human endothelial cells were derived from umbilical veins [19]. Human intestinal smooth muscle cells were obtained from Dr. H. Perr, Department of Pediatrics, Medical College of Virginia. Rat aorta smooth muscle cells were a gift of Dr. White, Department of Anesthesiology, Uniformed Services University for the Health Sciences (USUHS).

Human and rat smooth muscle cells behaved in a similar way in preliminary assays and consequently both lines were used. Fibrosarcoma cells (HT 1080), adenocarcinoma cells (SW 620), melanoma cells (Malme 3M), and a rhabdomyosarcoma cell line (A 204) were purchased from Am Type Culture Collection, Rockville, MD.

Matrigel Invasion Assay

This assay was performed in Boyden chambers, as previously described [20]. Polyvinylpyrrolidone-free polycarbonate filters (12 μm pore size) were coated with varying amounts of matrigel [21] (a gift from H. K. Kleinman, NIDR, NIH). Matrigel is a urea extract of the Englebrecht-Holm-Swarm tumor, containing laminin, type IV collagen, entactin, and heparan sulphate proteoglycan, the major components of basement membranes. When dialyzed against PBS or serum-free medium, it is liquid at 4°C and polymerizes in a three-dimensional matrix at 37°C. Fibroblast conditioned medium was placed in the lower compartment of Boyden chambers to stimulate migration. Cells were harvested with trypsin, resuspended in 0.1% bovine serum albumin (BSA) in Dulbecco's Minimum Essential Medium (DMEM), and placed in the upper compartment at 1.5 to 2 $\times$ 10^5 cells per chamber. The cells were allowed to migrate for 6 h at 37°C in air plus 5% CO_2 in a humidified incubator. At the end of the incubation period, the cells on the upper surface of the filter were wiped away, and the filters were fixed in methanol and stained with hematoxylin and eosin. The mean number of migrated cells per field was determined by counting five microscopic fields. All assays were run in duplicate.

Chemotaxis

The assay was run in Boyden chambers as previously described [22]. The filters were soaked in a diluted solution of collagen IV (50 μg/ml), which coats the surface and pores and promotes the adhesion and migration of cells. In some studies fibroblast-conditioned medium was used as a source of chemoattractants [22]. In addition, the following growth factors were used as chemoattractants at concentrations found to promote cell migration: platelet derived growth factor (PDGF), 1–10 ng/ml (Collaborative Research); epidermal growth factor (EGF), 5–50 ng/ml (Collaborative Research); endothelial cell growth factor (ECGF), 10–100 ng/ml (Meloy Labs., Springfield, MD); transforming growth factor, beta (TGFβ), 1–10 ng/ml (a gift of A. Roberts, NCI, NIH); transforming growth factor, alpha (TGFα), 1–10 ng/ml (a gift of G. Todaro, Seattle, WA). These were added, along with 0.1% BSA as carrier, to the lower compartment of the Boyden chamber. After the termination of the migration period, the filters were fixed, stained, and counted in the same way as for the invasion assays.

RESULTS

Invasion

Four cell lines were established from KS tissue from four patients and were selected by their ability to grow in culture at low serum levels. The ability of the KS culture to invade a matrix of basement membrane components reconstituted onto a porous filter was measured both before and after selection [20]. In these studies, fibroblast-conditioned media containing a mixture of potent chemoattractants was placed in the chambers below the filter. KS cells were able to invade through varying amounts of basement membrane matrix (Fig. 1–a,b). Normal human cells, including human fibroblasts, endothelial cells, and smooth muscle cells, were also studied, as well as malignant cells from various human tumors. The invasiveness of the KS cells varied among the different lines, but the range of activity was comparable to that observed with metastatic tumor cells, including those from a fibrosarcoma and a melanoma (Table I). Human intestinal and rat aorta smooth muscle cells, human umbilical vein endothelial cells, and human fibroblasts were not invasive when tested in this assay. However, they showed a significant migration through the filter in the absence of the layer of basement membrane (Fig. 1b).

To investigate the effect of the selection protocol, we compared the invasiveness of cells in the original outgrowth with those cells selected by growth in media with reduced serum content. The selected cultures were 3–7-fold more invasive than the original population of cells (Table II).

Chemotaxis

We also tested the chemotactic response of the most invasive KS cell strain (Patient C) to several growth factors as compared to primary fibroblasts, smooth muscle, and endothelial cells (Table III). These studies were performed in a manner similar to the invasion assays, but without the layer of basement membrane imposed as a barrier over the porous filter. To allow easier comparison, the data have been normalized to the response obtained using conditioned media as an attractant with each cell type studied. The absolute values varied, with the endothelial cells showing a much lower response than the other cells tested (i.e., 10 cells/field vs. 30 or 40 cells/field with the other cells). As shown in Table III, each cell type responded differently to this panel of attractants. For each growth factor a range of concentra-

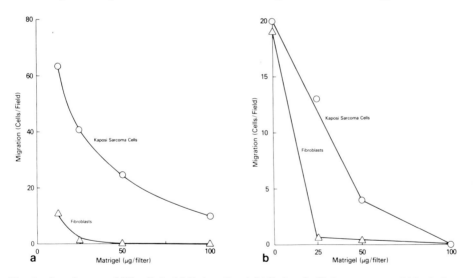

Fig. 1. Invasiveness of KS cells in **(a)** Patient C and **(b)** Patient L. Various amounts of Matrigel were coated onto porous filters. KS cells and fibroblasts were put in the upper compartment of the chemotaxis chamber and incubated for 6 h. Fibroblast-conditioned media were used as a source of chemoattractants. KS cells were more invasive than fibroblasts for all amounts of matrigel tested (**a** and **b**). In the absence of matrigel only chemotaxis is being assayed (**b**). Data are expressed as cells invaded/field. Five random fields per filter were counted and symbols represent average value of two experiments. Standard error was less than 5 cells.

TABLE I. Invasiveness of Kaposi's Sarcoma Cells as Compared to Normal Cells and to Human Tumor Cells*

Kaposi's Sarcoma cells	Patient L	$19^a \pm 3$
	Patient C	32 ± 4
	Patient B	7 ± 1
	Patient M	invasive[b]
Normal cells	Primary fibroblasts	0.5 ± 0.4
	Smooth muscle cells	1 ± 0.2
	Endothelial cells	0
Invasive tumor cells	Fibrosarcoma (HT-1080)	16 ± 3
	Melanoma (Malme 3M)	28 ± 6
	Rhabdomyosarcoma (A 204)	56 ± 8
	Adenocarcinoma (SW 620)	60 ± 7

*Cells derived from biopsy specimen of Kaposi's patients (as well as control cells) were tested for their ability to invade through a reconstituted basement membrane (Matrigel) in the chemoinvasion assay as adapted for the Boyden chamber (20). Fibroblast-conditioned medium was used as chemoattractant and was placed in the bottom chamber.
[a]Data are expressed as migrated cells/field, with the mean of 5 fields from each of 2 assays reported.
[b]This study was conducted in a separate experiment and showed invasive cells, but the data cannot be directly compared, and this cell line was subsequently lost.

TABLE II. Effect of Selection in Low Serum on the Invasiveness of KS Cells*

Cells	Unselected	Selected
Control fibroblasts	0.5 ± 0.4^a	NA[b]
Patient L	5 ± 2	17 ± 4
Patient B	1 ± 0.5	7 ± 1

*Cells derived from cultured biopsy specimens in 20% FBS were selected by growth in low serum (2.5% FBS) to enrich for tumor cells. Cultures of the original outgrowth and from the selected lines were tested for invasive activity in the chemoinvasion assay.
[a]Data are expressed as migrated cells/fields (mean of 5 fields from each of two assays).
[b]The control cells did not survive in the low serum media.

TABLE III. Chemotaxis of Kaposi's Sarcoma Cell to Growth Factors*

	Cell Type			
Attractant	Fibroblast	Endothelial	Smooth muscle	Kaposi's
BSA (1 mg/ml)	0	0	0	0
PDGF (10 ng/ml)	52 ± 9	0	179 ± 19	139 ± 18
ECGF (75 ng/ml)	8 ± 3	100 ± 19	85 ± 4	80 ± 5
EGF (50 ng/ml)	14 ± 2	40 ± 4	31 ± 1	71 ± 5
TGF α (10 ng/ml)	9 ± 4	3 ± 2	18 ± 3	36 ± 7
TGF β (10 ng/ml)	58 ± 8	0	19 ± 5	22 ± 4
CM	100	100	100	100

*Cells from the most invasive Kaposi's cell strain (Patient C) were tested for their chemotactic response to several growth factors in the Boyden chamber assay. A large range of concentrations was investigated in preliminary experiments (4–6 log). The responses to an optimal concentration in the active range are reported. Data are expressed as % of cells that migrated relative to the number of cells migrating toward fibroblast-conditioned medium (100%) and BSA (0%).

tions of 4–6 logs was tested in preliminary experiments, and the migration observed at an optimal concentration of each attractant is reported. Under these conditions, smooth muscle cells preferentially migrated to PDGF and to ECGF, and less to the other factors. As expected, endothelial cells migrated preferentially to ECGF, to a lesser extent to EGF, and not at all to PDGF or TGFβ. Fibroblasts were found to respond to PDGF, TGFβ, and only minimally to ECGF or TGFα. KS cells were highly responsive to PDGF, ECGF, and EGF, and showed a lesser response to TGFα. TGFβ exerted little attraction on the KS cells.

These data suggest that the selected KS cultures contain a mixed population of cells, with smooth muscle-like cells the most abundant. Alternatively, the KS cells may have originated from smooth muscle cells but later acquired some additional growth factor responsiveness.

DISCUSSION

Although generally thought to be a malignancy, KS exhibits certain features that are not typical of tumors; for example, KS may regress, it can present with multicentric lesions, and its cells are not always karyotypically abnormal [5], although they may show some instability [23]. We cultured cells from KS lesions obtained from AIDS patients and selected a subpopulation of cells by their ability to survive and proliferate at a lower serum concentration. The selected cells were shown to be capable of anchorage-independent growth and to be able to invade muscle tissue [17]. Such behavior is consistent with a transformed phenotype.

The appearance of the cells in culture and the presence of certain characteristic markers suggested a smooth muscle cell origin for the KS cells examined here, rather than an endothelial one [17]. These KS cells in culture stained with Masson trichrome. Dense bodies representing characteristics typical of myoblasts were observed by electron microscopy. The cells did not form capillary structures like endothelial cells, they lacked Weibel-Palade bodies, and did not express Factor VIII-related antigen or receptors for *Ulex europeaus* I-a lectin [17].

To characterize these cells further, we investigated their ability to invade through a reconstituted basement membrane barrier and the chemotactic response of the most invasive line to various growth factors. The breaching of basement membranes is an important step in the spread of malignant cells [24]. Such invasive activity is dependent on the ability of the cells to attach to the basement membrane, to produce enzymes that degrade this barrier, and to recognize chemoattractants which activate and direct their motile response [25]. Our assay uses a Boyden chamber with basement membrane proteins reconstituted onto the surface of a porous filter and chemoattractants placed in the lower chamber. The selectivity of the assay can be increased by using a thicker barrier, which requires longer periods for cells to cross. Using fibroblast-conditioned medium as a source of attractants, we assessed the invasiveness of cells cultured from Kaposi's lesions from four patients as well as normal cells and cells from metastatic cancers. The KS cells, selected by their ability to grow in media with a lower serum content, were invasive. Invasiveness varied among the cell lines, but all four cell lines showed a greater capacity for penetration of the barrier than normal cells, and in two cases their invasiveness was comparable to that observed with metastatic tumor cells used as a positive control. Normal cells, including fibroblasts, smooth muscle cells and endothelial cells, were not invasive.

Cells from two KS lesions were studied both before and after selection by growth at a lower serum concentration and showed a significant increase in invasiveness after selection. The most likely explanation for these results is that a mixed population of cells is obtained in the initial outgrowth from the lesions, and that the most invasive cells survive the selection process.

Since chemotaxis is a receptor-mediated event, considerable specificity is encountered in the response of cells to various attractants [see 26]. Recent studies indicate that certain growth factors exhibit chemotactic activity [see 27]. Thus, PDGF is both an attractant and a mitogen for fibroblasts and smooth muscle cells [28,29] and ECGF induces both the migration and proliferation of endothelial cells [30]. TGFβ has a higher chemotactic activity for fibroblasts [31] than for the other cell types studied here. The chemotactic response of the cells occurs prior to DNA synthesis and occurs even when DNA synthesis is inhibited [28,29], but it is thought to be mediated via similar initial reactions.

Here we tested several growth factors for chemotactic activity with a KS cell strain and with various normal cells. Distinctive patterns were observed with fibroblasts, endothelial cells, and smooth muscle cells. PDGF was a potent chemoattractant for fibroblasts, smooth muscle, and KS cells, but not endothelial cells. ECGF was active with endothelial cells, smooth muscle cells, and KS cells. TGFα induced a significant response for smooth muscle and KS cells, while TGFβ was very active for fibroblasts but only minimally for KS cells. Based on these observations (and particularly on their attraction toward PDGF, to which endothelial cells show no response) we suggest that the KS cells respond in this assay as smooth muscle cells. This is in agreement with previous work suggesting a smooth muscle cell-like phenotype for KS cells [17].

It should be noted, however, that the Kaposi cells showed quite a strong response to EGF, and in this regard differ from the adult smooth muscle cells studied here. While the lineage through which smooth muscle cells develop is not fully established, it is known that their phenotype can vary. Thus, the state to which the KS cells have developed may include the retention of EGF responsiveness and be related to their aberrant behavior in creating these lesions.

Current concepts suggest that the repertoire of receptors for mitogens and chemoattractants is related to a cell's function and therefore may represent a rather specific profile [27]. The studies reported in this paper support the previous suggestion [17] that the malignant cells in the Kaposi's lesions are a transformed mesenchymal cell resembling smooth muscle cells.

ACKNOWLEDGMENTS

We thank Dr. G. Todaro (Oncogene, WA) and Dr. A. Roberts (NIH, MD) for the gift of TGFα and TGFβ. We are grateful to Dr. Perr (Medical College of Virginia, VA) and Dr. White (USUHS, MD) for providing us with the smooth muscle cells. We thank Ms. S. Jacobs and Ms. L. Wepasnick for typing the manuscript.

REFERENCES

1. Jones RR, Spaull J, Spry C, Jones EW: J Clin Pathol 39:742, 1986.
2. Safai B, Johnson KG, Myokowsky PL, Koziner B, Yang SY, Cunningham-Rundles S, Godbold JH, Dupont B: Ann Intern Med 103:744, 1985.

3. Safai B, Sarngadharan MG, Koziner B, Godbold J, Myskowski PL, Cunningham-Rundles S, Johnson K, Gold J, Krown S, Dupont B: Cancer Research 45:4646s, 1985.
4. Petit JC, Ripamonti U, Hille J: J Periodontol 57:159, 1986.
5. Brooks JJ: The Lancet, 8519:1309, 1986.
6. Blayney DW, Ito JT, Jensen FC: Cancer 58:1583, 1986.
7. Janier M, Vignon MD, Cottentot F: N Engl J Med 312:1638, 1985.
8. Real FX, Krown SE: N Engl J Med 313:1659, 1986.
9. Leu HJ, Odermatt B: Virchows Arch A 408:29, 1985.
10. Braun-Falco, O, Schmoeckel C, Hubner G: Virchows Arch A 369:215, 1976.
11. Blumenfeld W, Egbert BM, Sagebiel RW: Arch Pathol Lab Med 109:106, 1985.
12. Costa J, Rabson AS: The Lancet 1:58, 1983.
13. Beckstead JH, Wood GS, Fletcher V: Am J Pathol 119:294, 1985.
14. Rutgers JL, Wieczorek R, Bonetti F, Kaplan KL, Posnett DN, Friedman-Kien AE, Knowles DM 2nd: Am J Pathol 122:493, 1986.
15. Schenk P, Konrad K: Arch Otolaryngol 242:305, 1985.
16. Harrison AC, Kahn LB: J Pathol 124:157, 1978.
17. Quinnan GV, Mitchell CD, Armstrong G, Albini A, Martin GR, Seeman R, Levenbook IS, Wierenga DE, Steis R, Dunlap RC, Wittek AE: Cancer Res (in review).
18. Mitsuyasu RT, Taylor JM, Glaspy J, Fahey JL: Cancer 15;56:1657, 1986.
19. Jaffe, EA, Nachman RL, Becker CG, Minick CR: J Clin Invest 52:2745, 1973.
20. Albini A, Iwamoto Y, Kleinman HK, Martin GR, Aaronson SA, Kozlowsky JM, McEwan RN: Cancer Research, 47:3239, 1987.
21. Kleinman HK, McGarvey ML, Hassel JR, Star VL, Cannon FB, Laurie GW, Martin GR: Biochemistry, 25:312, 1986.
22. Albini A, Allavena G, Parodi S, Santi L: Tumori, 71:97, 1985.
23. Delli-Boni P, Danti E, Knowles DM, Friedman-Kein A, Luciw PA, Dina D, Dalla-Favera R, Basilico C: Cancer Res 46:6333, 1986.
24. Terranova VP, Hujanen ES, Martin GR: J Natl Cancer Inst 77:311, 1986.
25. Liotta LA: Am J Pathol 117:339, 1984.
26. Albini A, Adelmann-Grill BC, Müller PK: Collagen Rel Res 5:283, 1985.
27. Grotendorst GR, Martin GR: Rheumatology 10:385, Karger, Basel, 1986.
28. Seppä H, Grotendorst G, Seppä S, Schiffmann E, Martin GR: J Cell Biol 92:584, 1982.
29. Grotendorst GR, Chang T, Seppä HE, Kleinman HK, Martin GR: J Cell Physiol 113:261, 1982.
30. Terranova VP, Di Florio R, Lyall RM, Hic S, Friesel R, Maciag T: J Cell Biol 101:23330, 1985.
31. Postlethwaite AE, Keski-Oja J, Moses HL, Kang AH: J Exp Med 165:251–256, 1987.

Growth Regulation of Cancer
145–150 (1988)

Tissue Organization and Cancer: Role of Autocrine Growth Factors in Extracellular Matrix Biosynthesis

W. R. Kidwell, S. Mohanam, B. Sanfilippo, and D. S. Salomon

Laboratory of Tumor Immunology and Biology, National Cancer Institute, Bethesda, Maryland 20892

The mammary glandular epithelium synthesizes and deposits an extracellular matrix, the basement membrane, between its basal surface and the surrounding stroma. Production of the basement membrane is of interest because it appears to serve as a barrier that restricts invasion and metastasis of tumors of the mammary gland and because contact with the basement membrane enhances mammary cell growth and differentiation. Recent findings of our laboratory indicate that basement membrane biosynthesis is regulated by both positive and negative factors: the positive factors are one or more growth factors made by mammary cells, and the negative controls are inhibitory factors from the mammary gland as well as the basement membrane itself. Comparative studies of well-differentiated, noninvasive mammary tumors making a basement membrane, and poorly differentiated, invasive ones that do not, have suggested new ways by which breast cancer progression to a more malignant state might occur. Confirmation of this process and the agents involved could, therefore, lead to the development of new tests for diagnosing metastatic potential. A model depicting the salient regulatory steps of basement membrane synthesis is given. From the proposed model, the future directions of our research will be evident.

Key words: mammary cells, growth factors, autocrine controls

Figure 1 shows three stages of basement membrane biosynthesis. In A, a nondividing cell is depicted as sitting on the basement membrane. Following a growth stimulus (i.e., estrogen), the cell produces autocrine growth factors (mammary-derived growth factor 1, or MDGFI; transforming growth factor alpha, or TGFα) [1,2]. Additionally the cell produces two proteolytic factors, procollagenase 1V [3] and plasminogen activator [4]. The latter converts plasminogen to plasmin, a protease that, in turn, converts inactive procollagenase 1V to active collagenase 1V [5]. The combined action of plasmin and collagenase 1V (and possibly other hydrolases)

Received February 17, 1987.

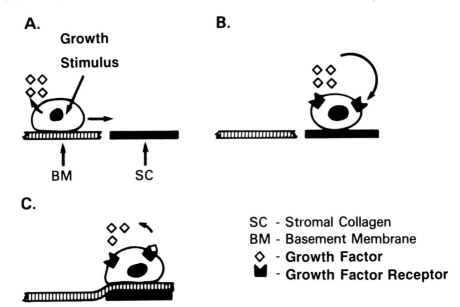

Fig. 1. Model depicting the various stages in normal mammary epithelial cell proliferation and accompanying regeneration of the basement membrane (see text for details).

enables the mammary cell to locally degrade the basement membrane and migrate into the stromal compartment.

In stage B of Figure 1, the migrated cell has come in contact with stromal elements (depicted as stromal collagen fibers). A consequence of this contact and accompanying cell shape change is the generation of additional growth factor receptors for the autocrine growth factors elaborated by mammary cells in response to a proliferative stimulus [2]. These latter factors (MDGFI and/or TGFα) then interact with their respective receptors, effecting a great and differential increase in production of basement membrane proteins—collagen 1V, proteoglycan, and laminin [1,6].

The completion of new basement membrane deposition as a layer intervening between the mammary cell surface and stromal collagen represents the progression to the third stage (c) of the model. Herein, the growth factor receptors are down-regulated and fail to up-regulate [2]. In this state, basement membrane deposition ceases, whether or not MDGFI or TGFα is present. Thus, basement membrane feedback-regulates its own synthesis via effecting changes in the expression of membrane receptors.

As indicated in the above references, most aspects of the model have been directly demonstrated. Estrogen is known to induce procollagen 1V and plasminogen activator release. The steroid also induces the production of TFGα and its mRNA in both rodent [7] and human [8,9] mammary tumor cells in vivo and in vitro. Withdrawal of estrogenic hormone support by ovariectomy also results in a desensitization of mammary epithelium for MDGFI responsiveness [1]. Chemically synthesized TGFα and MDGFI, purified to apparent homogeneity, have been shown to differentially amplify collagen 1V, laminin, and glycosaminoglycan synthesis in normal mammary cells in primary culture. Moreover, as indicated in the model, primary mammary cells responded dramatically to TGFα or MDGFI addition to the cultures if the cells were grown on stromal collagen. However, they were almost totally refractory to the factors when grown on basement membrane collagen [1,6]. Evaluation of cells grown on either collagen type revealed that TGFα receptors downregulated on stromal collagen and then up-regulated even in the presence of an excess of TGFα. In contrast, on type 1V the collagen TGFα receptor was down-regulated by its ligand but did not up-regulate [2]. Since continued expression of growth factor receptor is a requisite for continued growth factor responsiveness, it is likely that changes in growth factor receptors effected by contact with the extracellular matrix explain the large differences in mammary cell responsiveness to TFGα and MDGFI on collagen 1V and stromal collagen.

Other aspects of the model, although more speculative, are consistent with experimental observations. For example, direct proof of a transient break in the continuous basement membrane surrounding the glandular epithelium has not been seen during normal proliferation. However, we have shown that gaps in the basement membrane develop in the gland in vivo if, simultaneously with a proliferative stimulus, we administer cis-4-hydroxyproline, a drug that selectively blocks new collagen deposition. If cis-4-hydroxyproline is administered in the absence of a proliferative stimulus, no gaps in the basement membrane are generated [10].

Before considering the changes in basement membrane synthesis that accompany neoplastic transformation, it is important to mention two additional aspects of formation of the matrix by normal mammary cells. First, there is a large and differential increase in basement membrane protein synthesis accompanying accelerated mammary cell division in response to TGFα and MDGFI, as described. However, almost all factors that accelerate cell division rates in primary mammary cell cultures also evoke the same differential amplification of matrix synthesis [11]. This indicates that enhanced extracellular matrix production is tightly coupled to the division process and, in fact, may be a requisite for normal mammary cell growth. Consistent with this tenet is the fact that when cell division is inhibited (e.g., by a polypeptide inhibitor purified from milk), there is also a differential drop in the biosynthetic rates for basement membrane protein [12].

The second point is that collagen biosynthesis by normal mammary cells is dependent on an external supply of proline. In fact, if collagen synthesis rates are high (as is the case when mammary cells are plated on stromal collagen and stimulated with MDGFI), mammary cells actually become proline auxotrophs [13]. The reason for the proline auxotrophy seems to be explained by the fact that net synthesis of collagen, a very proline-rich protein, is a highly wasteful process. The protein turns over very rapidly within the cell so that only about 30% of the newly synthesized protein is secreted intact [6]. Proline in the degradation products is not readily reutilized by the cells because it is hydroxylated or it is in the form of relatively stable collagen fragments. We believe the additional proline requirements from exogenous sources, over and above the proline synthesized de novo, are obtained by growth factor (TGFα and/or MDGFI)-stimulated active transport of proline. The significance of these observations becomes more apparent as we consider the implications of altered basement membrane protein synthesis in breast cancer cells.

BASEMENT MEMBRANE PROTEIN BIOSYNTHESIS BY MAMMARY TUMORS

Comparative studies of normal, benign, and malignant (metastatic and invasive) mammary tumors have been made utilizing rat mammary tumor model systems.

Benign tumors are defined operationally here as tumors that are locally confined. Animals bearing such tumors are "cured" of their disease by surgical excision of their tumors. Metastatic and invasive tumors, on the other hand, kill their hosts whether or not the primary lesion is surgically removed because such tumors have become disseminated to various sites in the host. Examples of benign rat mammary tumors are primary tumors such as those induced by methylnitrosourea (NMU) and 7,12-dimethylbenz(α)anthracene (DMBA) as well as transplantable tumors, i.e., MTW9 and R3230AC tumors. Examples of metastatic tumors are transplantable tumors derived from primary NMU- or DMBA-induced rat mammary tumors following many transplant generations, or tumor lines established directly from metastatic lesions.

Benign rat mammary tumors produce large amounts of several growth factors (e.g., TGFα, TGFβ, and collagen synthesis stimulating factor (CSSF). CSSF greatly resembles a growth factor purified from human milk and human mammary tumors, namely MDGFI. Both factors are high molecular weight proteins (CSSF, Mr 68,000; MDGFI, Mr 62,000) and both are acidic (CSSF, pI 5.9; MDGFI, pI 4.8). In bioassays, both CSSF and MDGFI stimulate normal mouse or rat mammary cell division and greatly amplify collagen IV biosynthesis [1,6]. All benign tumors synthesize and deposit a continuous basement membrane between the stroma and the tumor epithelium. Basement membrane is not made by the malignant tumors. Nor are TGFα or CSSF made by any metastatic rat tumors studied by us (transplantable NMU-, DMBA-induced tumors; transplantable, poorly differentiated tumor line derived from the transplantable, well-differentiated MTW9 tumor). These observations provide the strongest evidence that CSSF and/or TGFα are involved in the regulation of basement membrane synthesis. Consistent with this observation is the fact that normal mammary epithelium synthesizes and releases CSSF (or MDGFI) and TGFα in primary cell cultures, albeit the production of these factors by normal cells is significantly lower than that of benign tumor cells [14].

As indicated, metastatic rat mammary tumor cells do not make TGFα or CSSF. They make large amounts of TGFβ, however. Bioassays of conditioned medium from primary cultures of rat and human mammary tumor cells have shown that TGFβ release is approximately the same for benign and malignant breast tumor cells [14]. This fact is significant because two groups have reported that TGFβ is a potent stimulator of extracellular matrix protein synthesis [15,16]. We can conclude from our observations that TGFβ cannot be a regulatory factor for basement membrane synthesis in the mammary system unless the metastatic cells have lost their responsiveness to TGFβ.

Loss of responsiveness to TGF has been demonstrated, in fact. Not only have the metastatic rat mammary tumors lost their ability to make TGF, they have also lost receptors for this growth factor (and EGF). From this we may conclude that the loss of capacity to form a basement membrane (with increased metastatic potential) may be a consequence of (1) decreased growth factor production, (2) decreased growth factor receptor production, and (3) both. A fourth possibility is that the capacity for synthesizing the basement membrane is intact but that metastatic cells produce so much basement membrane degrading activity that basement membrane deposition is effectively prevented. There is some experimental evidence for this proposition [3] as well as for (1) and (2).

Synthesis of basement membrane proteins by normal and benign rat mammary cells is associated with other properties of these cells, namely: (1) their sensitivity to proline analogs such as cis-4-hydroxyproline, (2) their production of growth factors that stimulate basement membrane biosynthesis, and (3) their proline auxotrophy under conditions of maximal basement membrane collagen synthesis. We believe that all three of these phenotypes are causally related as follows. As a fail-safe mechanism for maintenance of tissue organization (a normal regulatory mechanism retained by benign tumor cells), normal mammary cells produce growth factors that assure that basement membrane will be resynthesized, if breaks in that structure occur. In support of basement membrane collagen synthesis, the same growth factors activate the transport of proline and proline-related amino acid analogs. The amino acid analogs would, therefore, be taken up and kill the growth factor activated cell. Metastatic mammary tumor cells do not make basement membrane collagen; nor do they make growth factors, such as TGFα or MDGFI, that could facilitate proline analog transport. Consequently, the latter tumors exhibit little proline analog (e.g., cis-4-hydroxyproline) sensitivity [17].

A corollary is that cells that do not make TGFα or MDGFI-like growth factors may be sensitized to the killing effects of cis-4-hydroxyproline by exogenously supplying growth factors (if the growth factor receptor system is intact). In fact, we have recently shown that NRK cells (cells that produce little TGFα or little active TGFβ, but that possess receptors for both factors) are greatly sensitized to cis-4-hydroxyproline if TGFα and TGFβ are added to the cell growth medium. This is shown in Table I. This fact suggests the possibility that we will be able to predict which mammary tumors will respond to cis-4-hydroxyproline, namely those that produce MDGFI and/or TGFα (if the tumors also possess receptors for one or both of these growth factors). In the event that a class of tumors are found that do not produce either growth factor but do possess receptors, we may be able to block the growth of such tumors by administering both cis-4-hydroxyproline and TGFα or MDGFI. Tumors that do not express receptors for TGFα or MDGFI would likely be refractory to cis-4-hydroxyproline, regardless of whether the tumors produced growth factors that stimulated basement membrane biosynthesis. Our goal is to test these

TABLE I. Enhanced Sensitivity of NRK Cells to Cis-4-hydroxyproline (CHP) in the Presence of TGFα and TGFβ*

CHP conc. (μg/ml)	% Inhibition of NRK cell growth	
	+ TGFs	− TGFs
5	22	8
10	43	17
25	77	28
50	95	39
100	100	71

*Approximately 2×10^5 NRK cells in 2 ml culture medium (Dulbecco's modified Eagle's medium containing 20 mM HEPES buffer, pH 7.4, 5% fetal calf serum, and 2 mM glutamine) were plated in 35 mm culture dishes. One set of dishes also received 5 ng/ml TGFα and 2 ng/ml TGFβ. After 4 days incubation, the cells were removed from the dishes with trypsin and counted in a Coulter counter. Values are the average of four dishes. CHP was added at the indicated concentrations at the time of plating. Half-maximal inhibition of cell growth was seen at 12 μg CHP with TFGs present, and at 60 μg/ml in the absence of the two growth factors.

possibilities with the hope that our answers will lead to practical tests for predicting metastatic potential and also for predicting proline analog sensitivity in vivo.

ACKNOWLEDGMENTS

B.S. acknowledges the generous fellowship support by the Associazione Italiana Per la Ricerca Sul Cancro.

REFERENCES

1. Bano M, Salomon DS, Kidwell WR: J Biol Chem 260:5745–5752, 1985.
2. Liu S, Kidwell WR, Derynck R, Tam J, Salomon DS: J Cell Biol 103:443a, 1986.
3. Liotta LA, Tryggvason K, Garbisa S, Gehron-Robey P, Abe S: Biochem 20:100–104, 1981.
4. Thorgiersson U, Turpeenniemi-Huganen T, Liotta LA: In Mihich E (ed): "Biological Responses in Cancer." New York: Plenum, 1985, pp, 21–35.
5. Salomon DS, Liotta LA, Kidwell WR: Proc Natl Acad Sci (USA) 78:382–386, 1981.
6. Bano M, Zwiebel JA, Salomon DS, Kidwell WR: J Biol Chem 258:2729–2725, 1983.
7. Salomon DS, Kidwell WR, Liu S, Kim N, Callahan R, Theillet C, Lidearu R, Derynck R: Breast Cancer Res Treat 8:106, 1986.
8. Perroteau I, Salomon DS, DeBertoli M, Kidwell WR, Hazarika P, Pardue R, Dedman J, Tam J: Breast Cancer Res Treat 7:201–210, 1986.
9. Dickson RB, Huff KK, Spencer EM, Lippman ME: Endocrin 118:138–142, 1985.
10. Wicha MS, Liotta LA, Vonderhaar BK, Kidwell WR: Develop Biol 80:253–266, 1980.
11. Kidwell WR, Bano M, Taylor SJ: In Mihich E (ed): "Biological Responses in Cancer." New York: Plenum, 1985, pp 47–69.
12. Kidwell WR: In Rochefort H (ed): "Hormones, Oncogenes, Growth Factors." Paris: ISR, 1986, p 14.
13. Kidwell WR, Smith GS, Vonderhaar BK: In Murakami H (ed): "Growth and Differentiation of Cells in Defined Environments." Berlin: Springer-Verlag, 1985, pp 103–108.
14. Kidwell WR, Salomon DS, Mohanam S: In Goldman A (ed): "Effect of Human Milk on the Recipient Infant." New York: Plenum. 1987 (in press).
15. Ignotz RA, Massague J: J Biol Chem 261:4337–4345, 1986.
16. Sporn MB, Roberts AB: Science 233:532–534, 1986.
17. Lewko W, Liotta LA, Wicha MS, Vonderhaar BK, Kidwell WR: Cancer Res 41:2855–2862, 1981.

Growth Regulation of Cancer
151–155 (1988)

Expression and Function of the PDGF Receptor in Normal and Transformed Cells

Lewis T. Williams, Jaime A. Escobedo, Shaun R. Coughlin, and Mark T. Keating

Department of Medicine, Cardiovascular Research Institute, and Howard Hughes Medical Institute, University of California, San Francisco, California 94143

Platelet-derived growth factor (PDGF) is a potent mitogen for mesenchymal cells. Early studies on PDGF focused on its role in stimulating proliferation of vascular smooth muscle cells in atherosclerotic plaques [1]. With the discovery by a number of investigators of the existence of PDGF-like compounds in a variety of normal and pathological tissues, there was a realization that the PDGF system is likely to play a role in normal development, wound healing, fibrotic diseases, and cancer. PDGF, purified from human platelets, is a 32 kDa heterodimer consisting of two chains, A and B, that are disulfide-linked. These chains are homologous but are not identical. In addition to the heterodimeric form of PDGF, homodimers of A-chains or B-chains are expressed in several types of cells [2]. Another form of PDGF-like compound is the homodimer encoded by the v-*sis* gene, which is the oncogene of the simian sarcoma virus and is highly homologous to the c-*sis* gene that encodes the B-chain of PDGF (3,4). All of these forms of PDGF-like compounds stimulate DNA synthesis by first interacting with the PDGF receptor, a 180 kDa single monomeric membrane protein. Much of the recent work on the PDGF system has focused on the regulation of the expression of PDGF-like growth factors, the interaction of these factors with the PDGF receptor, the structure and function of the receptor, and the mechanism by which the receptor stimulates cell replication.

PDGF receptors can be activated in three distinct ways. First, PDGF-like compounds can be carried in circulating cells, e.g., platelets or monocytes, and released locally near responsive tissue such as vascular smooth muscle cells in an injured blood vessel. In this mode of action, PDGF acts as a locally released hormone. The second mode of PDGF is in paracrine processes. For example, endothelial cells that line the inner surface of blood vessels release biologically active B-chain and A-

Received February 15, 1987.

chain homodimers, which can stimulate the adjacent smooth muscle cells of the vessel wall. A third mode of action of PDGF-like compounds is an autocrine mechanism by which a PDGF-like compound is produced by a tumor cell and acts on the same cell to stimulate its receptors. In each of these modes of action, the PDGF receptor plays a pivotol role.

PARACRINE ACTION OF PDGF-LIKE COMPOUNDS: ENDOTHELIAL CELLS AND SMOOTH MUSCLE CELLS

Recent studies by a number of groups have shown that PDGF-like growth factors are produced by endothelial cells (5,6,7). Endothelial cells lack PDGF receptors and therefore cannot respond to the PDGF-like mitogens that they produce. By contrast the adjacent cells in the vessel wall, the vascular smooth muscle cells, are replete with PDGF receptors and are extraordinarily responsive to PDGF. Thus this system appears to act by a paracrine mechanism in which the endothelial cells produce mitogens that act directly on vascular smooth muscle cells. It seems likely that the production of these mitogens by endothelial cells is not constitutive but is highly regulated since a proliferative response should be required only at specific times, e.g., when there is injury to the blood vessel or surrounding tissues. For this reason we have studied the regulation of the expression of PDGF-like compounds by endothelial cells. In the initial studies we screened a variety of substances that were likely to play a role in tissue response to injury. We found two, thrombin and transforming growth factor-beta (TGF-beta), that elicited a dramatic increase in the expression of the gene (*sis* gene) that encodes the B-chain of PDGF (7,8). Thrombin exposure of renal microvascular endothelial cells increases the levels of *sis* message by 3–5-fold over a time course that peaks 4 hours after exposure. Similarly, thrombin-stimulated microvascular cells release increased amounts of PDGF activity into their media. This effect of thrombin may be important in vivo since thrombin production would be expected to occur at sites of tissue injury. Another factor that may be involved in the response to injury, TGF-beta, is released by activated platelets. TGF-beta, like thrombin, enhances the expression and the release of PDGF activity from endothelial cells, although the time course of the TGF-beta effect is significantly longer than that of the thrombin effect [8]. Recently, Tom Daniel, Griff Harsh, and Niel Starksen in our lab have found that agents that elevate cyclic AMP dramatically reduce the expression of PDGF-like growth factor genes in a variety of cell types, including endothelial cells (8). Thus the expression of these mitogens by endothelial cells is regulated both in a positive sense, by thrombin and TGF-beta, and in a negative sense, by cyclic AMP-elevating agents. The molecular mechanism that mediates these regulatory effects on the *sis* gene is currently under investigation.

AUTOCRINE ACTIVATION OF PDGF RECEPTORS IN CELLS TRANSFORMED BY THE V-SIS ONCOGENE

Many investigators have recently studied cells transformed by simian sarcoma virus (SSV) as a model system for the autocrine stimulation of PDGF receptors. The SSV-transforming gene, the v-*sis* gene, is known to encode a protein that is processed to homodimeric form that are similar to homodimers of the B-chain of PDGF [9]. When the v-*sis* gene is expressed in cells that have PDGF receptors, the cells become transformed [10]. Normal rat kidney cells transformed by the SSV have few if any PDGF receptors expressed at the cell surface, whereas their normal counterparts express approximately 80,000 PDGF receptors at the surface. The absence of receptors in the SSV-transformed cells appears to be due to the internalization and degradation of the receptors caused by the v-*sis* gene product. This process can be mimicked in normal cells by adding a large amount of PDGF, which is known to elicit this down-regulation phenomenon. How is the PDGF receptor activated in these SSV-transformed cells? Is the v-*sis* gene product released to the outside of the cell where it can activate cell surface receptors? Or does the v-*sis* product act on intracellular receptors? We and other investigators have been studying these questions during the last three years. Although most of the v-*sis* encoded protein remains cell-associated [11], there is enough released into the media of SSV-transformed cells to activate and down-regulate all of their PDGF receptors [12]. If SSV-transformed cells are treated with suramin, an agent that blocks the interaction of the v-*sis* gene product with PDGF receptors, then a normal number of receptors are expressed at the cell surface [12]. These and other data have suggested that in the SSV-transformed cells the receptors are down-regulated by the action of the v-*sis* gene product at the surface. However, other findings have suggested the possibility that intracellular receptors are activated as well [11,13]. To examine this issue further, we needed to know more about the receptor. How is the receptor processed? When is it activated? What is the fate of the activated receptor? How does activation of the receptor lead to cell transformation? Studies of these issues have recently been facilitated by two useful reagents: antibodies directed at the PDGF receptor sequences [14] and antibodies that specifically recognize phosphotyrosine residues and thus bind to the activated auto-phosphorylated receptors [15]. By the use of these reagents we have been able to study the processing of the PDGF receptor and the activation of the receptor in normal and transformed cells.

In normal rat kidney cells the 5.2 kb PDGF receptor mRNA is translated to a distinct 160 kDa precursor that contains oligosaccharides sensitive to endoglycosidase H (endo H) [14]. This precursor is not expressed at the cell surface and is resistant to the effects of trypsin on intact cells. The precursor rapidly matures to a 175–180 kDa mature receptor, which is resistant to endo H and is expressed at the surface. The mature form of the receptor has a half-life of approximately 3 hr in the absence of PDGF. Addition of PDGF reduces the receptor of half-life to approximately 45 min. Thus even in normal cells the receptors turn over rapidly. There are two important issues in receptor processing in SSV-transformed cells. First, since the mature receptor is not expressed at the cell surface, it is important to know whether the precursors of the receptor are formed normally in these cells. Recent studies have shown that the 160 kDa precursor is in fact normally expressed in SSV-transformed cells and that it matures to a 170–180 kDa receptor that appears to be normal except that it is expressed only transiently and it is slightly more heterogeneous in apparent size than the receptor in normal cells. A second issue of receptor processing in SSV-transformed cells is to determine the cellular compartment where the receptor is activated by autocrine mechanisms in these cells. Currently Mark Keating in our laboratory using antiphosphotyrosine antibodies has been able to demonstrate that only the more mature forms of the receptor, and not the precursors, are activated in SSV-transformed cells. Further studies should determine the exact localization of receptor activation in these cells. The results will provide basic insight into the relationship between processing and activation of receptors, and may also have therapeutic implications.

What is the relevance of autocrine activation of PDGF receptors to human tumor formation? Obviously a prerequisite for autocrine activation of a cell is that both the growth factor and receptor be expressed by the same cell. Griff Harsh in our lab has screened a number of human tumors for the expression of PDGF-like growth factors and PDGF receptors. These studies have revealed that a number of human tumors at least potentially could involve autocrine mechanisms since both the factors and receptors are expressed by these cells. However, there clearly are some cells that express PDGF-like factors at high levels but lack PDGF receptor mRNA. Thus for these particular cells, the relevance of the expression of PDGF-like factors in tumor formation can be questioned.

THE MOLECULAR MECHANISM OF ACTION OF PDGF AND PDGF-LIKE COMPOUNDS

Whether PDGF-like compounds act through endocrine, paracrine, or autocrine mechanisms, their effects are mediated by interaction with the PDGF receptor. The mechanism by which this receptor stimulates the proliferation of mesenchymal cells is unknown. The interaction of PDGF with its receptor elicits a diverse group of responses including enhanced expression of the c-*myc* and c-*fos* genes [16,17], increase in cyclic AMP levels [18], activation of tyrosine kinase, stimulation of protein kinase C, changes in cell shape [19], alterations in ion flux [20], and a characteristic change in cellular pH [21]. We have shown that one pathway that mediates PDGF-stimulated c-*myc* gene expression involves receptor-mediated phosphoinositide turnover and activation of protein kinase C [22]. When protein kinase C is depleted by chronic exposure of the cells to phorbol esters and c-*myc* induction by subsequent phorbol ester exposure is abolished, PDGF-stimulated c-*myc* expression is attenuated by 60% [22]. Thus the phosphoinositide turnover-protein kinase C pathway is involved in a pathway from PDGF receptor to c-*myc* gene expression. Recently, Shaun Coughlin and Ray Kacich in our lab have shown that PDGF can activate c-*myc* and c-*fos* expression by a seperate pathway involving activation of phospholipase A_2 with the consequent release of arachidonic acid, formation of prostaglandins, and elevation of cyclic AMP levels. Thus elevation of cyclic AMP in Swiss 3T3 cells by forskolin, prostaglandin E_1, or arachidonic acid causes a dramatic enhancement in c-*myc* and c-*fos* expression [23]. The molecular mechanism of this effect of cyclic AMP on the c-*fos* and c-*myc* genes is under investigation, and the relation of this pathway to the protein kinase C and other pathways stimulated by growth factors is also under study.

Although the expression of the c-*myc* and c-*fos* genes may be necessary for the mitogenic response to PDGF, it is not sufficient because some agents that stimulated phosphoinositide turnover and c-*myc* expression to the same extent as PDGF are poor mitogens [22]. Furthermore, when cells are depleted of protein kinase C, the stimulation of c-*myc* expression by PDGF is significantly attenuated, whereas the mitogenic response to PDGF is unchanged [22]. Thus there is at least one pathway involved in PDGF action that is independent of c-*myc* and c-*fos* expression.

The PDGF receptor has a large cytoplasmic region that mediates the effects of PDGF on c-myc expression and activates the other pathways necessry for PDGF-stimulated proliferation [24]. To determine the role of the tyrosine kinase domain and nonkinase domains in these responses, Jaime Escobedo in our lab has expressed the PDGF receptor cNDA in Chinese hamster ovary (CHO) cells that normally lack PDGF receptors. Stable transfectants of the cDNA expressed under the control of the SV40 early promotor expressed receptor mRNA that is translated and processed to a mature cell surface receptor protein. The transfected receptor mediates a number of PDGF-stimulated responses. This CHO expression system for the PDGF receptor provides an approach to the study of the pathways that mediate c-*myc* and c-*fos* gene expression and other pathways involved in the mitogenic response to PDGF. These studies in combination with the findings from other growth factor systems should provide insight into the mechanisms by which growth factors stimulate proliferation.

REFERENCES

1. Ross R, Glomset JA: New Eng J Med 295:369–377, 1976.
2. Betsholtz C, Johnsson A, Heldin C-H, Westermark B, Lind P, Urdea MS, Eddy R, Shows TB, Philpott K, Mellor AL, Knott TJ, Scott J: Nature 320:695–699, 1986.
3. Waterfield MD, Scrace T, Whittle N, Stroobant P, Johnsson A, Wasteson A, Westermark B, Heldin C-H, Huang JS, Deuel TF: Nature 304:35–39, 1983.
4. Doolittle RF, Hunkapiller MW, Hood LE, Devare SG, Robbins KC, Aaronson SA, Antonaides HN: Science 221:275–277, 1983.
5. Dicorleto PE, Bowen-Pope DF: Proc Natl Acad Sci USA 80:1919–1923, 1983.
6. Barrett TB, Gajduseck CM, Schwartz SM, et al.: Proc Natl Acad Sci USA 81:6772–6774, 1984.
7. Daniel TO, Milfay DF, Gibbs VG, Garovoy MR, Williams LT: J Biol Chem 261:9579–9582, 1985.
8. Daniel TO, Gibbs V, Milfay DF, Williams LT: Clin Res (in press).
9. Robbins KC, Leal F, Pierce JH, Aaronson SA: EMBO J 4:1783–1793, 1985.
10. Leal F, Williams LT, Robbins KC, Aaronson SA: Science 230:327–330, 1985.
11. Robbins KC, Leal F, Pierce JH, Aaronson SA: EMBO J 4:1783–1792, 1985.
12. Garrett JS, Coughlin SR, Niman HL, Tremble PM, Giels GM, Williams LT: Proc Natl Acad Sci USA 81:7466–7470, 1984.
13. Huang JS, Huang SS, Deuel TF: Cell 39:79–87, 1984.
14. Keating MT, Williams LT: J Biol Chem (submitted).
15. Frackelton AR Jr, Tremble PM, Williams LT: J Biol Chem 12:7907–7915, 1984.
16. Kelly K, Cochran BH, Stiles CD, Leder P: Cell 35:603–610, 1983.
17. Cochran BH, Zullo J, Verma IM, Stiles CD: Science 226:1080–1082, 1984.
18. Rozengurt E, Stroobant P, Waterfield MD, Deuel TF, Keehan M: Cell 34:265–272, 1983.
19. Mellstrom K, Hoglund AS, Nister M, Heldin C-H, Westermark B, Lindberg U: J Muscle Res Cell Motil 4:589–609, 1983.
20. Ives HE, Daniel TO: Proc Natl Acad Sci (in press).
21. Cassel D, Rothenburg P, Zhuang Y, Deuel T, Glaser L: Proc Natl Acad Sci USA 80:6224–6228, 1983.
22. Coughlin SR, Lee WMF, Williams PW, Giels GM, Williams LT: Cell 43:243–251, 1985.
23. Coughlin SR, Kacich RL, Williams LT (submitted).
24. Yarden Y, Escobedo JA, Kuang W-J, Yang-Feng TL, Daniel TO, Tremble PM, Chen EY, Ando ME, Harkins RN, Francke U, Fried VA, Ullrich A, Williams LT: Nature 323:226–232, 1986.

Growth Regulation of Cancer
157–167 (1988)

Epidermal Growth Factor Receptor: Structure and Regulation by Self-Phosphorylation

Paul J. Bertics, Laura Hubler, William S. Chen, Cliff D. Carpenter, Michael G. Rosenfeld, and Gordon N. Gill

Department of Physiological Chemistry, University of Wisconsin-Madison, Madison, Wisconsin 53706 (P.J.B., L.H.) and the Department of Medicine, Division of Endocrinology and Metabolism, University of California-San Diego, La Jolla, California 92093 (W.S.C., C.D.C., M.G.R., G.N.G.)

Epidermal growth factor (EGF) binds specifically and with high affinity to a single site on the extracellular domain of its receptor, which is a transmembrane glycoprotein exhibiting EGF-stimulable, protein-tyrosine kinase activity. The EGF receptor is homologous to the erb B oncogene product but is under extensive regulation. On activation by EGF, the receptor undergoes a rapid, intramolecular, self-phosphorylation reaction. The principal sites of tyrosine self-phosphorylation are located in the extreme carboxyl-terminal region of the molecule, which is one of the regions truncated in erb B. These self-phosphorylation sites act as competitive inhibitors/alternate substrates versus exogenous peptide substrates. Self-phosphorylation decreases the ability of the carboxyl-terminal region to compete with exogenous substrates, thereby leading to enhanced protein-tyrosine kinase activity at nonsaturating substrate levels. Mutation of tyrosine 1173, the major self-phosphorylation site, to a phenylalanine residue results in decreased protein-tyrosine kinase activity at low substrate concentrations, but normal kinase activity at saturating substrate levels. This mutation also attenuates the ability of the receptor to mediate cell growth in response to EGF, suggesting that this site of self-phosphorylation is important in modulating the maximal activity of the EGF receptor.

Key words: epidermal growth factor, protein-tyrosine kinase, growth factors, oncogenes

In recent years, numerous investigations centering on cell growth control and transformation have shown that many retroviral transforming proteins are themselves protein-tyrosine kinases or are ligands for receptors exhibiting protein-tyrosine kinase

Received March 17, 1987.

activity [1–3]. These studies have highlighted the importance of this type of enzyme activity in the regulation of cell proliferation. The epidermal growth factor (EGF) receptor, which is one of the better characterized enzyme/receptor systems involved in growth control, is a 170 kDa transmembrane glycoprotein possessing EGF-stimulable, protein-tyrosine kinase activity [3–5]. EGF binding to the extracellular receptor domain activates its tyrosine kinase activity and leads to increased intracellular substrate phosphorylation as well as self-phosphorylation [4,6]. The cytoplasmic protein-tyrosine kinase domain of the EGF receptor is homologous to erb B, the transforming protein of the avian erythroblastosis virus [7–10], and is structurally similar to other cellular tyrosine kinases identified as the proto-oncogene products of certain retroviruses [1–3,9]. In this review, we detail our present understanding of EGF receptor structure and provide evidence for regulation of receptor function by self-phosphorylation.

EGF RECEPTOR STRUCTURE AND BIOCHEMICAL PROPERTIES

Analysis of the nucleotide sequence of EGF receptor cDNA predicts an 1186 amino acid protein consisting of an extracellular and an intracellular domain separated by a single hydrophobic transmembrane region [11–13]. The amino-terminal extracellular domain is made up of approximately 621 amino acids and is glycosylated at 11–12 asparagine residues [14,15]. Glycosylation appears to be a maturation process that is critical for the proper expression of the EGF receptor on the cell surface [15–17]. The extracellular region of the EGF receptor contains 51 cysteine residues that are preferentially localized in two regions, i.e., residues 134–313 and 446–612 [11], whereas only nine cysteine residues are located in the remaining intracellular carboxyl-terminal domain. These two cysteine-rich regions appear to cooperate to produce a single high affinity EGF binding site [18,19]. Several other recently characterized cell surface receptors, such as those for LDL [20] and insulin [21,22], also have a high cysteine content in their extracellular domains, a feature that may be important for maintaining the structural integrity of these binding sites. Although the PDGF and CSF-1 receptors are devoid of regions of high cysteine content, these proteins do contain a highly conserved spacing of cysteine residues in their extracellular domains [23,24].

The intracellular portion of the EGF receptor is separated from the ligand binding domain by a hydrophobic membrane-spanning region consisting of approximately 23 amino acids [11]. The carboxyl-terminal domain contains structural features analogous to those of other oncogene products possessing protein-tyrosine kinase activity, such as src and erb B [2,8–12]. The EGF receptor homology with other tyrosine kinases starts in the region of residue 694 and extends for approximately 50 amino acids. The remainder of the carboxyl-terminal domain, which contains the primary sites of self-phosphorylation, does not appear homologous to other known proteins [3]. Examination of the nucleotide sequence of the receptor reveals that the common ATP binding sequence G-X-G-X-X-G starts at amino acid 700 [3]. Furthermore, the ATP affinity label, 5′-p-fluorosulphonylbenzoyl adenosine, labels the receptor in the region of lysine-721 [25,26], an area that exhibits strong homology with other nucleotide binding sites [27], including the ATP binding site of the cAMP-dependent protein kinase [28]. The ATP binding site of all receptor/protein-tyrosine kinases is located around 50 residues from the inner boundary of the transmembrane domain as defined by the "stopper" sequence of three consecutive dibasic amino acids.

The domain structure of the EGF receptor has also been studied using mild tryptic digestion [29,30]. In these experiments, the 170 kDa form can be clipped to a 150 kDa fragment, which exhibits EGF-dependent tyrosine kinase activity, and a 15–20 kDa carboxyl-terminal fragment, which contains the major self-phosphorylation sites [5,29–31]. The 150 kDa fragment can be further digested to produce a 108 kDa fragment and a 42 kDa piece, which exhibits about 30% of the tyrosine kinase activity of the intact receptor. This 42 kDa piece contains the ATP binding site and most of the phosphoserine and phosphothreonine phosphorylation sites [3,30]. It is of interest that the production of erb B from the proto-oncogene EGF receptor occurs via a deletion/truncation of the cell surface EGF binding domain as well as the carboxyl-terminal self-phosphorylation sites [3,8,11]. As discussed below, both of these regions are important regulatory domains and their deletion by erb B appears crucial for its transforming activity [2,32]. In terms of evolution, it is noteworthy that the Drosophila EGF receptor homologue has both EGF binding and tyrosine kinase domains, suggesting that these two activities have existed in the same molecule for over 800 million years [33].

Kinetic analyses of EGF-stimulated tyrosine kinase activity of the receptor have indicated that relatively low levels of Mn^{++} (1–5 mM) or higher levels of Mg^{++} (10–20 mM) are required for maximal enzyme activity [34,35]. The receptor can utilize either ATP or GTP as the phosphate source, although ATP is the favored substrate [34,35]. Using a variety of peptide substrates, the K_m for ATP calculated for the receptor is generally 1–3 μM [35,36]. The kinetic mechanism for the phosphorylation of exogenous substrates appears as a Bi Bi ordered sequential mechanism wherein the binding of the protein/peptide substrate precedes that of ATP [36]. Product release is also ordered with the dissociation of phosphopeptide preceding that of ADP. This kinetic mechanism is of interest because other protein kinases, both serine/threonine [37] and tyrosine kinases [38], have generally been found to have an ordered mechanism, wherein ATP, not the protein substrate, binds to the enzyme first. These unusual kinetics may be a critical feature of the primary structure of the EGF receptor in that this reaction mechanism may play an important role in the suppression of EGF receptor tyrosine kinase activity via competition with the self-phosphorylation site.

EGF RECEPTOR SELF-PHOSPHORYLATION

Although ligand binding appears as the major regulator of enzyme activity, comparatively little is known of the molecular mechanisms involved in EGF receptor activation. Structural information on the EGF receptor indicates a single binding site per molecule [18,19], but studies on EGF binding to its receptor in vivo suggest the presence of two classes of binding sites in many cell types [39,40]. Both high affinity (K_d = 0.1–0.2 nM) and low affinity (K_d = 1 nM) sites have been reported [39–41]. Because there appears to be a single EGF receptor gene, these receptor classes could be the result of posttranslational events (e.g., phosphorylation, receptor-receptor interactions, or possibly receptor-membrane interactions [41,42]). One process that the EGF receptor is well characterized to undergo is a rapid agonist-induced, self-phosphorylation reaction [3,18].

Previous studies have shown that the EGF receptor is a phosphoprotein in vivo, containing 2–3 mol of phosphate per mol of receptor protein [43]. Using tryptic phosphopeptide mapping, these phosphates have been found to be primarily distributed into serine- and threonine-containing peptides [6,43]. Activation by EGF results in receptor self-phosphorylation on tyrosine residues located in the extreme carboxyl-terminal region of the molecule [44]. The major site of EGF-enhanced self-phosphorylation is tyrosine 1173, but receptor phosphorylation on tyrosines 1068 and 1148 also occurs [44,45]. In light of the fact that self-phosphorylation can regulate several tyrosine kinases [46–50] as well as the cAMP-dependent kinase [51], calmodulin kinase II [52–54], phosphorylase kinase [55,56], and protein kinase C [57–59], it may be that this type of "auto" regulation serves as an important general control mechanism for protein kinases. There is evidence that self-phosphorylation has a biological role in modulating EGF receptor activity [60; Bertics et al., in press], although it does not appear to be required for receptor internalization [61].

The properties and function of the EGF receptor self-phosphorylation reaction have been studied using purified receptor protein isolated from A431 human epidermoid carcinoma cells by immunoaffinity chromatography [18,19,60,62]. These investigations and others have shown that the self-phosphorylation reaction proceeds as a rapid, intramolecular process [18,63], which is maximal at 30–37°C and exhibits a K_m for ATP (200 nM) that is severalfold less than that calculated for exogenous substrate phosphorylation [18,35,36,62].

When the phosphorylation of exogenous peptide substrates is measured as a function of receptor self-phosphorylation, tyrosine kinase activity is enhanced 2–3-fold at 1–2 mol of phosphate per mol of EGF receptor at nonsaturating substrate levels [19,60,62]. Significant differences between unphosphorylated and phosphorylated enzyme can be seen when their tyrosine kinase activity is compared at various ATP concentrations. At low ATP levels, a double reciprocal plot of the tyrosine kinase activity of the unphosphorylated enzyme is hyperbolic, suggesting that ATP is an enzyme activator and/or that the self-phosphorylation site(s) is an alternate substrate [64,65]. At high ATP levels, where more self-phosphorylation occurs during the reaction, the kinetics appear linear and similar to that of the phosphorylated enzyme. As shown in Figure 1, dose response studies using three different peptide substrates (angiotensin II, gastrin, and a peptide corresponding to the self-phosphorylation site of p60v-src) indicate that exogenous substrates can inhibit the EGF receptor self-phosphorylation reaction [60]. In each case, half-maximal inhibition is seen at a peptide level approximately equal to that substrate's steady state affinity (K_m).

These data were consistent with the idea that the self-phosphorylation sites act as alternate substrates for the receptor and that the inhibition of self-phosphorylation by exogenous substrates is a result of competition for the enzyme active site. To determine whether the enhanced tyrosine kinase activity of the phosphorylated receptor was due to the removal of a competitive/alternate substrate (the self-phosphorylation site), the initial rate of angiotensin II phosphorylation was assayed over a large substrate concentration range using either phosphorylated or unphosphorylated EGF receptor [60]. If the self-phosphorylation site is a competitive inhibitor versus exogenous substrates, the phosphorylated receptor would be expected to possess a lower effective inhibitor level (assuming the phosphorylated site has a lower affinity for the enzyme). During the short time course of the assay, the prephosphorylated receptor

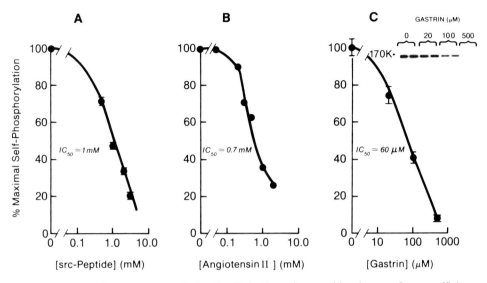

Fig. 1. Inhibition of EGF receptor self-phosphorylation by various peptide substrates. Immunoaffinity-purified receptor was mixed with the indicated level of peptide before the reactions were initiated via the addition of ATP, and phosphate incorporation into the receptor was generally determined using a filtration assay. A) Inhibition of self-phosphorylation by the src peptide. The reactions were performed at 30°C for 30 sec using 5.0 μM [γ-^{32}P]-ATP and 0.51 pmol EGF receptor. B) Angiotensin II inhibition of self-phosphorylation. The incubations were run at 0°C for 30 sec using 0.2 μM [γ-^{32}P]-ATP and 0.68 pmol EGF receptor. C) Inhibition of self-phosphorylation by gastrin. The incubations were performed at 30°C for 30 sec using 5.0 μM [γ-^{32}P]-ATP and 0.74 pmol EGF receptor. The reactions were stopped with SDS gel electrophoresis sample buffer, and 0.12 pmol of EGF receptor (in each lane) were analyzed on a 20% SDS-polyacrylamide gel (autoradiograph shown in inset). Phosphate incorporation was measured by excising the EGF receptor band from the gel and counting the associated radioactivity. Reprinted with permission from Bertics and Gill [60].

would exhibit a higher tyrosine kinase activity than the unphosphorylated receptor at nonsaturating substrate levels, but this effect would be overcome at high substrate levels via competition against the self-phosphorylation site. Thus, either a competitive or noncompetitive profile on a double reciprocal plot would be expected depending on the number of points in the reaction pathway at which the "inhibitor" combines [65]. However, if self-phosphorylation is obligatory and causes substantial enzyme activation, then one would predict that increasing substrate concentrations would not overcome the low activity of the unphosphorylated receptor, and the phosphorylated receptor would exhibit an appreciably larger V_{max}, a lower K_m, or possibly both. The double reciprocal plot in Figure 2 shows that both the phosphorylated and the unphosphorylated receptors exhibit comparable V_{max} values and slightly different K_m values for the peptide substrate. These data indicate that the self-phosphorylation sites serve as alternate/competitive substrates.

As stated above, the 170 kDa EGF receptor can be converted to a 150 kDa protein by a Ca^{++}-dependent protease by the removal of a 20 kDa piece from the carboxyl-terminus. The 150 kDa kinase has been reported by Cohen et al. [5] to be more active against some exogenous substrates but exhibits reduced self-phosphorylation activity. Recently, Livneh et al. [66] have found that a carboxyl-terminal truncated EGF receptor devoid of two of the major self-phosphorylation sites also lacks high affinity EGF binding. These findings support the concept that the carboxyl-

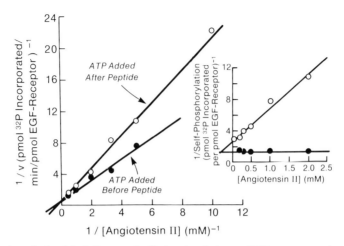

Fig. 2. Kinetic analysis of the influence of self-phosphorylation on EGF receptor-catalyzed angiotensin II phosphorylation. Purified EGF receptor (0.68 pmol/assay) was incubated with 1.0 [γ-^{32}P]-ATP at 0°C for 1 min before the addition of the indicated amounts of angiotensin II (●), or angiotensin II was added to the enzyme before ATP (○). The final ATP concentration after addition of the peptide was 0.2 μM, and the reactions were run at 0°C for 30 sec. Phosphate incorporation into angiotensin II and the EGF receptor was determined by phosphocellulose binding or filtration assays. The data are plotted in double reciprocal form and represent the averages of two experiments. Inset: Dixon plot of the self-phosphorylation inhibition by angiotensin II. The graph shows the self-phosphorylation states of both the enzyme that was first incubated with 1 μM ATP before peptide addition (●) and the enzyme that was combined with the peptide before ATP addition (○). Reprinted with permission from Bertics and Gill [60].

terminus, which contains the major self-phosphorylation sites, can modulate receptor function. Changes in the regulatory region of the molecule, by either phosphorylation or protease action, can result in altered receptor activity. Because erb B lacks the major carboxyl-terminal self-phosphorylation site of the proto-oncogene EGF receptor [2,3,67], it would not be influenced by this regulatory domain. In this regard, analyses of the effects of viruses recovered following avian leukosis and Rous-associated virus type 1 infection clearly indicate a functional role of the carboxyl-terminal domain of the EGF receptor, i.e., the region that is truncated in the erb B gene product. The avian leukosis virus results in the production of an erb B product via insertional mutagenesis, which consistently truncates the amino-terminal EGF binding domain but variably deletes the carboxyl-terminal region [68,69]. Following infection with the recovered viruses, erythroblastosis has been found to occur independent of the degree of carboxyl-terminal truncation, but the generation of sarcomas is detected only with mutants lacking the carboxyl-terminal region [32].

Several studies on the insulin receptor [46,47,70] and transforming proteins of the Rous [48,49] and Fujinami sarcoma viruses [50] have shown that self-phosphorylation enhances their protein-tyrosine kinase activity, although the exact mechanism of this activation is unknown. In the case of the EGF receptor, self-phosphorylation appears to remove a competitive constraint so that the enzyme active site can be more freely accessible to certain exogenous substrates. Thus, the site(s) of self-phosphorylation can be viewed as an alternate substrate for the EGF receptor, and the removal of this competitive/alternate substrate by self-phosphorylation may be the mechanism by which the receptor achieves maximal activity [60]. A similar effect has been proposed for the type II cAMP-dependent protein kinase where the self-phosphorylation of a substratelike region of the regulatory subunit favors the formation of a free catalytic subunit that is enzymatically active [51,71,72].

With the EGF receptor, ligand binding is the major regulator of enzyme activity. However, it appears that self-phosphorylation acts as a mechanism for the suppression of basal tyrosine kinase activity so that undesired tyrosine phosphorylation of intracellular substrates is dampened in the unstimulated state. The kinetic mechanism of the receptor is such that the self-phosphorylation site would be bound before ATP; therefore the receptor would be subject to competitive binding of the self-phosphorylation site regardless of the intracellular ATP level, thereby allowing for a continual and potent blockade of enzyme activity. In this case, the basal tyrosine kinase activity of the receptor would result in self-phosphorylation in preference to the phosphorylation of exogenous substrates. In the absence of EGF, the slow rate of self-phosphorylation would be rapidly offset by phosphotyrosyl phosphatase activities present within the cell [6,73], a process that would regenerate the less active receptor via competitive inhibition by the self-phosphorylation site. Full enzyme activation would require EGF binding as the primary signal, and self-phosphorylation would occur as a rapid secondary response. The activated receptor would exhibit a tyrosine kinase activity in excess of the phosphotyrosyl phosphatase activities, thus leading to increased intracellular phosphorylation.

According to this model, the phosphorylation rate of a given substrate would depend in part on its concentration and relative affinity for the enzyme relative to that of the self-phosphorylation site. At low substrate levels, the phosphorylation rate would be slowed by competition with self-phosphorylation. At high substrate levels, the phosphorylation rate would appear maximal since the substrate could now completely compete with the self-phosphorylation site. The fact that self-phosphorylation occurs in vivo shows that the receptor is not saturated with high affinity substrates in the cell, suggesting this reaction may play a role in receptor regulation in vivo. A model incorporating current data on the influence of self-phosphorylation on EGF receptor tyrosine kinase activity is shown in Figure 3. Ligand binding causes an enzyme conformational change that increases the tyrosine kinase catalytic rate and/or substrate binding, e.g., higher affinity binding of ATP has been reported [74]. The activated receptor can then self-phosphorylate tyrosine residues located in its extreme carboxyl-terminus. This region can reversibly interact with the enzyme active site allowing for self-phosphorylation to be competitively inhibited at high levels of exogenous substrates. Phosphorylation of the carboxyl-terminal domain decreases its affinity for the enzyme active site, and/or results in an additional conformational change, thereby permitting exogenous substrates greater access to the substrate binding domain and enhanced tyrosine kinase activity.

The model for the effect of self-phosphorylation on EGF receptor activity presented above would initially appear to be in opposition to that of Downward et al. [45] who found no effect of self-phosphorylation on the maximal catalytic rate of the receptor in vitro. Both this study [45] and our own [60] agree that there is no influence of self-phosphorylation on the V_{max} of the reaction where high saturating levels of exogenous substrates effectively compete with the self-phosphorylation site. Our studies emphasized the competitive nature of the self-phosphorylation site, a phenomenon that is most easily seen at lower nonsaturating substrate levels.

To clarify the role of self-phosphorylation in the regulation of EGF receptor activity, a mutant EGF receptor was prepared via site-directed mutagenesis of the

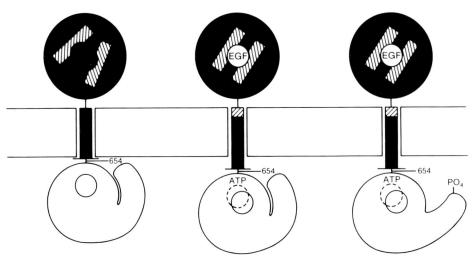

Fig. 3.   Proposed model of EGF receptor activation and self-phosphorylation. See text for explanation.

human protein [Bertics et al., in press]. This mutant contains a phenylalanine residue instead of a tyrosine residue at amino acid 1173 (the major in vivo site of self-phosphorylation). We postulated that the substitution of a structurally similar amino acid might allow this region to still serve as a competitive inhibitor versus exogenous substrates, but that it could not be "removed" via phosphorylation. Likewise, if the mechanism of action of self-phosphorylation is consistent with the above model, then one would predict that the receptor would exhibit impaired kinase activity at low substrate levels but essentially normal kinase activity at saturating substrate levels, thereby indicating that the mutation did not merely generate some nonspecific enzyme inactivation.

cDNA constructs containing the human EGF receptor with tyrosine 1173 or phenylalanine 1173 were prepared and transfected into recipient rodent cells that do not express endogenous EGF receptors (e.g., Chinese hamster ovary (CHO) and mouse B82L cells), and cells expressing human EGF receptors were grown under appropriate selection conditions. A comparison of some of the properties of the control and mutant EGF receptor is shown in Table I.

Kinetic analyses of the mutant receptor indicate that although the major site of self-phosphorylation has been removed, this enzyme can still phosphorylate at least two other principal sites, probably tyrosines 1068 and 1148 [44,45]. For self-phosphorylation, the mutant receptor still exhibits a very low K_m for ATP (200 nM) and the reaction still proceeds intramolecularly, indicating that the receptor has not been grossly altered by the mutation. Although mutant receptors containing phenylalanine 1173 are as active as control receptors at saturating substrate levels, where effective competition occurs, they exhibit greatly reduced protein-tyrosine kinase activity at low, nonsaturating levels of substrate. This effect is due to the fact that the self-phosphorylation site, which may act as a tight binding inhibitor, cannot be removed by phosphorylation. These studies provide additional support for the mechanistic model shown in Figure 3. Of particular interest are the effects of this mutation on cell growth. When EGF-dependent growth of CHO cells expressing comparable levels of

TABLE I. Characteristics and Comparison of the Normal EGF Receptor (Tyr 1173) and a Mutant EGF Receptor (Phe 1173) Lacking the Major Self-Phosphorylation Site

Receptor property	Normal (Tyr 1173) EGF receptor	Mutant (Phe 1173) EGF receptor
Major sites of self-phosphorylation	Tyrosines 1173, 1148, 1068	Tyrosines 1148, 1068
Km for ATP with self-phosphorylation	200 nM	200 nM
Mechanism of self-phosphorylation	Intramolecular	Intramolecular
Kinetics of protein-tyrosine kinase activity	Exhibits linear kinetics in a double reciprocal plot with peptide substrates	Same Vmax as normal receptor but reduced activity at low substrate levels: competitive inhibition
In vitro stimulation of kinase activity by EGF	Yes ED (50) $\approx$ 20–30 nM	Yes ED (50) $\approx$ 10–30 nM
Ability to mediate cell growth in response to EGF	Yes ED (50) $\approx$ 0.01 nM	Reduced >50% compared to control ED (50) $\approx$ 0.01 nM

control or mutant EGF receptor is measured, one observes that the ability of the mutant receptor to mediate cell growth in response to EGF is reduced by over 50%, yet both receptors exhibit a similar affinity and ED_{50} for EGF.

In summary, these studies indicate that the EGF receptor self-phosphorylation sites act as competitive inhibitors versus exogenous substrates. Self-phosphorylation under certain conditions enhances the tyrosine kinase activity of the receptor via the removal of these competitive substrates. Also, the inhibition of the maximal response to EGF by the mutant receptor (phenylalanine 1173) suggests that the carboxyl-terminus may have a functional, regulatory role in vivo, but that it is quantitatively smaller than that of EGF itself. Because self-phosphorylation of tyrosines 1148 and 1068 also occurs via an intramolecular process, these residues may also serve as effective competitive inhibitors with exogenous substrates. To test this possibility, we are currently using site-directed mutagenesis to convert these residues to phenylalanines as well.

Self-phosphorylation accounts for only a fraction of total EGF receptor phosphorylation in vivo [6,43], and it appears that other protein kinases, such as the cAMP-dependent protein kinase [35,75,76], can phosphorylate the receptor. The function of these other phosphorylations is unclear, although they may directly exert additional controls on receptor activity or may function indirectly by targeting the receptor for interaction with other intracellular components or pathways such as internalization and turnover.

ACKNOWLEDGMENTS

These studies were supported by research grants to G.N.G. from the American Cancer Society, the National Institutes of Health, and the Council for Tobacco Research-USA, Inc., and by awards to P.J.B. from the Life and Health Insurance Medical Research Fund and the Medical and Graduate Schools of the University of Wisconsin-Madison. L.H. is a predoctoral student supported in part by the Markey Trust Fund.

REFERENCES

1. Bishop JM: Ann Rev Biochem 52:301–354, 1983.
2. Bishop JM: Cell 42:23–38, 1985.
3. Hunter T, Cooper JA: Ann Rev Biochem 54:897–930, 1985.
4. Ushiro H, Cohen S: J Biol Chem 255:8363–8365, 1980.
5. Cohen S, Ushiro H, Stoschek C, Chinkers M: J Biol Chem 257:1523–1531, 1982.
6. Hunter T, Cooper JA: Cell 24:741–752, 1981.
7. Yamamoto T, Nishida T, Miyajima N, Kawai S, Ooi T, Toyoshima K: Cell 35:71–78, 1983.
8. Downward J, Yarden Y, Mayes E, Scrace G, Totty N, Stockwell P, Ullrich A, Schlessinger J, Waterfield MD: Nature 307:521–527, 1984.
9. Privalsky ML, Ralson R, Bishop JM: Proc Natl Acad Sci USA 81:704–707, 1984.
10. Frykberg L, Palmieri S, Beug H, Graf T, Hayman MJ, Vennstrom B: Cell 32:227–238, 1983.
11. Ullrich A, Coussens L, Hayflick JS, Dull TJ, Gray A, Tam AW, Lee J, Yarden Y, Libermann TA, Schlessinger J, Downward J, Mayes ELV, Whittle N, Waterfield MD, Seeburg PH: Nature 309:418–425, 1984.
12. Xu Y-H, Ishii S, Clark AJL, Sullivan M, Wilson RK, Ma DP, Roe BA, Merlino GT, Pastan I: Nature 309:806–810, 1984.
13. Lin CR, Chijen WS, Kruijer W, Stolarsky LS, Weber W, Evans RM, Verma IM, Gill GN, Rosenfeld MG: Science 224:843–848, 1984.
14. Weber W, Gill GN, Spiess J: Science 224:294–297, 1984.
15. Mayes ELV, Waterfield MD: EMBO J 3:531–537, 1984.
16. Cummings RD, Soderquist AM, Carpenter G: J Biol Chem 260:11944–11952, 1985.
17. Soderquist AM, Carpenter G: J Biol Chem 259:12586–12594, 1984.
18. Weber W, Bertics PJ, Gill GN: J Biol Chem 259:14631–14636, 1984.
19. Gill GN, Bertics PJ, Thompson DM, Weber W, Cochet C: Cancer Cells 3:11–18, 1985.
20. Yamamoto T, Davis CG, Brown MS, Schneider WJ, Casey ML, Goldstein JL, Russell DW: Cell 39:27–38, 1984.
21. Ullrich A, Bell JR, Chen EY, Herrera R, Petruzzelli LM, Dull TJ, Gray A, Coussens L, Liao Y-C, Tsubokawa M, Mason A, Seeburg PH, Grunfeld C, Rosen OM, Ramachandran J: Nature 313:756–761, 1985.
22. Ebina Y, Ellis L, Jarnagin K, Edery M, Graf L, Clauser E, Ou J, Masiarz F, Kan YW, Goldfine ID, Roth RA, Rutter WJ: Cell 40:747–758, 1985.
23. Coussens L, Van Beveren C, Smith D, Chen E, Mitchell RL, Isacke CM, Verma IM, Ullrich A: Nature 320:277–280, 1986.
24. Yarden Y, Escobedo JA, Kuang W-J, Yang-Feng TL, Daniel TO, Tremble PM, Chen EY, Ando ME, Harkins RN, Francke U, Fried VA, Ullrich A, Williams LT: Nature 323:226–232, 1986.
25. Buhrow SA, Cohen S, Garbers DL, Staros JV: J Biol Chem 258:7824–7827, 1983.
26. Kudlow JE, Leung Y: Biochem J 220:677–683, 1984.
27. Sternberg M, Taylor W: FEBS Lett 175:387–392, 1984.
28. Shoji S, Ericsson LH, Walsh KA, Fischer EH, Titani K: Biochemistry 22:3702–3709, 1983.
29. Chinkers M, Brugge JS: J Biol Chem 259:11534–11542, 1984.
30. Basu M, Biswas R, Das M: Nature 311:477–480, 1984.
31. Yeaton RW, Lipari MT, Fox CF: J Biol Chem 258:9254–9261, 1983.
32. Gamett DC, Tracy SE, Robinson HL: Proc Natl Acad Sci USA 83:6053–6057, 1986.
33. Livneh E, Glazer L, Segal D, Schlessinger J, Shilo B-Z: Cell 40:599–607, 1985.
34. Carpenter G, King L Jr, Cohen S: J Biol Chem 254:4884–4891, 1979.
35. Pike LJ, Krebs EG: The Receptors 3:93–134, 1986.
36. Erneux C, Cohen S, Garbers DL: J Biol Chem 258:4137–4142, 1983.
37. Whitehouse S, Feramisco JR, Casnellie JE, Krebs EG, Walsh DA: J Biol Chem 258:3693–3701, 1983.
38. Wong TW, Goldberg AR: J Biol Chem 259:3127–3131, 1984.
39. King AC, Cuatrecasas P: J Biol Chem 257:3053–3060, 1982.
40. Kawamoto T, Sato JD, Le A, Polikoff J, Sato GH, Mendelsohn J: Proc Natl Acad Sci USA 80:1337–1341, 1983.
41. Lin CR, Chen WS, Lazar CS, Carpenter CD, Gill GN, Evans RM, Rosenfeld MG: Cell 44:839–848, 1986.

42. Sargent DF, Schwyzer R: Proc Natl Acad Sci USA 83:5774–5778, 1986.
43. Cochet C, Gill GN, Meisenhelder J, Cooper JA, Hunter T: J Biol Chem 259:2553, 1984.
44. Downward J, Parker P, Waterfield MD: Nature 311:483, 1984.
45. Downward J, Waterfield MD, Parker PJ: J Biol Chem 260:14538, 1985.
46. Rosen OM, Herrera R, Olowe Y, Petruzzelli L, Cobb M: Proc Natl Acad Sci USA 80:3237, 1983.
47. Yu KT, Czech MP: J Biol Chem 259:5277, 1984.
48. Purchio AF, Well SK, Collett MS: Mol Cell Biol 3:1589, 1983.
49. Collett MS, Belzer SK, Purchio AF: Mol Cell Biol 4:1213, 1984.
50. Weinmaster G, Zoller MJ, Smith M, Hinze E, Pawson T: Cell 37:559, 1984.
51. Rangel-Aldao R, Rosen OM: J Biol Chem 251:3375, 1976.
52. Shields SM, Vernon PJ, Kelly PT: J Neurochem 43:1599, 1984.
53. Miller SG, Kennedy MB: Cell 44:861–870, 1986.
54. Schworer CM, Colbran RJ, Soderling TR: J Biol Chem 261:8581–8584, 1986.
55. King MM, Fitzgerald TJ, Carlson GM: J Biol Chem 258:9925, 1983.
56. Hallenbeck PC, Walsh DA: J Biol Chem 258:13493, 1983.
57. Huang K-P, Chan K-FJ, Singh TJ, Nakabayashi H, Huang FL: J Biol Chem 261:12134–12140, 1986.
58. Wolf M, Cuatrecasas P, Sahyoun N: J Biol Chem 260:15718–15722, 1985.
59. Walton GM, Bertics PJ, Hudson LG, Vedvick TS, Gill GN: Anal Biochem (in press).
60. Bertics PJ, Gill GN: J Biol Chem 260:14642, 1985.
61. Sunada H, Magun BE, Mendelsohn J, MacLeod CL: Proc Natl Acad Sci USA 83:3825–3829, 1986.
62. Bertics PJ, Weber W, Cochet C, Gill GN: J Cell Biochem 29:195, 1985.
63. Biswas R, Basu M, Sen-Majumdar A, Das M: Biochemistry 24:3795–3802, 1985.
64. Dixon M, Webb EC: "Enzymes," 3rd ed. New York: Academic Press, 1979.
65. Cleland WW: Adv Enzymol 45:273, 1977.
66. Livneh E, Prywes R, Kashles O, Reiss N, Sasson I, Mory Y, Ullrich A, Schlessinger J: J Biol Chem 261:12490–12497, 1986.
67. Kris RM, Lax I, Gullick W, Waterfield MD, Ullrich A, Fridkin M, Schlessinger J: Cell 40:619–625, 1985.
68. Fung Y-KT, Lewis WG, Crittenden LB, Kung H-J: Cell 33:357–368, 1983.
69. Nilsen TW, Maroney PA, Goodwin RG, Rottman FM, Crittenden LB, Raines MA, Kung H-J: Cell 41:719–726, 1985.
70. Ellis L, Clauser E, Morgan DO, Edery M, Roth RA, Rutter WJ: Cell 45:721–732, 1986.
71. Corbin JD, Sugden PH, West L, Flockhart DA, Lincoln TM, McCarthy D: J Biol Chem 253:3997, 1978.
72. Gill GN, Garren LD: Proc Natl Acad Sci 68:786, 1971.
73. Sparks JW, Brautigan DL: J Biol Chem 260:2042, 1985.
74. Das M, Knowles B, Biswas R, Bishayee S: Eur J Biochem 141:429–434, 1984.
75. Ghosh-Dastidar P, Fox CF: J Biol Chem 259:3864–3869, 1984.
76. Rackoff WR, Rubin RA, Earp HS: Mol Cell Endocr 34:113–119, 1984.

Growth Regulation of Cancer
169–173 (1988)

Epidermal Growth Factor Receptors as Potential Targets for Antitumor Therapy With Monoclonal Antibodies

John Mendelsohn

Department of Medicine, Memorial Sloan-Kettering Cancer Center and Cornell University Medical College, New York, New York 10021

During recent years at least four lines of evidence have demonstrated that growth factors play a central role in controlling cell proliferation. One, factors such as epidermal growth factor (EGF) and Interleukin-2, purified from active tissue extracts and conditioned cell culture medium, were found to bind to specific receptors on cell surface membranes and stimulate cell proliferation. Two, studies from a number of laboratories have demonstrated that cells can be cultured in defined medium in the absence of serum if necessary growth factors and hormones are provided [1,2]. Three, some retroviral oncogenes code for polypeptides that are similar to growth factors or portions of their receptors [3], with three examples of this homology to date: the product of the v-sis oncogene is homologous to the beta-chain of platelet-derived growth factor [4], the product of v-erb-B is homologous to the cytoplasmic portion of the receptor for epidermal growth factor [5], and the product of the fms oncogene is homologous to the receptor for colony stimulating factor 1 [6]. Four, transforming growth factors have been discovered that can bind to specific receptors on the surfaces of the very tumor cells that produce them, thereby stimulating self-activation through an "autocrine" mechanism [7]. The best character- ized of the transforming growth factors is TGFα, which is synthesized by a variety of tumor cell lines and by cells transformed with certain retroviruses. TGFα binds to and activates EGF receptors in a manner indistinguishable from EGF [8].

The evidence from this group of independent but related studies strongly suggests that receptors for certain essential growth factors are opportune targets for potential anticancer agents. Since these receptors are polypeptides in the cell surface

Received June 8, 1987.

membrane, they can serve as antigens for monoclonal antibodies that have the potential to alter receptor function by binding to their target antigens.

ANTIRECEPTOR ANTIBODIES

There is strong precedent for the expectation that antireceptor monoclonal antibodies can alter cellular function by binding to receptors on the cell surface. The evidence is provided by "experiments of nature," in which autoimmune reactions against receptors have resulted in the production of autoantibodies with the capacity for sustained biologic activity, resulting in human disease. The best studied autoimmune disorder involving antireceptor antibodies is myasthenia gravis, which is caused by the production of circulating antibodies against the acetylcholine receptor [9–11]. Two forms of autoimmune thyroid disorders are characterized by production of autoantibodies against the receptor for thyroid-stimulating hormone (TSH), acting as agonists [12], or as antagonists of TSH binding [13]. Autoantibodies to the insulin receptor have been found in the serum of patients with a rare form of insulin resistance, which presents clinically as diabetes accompanied by a number of additional abnormalities [14]. The occurrence of these clinical syndromes clearly demonstrates that circulating antireceptor antibodies may produce significant physiologic changes in vivo.

EGF AND THE EGF RECEPTOR

EGF is a mitogenic polypeptide that can alter the proliferation and function of a variety of cells [15]. Its effects are mediated through binding to a specific 170 Kd glycoprotein receptor in the plasma membrane. The receptor is composed of an extracellular binding domain, a transmembrane lipophilic segment, an intracellular tyrosine protein kinase domain, and a regulatory carboxyl-terminal segment that is autophosphorylated on tyrosine residues when the receptor is activated by EGF. The receptor-ligand complex is rapidly internalized into endosomes following EGF binding, and in most tissues this complex is transported into the lysosomal compartment where both EGF and the receptor are catabolized. In addition to expressing a tyrosine kinase activity intrinsic to the receptor molecule, receptor activation can produce secondary activation of protein kinase C, Na^+/H^+ exchange, and phosphoinositol turnover [16].

Two mechanisms have been identified by which tumor cells appear to improve their capacity to respond to EGF. A substantial portion of tumors with certain histological subtypes express increased numbers of EGF receptors on their cell surface membranes. The increase may involve up to a 2 log increment, compared with receptor numbers on normal cells. Examples of this phenomenon have been reported for a variety of tumors, including virtually all squamous lung cancers [17,18], some glioblastomas [19] and breast carcinomas [20], and immature melanomas [21]. The increased expression may be due to gene amplification or augmented transcription, and it appears to confer growth advantage in studies of tumor xenografts [22]. However, paradoxically, cells with increased EGF receptors may be inhibited in culture by nanomolar quantities of EGF, which can stimulate proliferation of cells with normal receptor numbers [23,24]. In a recent study examining a panel of human tumor cell lines expressing increased EGF receptors at varying levels, a strong correlation was observed between the degree of growth inhibition produced by EGF and the absolute number of receptors expressed [25]. The mechanism of growth inhibition (like the mechanism of growth stimulation) remains to be elucidated. Excessive activation of receptor tyrosine kinase activity may play a role, but this is only conjectural.

A second mechanism by which tumor cells may obtain selective advantage over other cells bearing EGF receptors is through secretion of $TGF\alpha$, which can activate the EGF receptor through an autocrine pathway [7,8].

ANTI-EGF RECEPTOR MONOCLONAL ANTIBODIES

Our laboratory has produced a panel of monoclonal antibodies against the EGF receptor; 225 IgG1 and 528 IgG2a are similar in that they bind to the EGF receptor with affinity comparable to the natural ligand (K_D = 3 nM), compete with EGF binding, precipitate the receptor, and block EGF-induced tyrosine kinase activity [26,27]. The initial rates of internalization of EGF receptors into endosomes are the same in the presence of EGF or antireceptor monoclonal antibody [28], but subsequent receptor processing and catabolism appear to be through a slower pathway when the receptor is bound to antibody [29]. It is likely that the monoclonal antibodies do not react with the actual EGF binding site, but near enough to it on the receptor to prevent EGF from binding, since they react with a human-specific sequence and do not recognize EGF receptors on rodent cells. The binding of EGF is known not to be species-specific.

The monoclonal antibodies do not have intrinsic inhibitory activity against normal human cells in culture. However, they can block EGF-induced stimulation of growth rate. This has been demonstrated in cultures of human foreskin fibroblasts, which grow with a doubling time of 5–7 days in serum-free medium supplemented only with insulin and transferrin. The marked increase in proliferation rate that is induced by addition of EGF can be blocked in a concentration-dependent manner by concurrent addition of antireceptor monoclonal antibody [27]. Similar effects are observed when a number of tumor cell lines are cultured in the presence of monoclonal antibody.

Monoclonal antibodies 225 IgG1 and 528 IgG2a at a concentration of 20 nM reduce the rate of proliferation of A431 human epidermoid carcinoma cells cultured in the absence of EGF [26,27]. A comparable direct inhibitory effect has been observed against some, but not all, epidermal tumor cell lines tested and against human mammary adenocarcinoma cell line MCF-7. The antibody-inhibited cell lines were those that were also inhibited by 5–20 nM EGF. The mechanism of monoclonal antibody-induced growth inhibition is probably different from the mechanism of EGF-induced reduction in growth rate, based on a number of observations: 1) EGF in picomolar concentrations stimulates A431 proliferation, unlike monoclonal antibody [26]; 2) antireceptor monoclonal antibody, in concentrations that compete for most, but not all, of EGF binding, can prevent EGF-induced inhibition of proliferation, and thereby enhance growth in the presence of EGF, whereas at higher concentrations the monoclonal antibody exerts its intrinsic inhibitory effect [30] (consistent with our observation that low (pM) concentrations of EGF can stimulate A431 cell proliferation in culture), and 3) unlike EGF, monoclonal antibody does not activate tyrosine kinase upon binding to the EGF receptors of intact cells [31].

In vivo effects of treatment with anti-EGF receptor monoclonal antibodies were assayed against xenografts of human A431 tumors in athymic mice. A treatment schedule of intraperitoneal injections twice weekly was selected, based on a measured monoclonal antibody half-life in serum of 3 days. Administration of either monoclonal antibody intraperitoneally, concurrent with tumor cell implantation subcutaneously, resulted in a dose-dependent inhibition of tumor growth [32]. A concentration of 2 mg per injection twice weekly for 3 weeks resulted in total suppression of tumor growth, which persisted for 3 months after completion of a 3-week course of therapy. Comparable inhibition of xenograft tumor growth was observed with two additional squamous cell carcinomas, which were also inhibited in culture, but was not observed against five other tumor cell lines, which were not inhibited in culture [32].

It could be argued that the antitumor effect in vivo might be mediated by an immune mechanism, rather than by a physiologic effect upon the receptor molecule. However, three lines of evidence support an alternative interpretation, that the antitumor effect was due to the capacity of monoclonal antibodies to block the function of the EGF receptor [33]. First, both an IgG1 and IgG2a antibody produced comparable inhibition of A431 cell proliferation, in culture and in xenografts. Complement and lymphocyte mediation of toxicity upon antibody-coated cells is far more efficient with the IgG2a isotype. Second, an $F(ab')_2$ fragment administered in vivo could produce antitumor activity, although requiring higher concentrations than needed with complete antibody (unpublished observations). Third, a number of EGF receptor-bearing tumor xenografts were not inhibited by monoclonal antibodies, suggesting that the antibodies were active against a subclass of tumors with particular susceptibility to blockage of the EGF receptor. The evidence for physiologic effects of anti-EGF receptor monoclonal antibodies does not rule out the possible concurrent activity of these antibodies as immune effector agents.

We postulate that the characteristic defining the subclass of tumor cells susceptible to inhibition by anti-EGF receptor monoclonal antibodies is those cells that produce $TGF\alpha$ and respond to it in an autocrine fashion. By adding sufficient quantities of monoclonal antibody to cultures of A431 cells, the capacity to bind growth factors in the culture medium is blocked, and under these conditions we were able to demonstrate accumulation of $TGF\alpha$ in the medium in preliminary studies. Other cell lines must be tested for $TGF\alpha$ production and quantitative studies of $TGF\alpha$ binding to receptors must be performed in order to validate the hypothesis that the direct antiproliferative activity of anti-EGF receptor monoclonal antibodies against some, but not all, EGF receptor bearing tumor cells is attributable to inhibition of access to an EGF-like growth factor produced by the cells.

SUMMARY

Monoclonal antibodies that bind to the EGF receptor have the capacity to inhibit EGF-induced effects upon proliferation and biochemical functions in cultured human cells. Some EGF-receptor bearing tumor cells are prevented from growth by treatment with antireceptor antibody. Evidence is presented that suggests that antibody mediated antiproliferative activity may result from effects upon growth factor-dependent processes in the receptor-bearing cells.

ACKNOWLEDGMENTS

The author wishes to acknowledge his collaborators in studies of monoclonal antibodies against the EGF receptor: G. Sato, H. Masui, T. Kawamoto, H. Sunada, D. Sato, A. Le, G. Gill, C. McLeod, J. Castagnola, A. Goldenberg, and P. Yu. This work was supported in part by grants R01 CA42060 and U01 CA37641 from the National Cancer Institute.

REFERENCES

1. Barnes D, Sato G: Cell 22:649, 1980.
2. Sato G, Pardee AB, Sirbasku D (eds): "Growth of Cells in Hormonally Defined Media," Cold Spring Harbor Conferences on Cell Proliferation, Vol. 9. Cold Spring Harbor, NY: Cold Spring Harbor Laboratory, 1982.
3. Hunter T: Sci Am 251:70–79, 1984.
4. Doolittle RF, Hunkapiller MW, Hood LE, Devare SA, Robbins KC, Aaronson SA, Antoniades MN: Science 221:275–277, 1983.
5. Downward J, Yarden Y, Mayes E, Scrace G, Totty N, Stockwell P, Ullrich A, Schlessinger J, Waterfield M: Nature 307:521–527, 1984.
6. Sherr CJ, Rettenmier CW, Sacca R. Roussel MF, Look AT, Stanley ER: Cell 41:665–671, 1985.
7. Sporn MB, Todaro GJ: N Engl J Med 303:898, 1980.
8. Todaro GJ, Fryling C, DeLarco JE: Proc Natl Acad Sci USA 77:5258–5262, 1980.
9. Lindstrom JM, Seybold ME, Lennon VA, et al: Neurology 26:1054–1059, 1970.
10. Appel SM, Anwyl R, McAdams MW, Elias SB: Proc Natl Acad Sci USA 74:2130, 1977.
11. Lewin R: Science 211:38, 1981.
12. Volpe R: Clin Endo Metab 7:3, 1978.
13. Dexhage HA, Bottazzo GF, Bitensky L, Chayen J, Doniach D: Nature 289:594, 1981.
14. Flier JS, Kahn CR, Jarrett DB, Roth J: J Clin Invest 58:1442, 1976.
15. Carpenter A, Cohen S: Ann Rev Biochem 48:193–216, 1979.
16. Thompson DM, Gill GN: Cancer Surveys 4:767–788, 1985.
17. Ozanne BW, Richards CS, Hendler FJ, Burns D, Gusterson B: J Path 149:9–14, 1986.
18. Hendler FJ, Ozanne BW: J Clin Invest 74:647–651, 1984.
19. Libermann TA, Razon N, Bartal AD, Yarden Y, Schlessinger J, Soreq H: Cancer Res 44:753–760, 1984.
20. Filmus J, Pollack MN, Cailleau R, Buick RM: Biochem Biophys Res Can 128:898, 1985.
21. Real FX, Rettia WJ, Chesa PG, Melamed MR, Old LJ, Mendelsohn J: Cancer Res 46:4726–4731, 1986.
22. Santon JB, Cronin MT, MacLeod CL, Mendelsohn J, Masui H, Gill GN: Cancer Res 46:4701–4705, 1986.
23. Gill GN, Lazar CS: Nature 292:305, 1981.
24. Barnes DW: J Cell Biol 93:1–4, 1982.
25. Kamata N, Kazuhiro C, Rikimaru K, Horikoshi M, Enomoto S, Kuroki T: Cancer Res 46:1648–1653, 1986.
26. Kawamoto T, Sato JD, Le A, Polikoff J, Sato GH, Mendelsohn J: Proc Natl Acad Sci USA 80:1337–1341, 1983.
27. Sato JD, Kawamoto T, Le AD, Mendelsohn J, Polikoff J, Sato GH: Mol Biol Med 1:511–529, 1983.
28. Sunada H, Magun B, Mendelsohn J, MacLeod CL: Proc Natl Acad Sci USA 83:3825–3829, 1986.
29. Sunada H, Yu P, Peacock JS, Mendelsohn J: (submitted).
30. Kawamoto T, Mendelsohn J, Le A, Sato GH, Lazar CS, Gill G: J Biol Chem 259:7761–7766, 1984.
31. Gill GN, Kawamoto T, Cochet C, Le A, Sato JD, Masui H, McLeod C, Mendelsohn J: J Biol Chem 259:7755–7760, 1984.
32. Masui H, Kawamoto T, Sato JD, Wolf B, Sato GH, Mendelsohn J: Cancer Res 44:1002–1007, 1984.
33. Masui H, Morayama T, Mendelsohn J: Cancer Res 46:5592–5598, 1986.

Growth Regulation of Cancer
175–188 (1988)

Product and Transcription of the *Fos* Gene

J.R. Barber, P. Sassone-Corsi, and I.M. Verma

Molecular Biology and Virology Laboratory, The Salk Institute, San Diego, California 92138-9216

The nuclear protein products of the resident oncogene of the FBJ-murine osteosarcoma virus (v-*fos*) and its corresponding cellular proto-oncogene (c-*fos*) are stoichiometrically phosphorylated on serine and threonine residues. The c-*fos* protein is more highly phosphorylated than the v-*fos* protein due to the phosphorylation of unique sites tentatively localized to the c-terminal 20 amino acid residues. The protein kinase C agonist, TPA, stimulates phosphorylation of the c-*fos*, but not the v-*fos* protein.

Expression of proto-oncogene *fos* is induced in response to a variety of growth factors and differentiation-specific agents. However, the induction of *fos* gene expression is not influenced by inhibition of protein synthesis. We therefore entertained the notion that expression of the *fos* gene may be governed by posttranslational modification of cellular transcriptional factors. We report here that transcription of the human c-*fos* gene is modulated by negatively and positively acting cellular factors.

Key words: C-terminal phosphorylation, TPA stimulation, regulation

The realization that normal cells harbor genes that have the potential to induce neoplasia has been a turning point in modern cancer research. Such genes are commonly called proto-oncogenes (c-*onc*) since they are the progenitors of the viral oncogenes (v-*onc*) that were first discovered in transforming retroviruses [1,2]. DNA transfection techniques have facilitated the isolation of additional transforming genes not found in retroviruses. To date, nearly two score of oncogenes have been identified, and the list is growing [3–5]. It thus seems paradoxical that the cell remains normal in the face of such potential adversity. Why has the cell not lost these potentially lethal genes during the course of evolution? As we decipher the functions of oncogenes, their conservation during evolution becomes less enigmatic. To cite an example, proto-oncogene *fms* protein is likely to be the receptor for macrophage colony stimulating factor (CSF-1), and hence it has a pivotal role in the proliferation and differentiation of macrophage precursors [6]. Similarly, proto-oncogene *sis* encodes the β-chain of platelet-derived growth factor (PDGF), a potent mitogen involved in connective tissue repair and wound healing [7–9].

Received March 24, 1987.

What events conspire to convert these essential cellular genes to acquire transforming potential? We have used proto-oncogene *fos* as a model system to understand the precarious balance between essential cellular functions and cellular transformation. The viral cognate of the *fos* gene is the resident transforming gene of FBJ murine osteosarcoma virus (FBJ-MSV). It is an acutely oncogenic retrovirus that gives rise to bone tumors when inoculated into newborn mice [10] and transforms fibroblasts in tissue culture [11,12]. The DNA sequence of the v-*fos* and c-*fos* genes predicts protein products of 381 and 380 amino acids, respectively, with greater than 85% homology in amino acid sequence [13]. Most of the differences in the predicted primary structure of the proteins are the result of a 104 bp deletion in the provirus, which alters the reading frame of the v-*fos* protein. The c-terminal 49 amino acids of v-*fos* are thus entirely unrelated to the c-terminal 48 amino acids of c-*fos*. Despite these structural alterations, both the v-*fos* and c-*fos* proteins are localized in the nucleus [14].

Transfection with the FBJ-MSV proviral DNA can induce focus formation in cultured rat fibroblasts [15]. In contrast, transfection of fibroblasts with c-*fos* DNA does not result in cellular transformation [15]. Genetic chimeras constructed between the v-*fos* and c-*fos* genes reveal that the protein product encoded by the c-*fos* gene can, however, lead to focus formation provided two manipulations are made: 1) linking viral LTR sequences, presumably to enhance transcription, and 2) removal of sequences downstream of the coding domain of the c-*fos* gene [15]. Thus a chimera between c-*fos* and FBJ-MSV that replaces the 3'-untranslated region of c-*fos* with the 3'-LTR of FBJ-MSV ["MMV," ref. 15] produces foci by DNA transfection of cultured fibroblasts. However, a chimera that contains the 5' viral LTR, and both the c-*fos* protein coding domain and 3'-untranslated regions ["VMM," ref. 15] is not transforming. The transforming potential of this construct can be activated by deleting as little as 67 bp from the c-*fos*-specific sequences downstream from the coding region [16]. Constructs in which these 3'-untranslated c-*fos* sequences are linked to the protein-coding domains of the FBJ-MSV provirus still result in focus formation after DNA transfection ["VMM," ref. 15]. Thus, the transforming potential of the protein coding domain of the FBJ-MSV provirus is dominant over the effect of these 3'-untranslated sequences, but the coding domain of the c-*fos* gene is not.

c-*fos* is an inducible gene that responds to a wide variety of mitogenic and differentiation specific agents as well as to external physiological stimuli. If both v-*fos* and c-*fos* gene products can induce cellular transformation of at least fibroblasts, how does the cell manage to escape transformation from c-*fos* protein synthesized upon induction? We suspect the answer to this enigma lies in its exquisite regulation at the posttranscriptional and posttranslational levels. In this work we describe the nature of the *fos* product, its modifications, and transcriptional regulation.

RESULTS

Fos proteins are posttranslationally modified. Cells transformed by either the c-*fos* or v-*fos* DNA constructs constitutively produce the corresponding *fos* proteins. In Figure 1, *fos* proteins were identified by metabolic labeling and immunoprecipitation of denatured lysates using *fos*-specific antisera [17]. Figure 1a shows the profile of c-*fos* and v-*fos* proteins. In addition to the *fos* specific proteins, in the c-*fos* protein lane there are other proteins ranging from 35–45 kda. None of them appears to be related to p39, a protein that has been shown to be noncovalently bound to *fos* proteins [17]. Pulse-chase analysis indicates that the primary translation products of c-*fos* and v-*fos* begin as forms with relatively high electrophoretic mobility (Fig. 1, lanes 2,6) that are rapidly modified to forms with lower mobility (lanes 4,8).

Since it had previously been shown that [^{32}P]phosphate could be incorporated into both c-*fos* and v-*fos* proteins [14,19] and since phosphorylation often affects the electrophoretic mobility of proteins in SDS gels, it was possible that phosphorylation of the proteins might account for part of this posttranslational processing. To test this, c-*fos* and v-*fos* proteins were purified by immunoprecipitation from cells metabolically labeled with [^{32}P]phosphate or L-[^{35}S]methionine. Both proteins were then treated for various times with the enzyme, alkaline phosphatase (AP), which hydrolyzes organic phosphoesters. The data in Figure 1B indicate that enzymatic removal of metabolically incorporated [^{32}P]phosphate was very efficient for both c-*fos* and v-*fos* proteins. Enzymatic phosphoester hydrolysis was inhibited by the specific phosphatase inhibitor, para-nitrophenylphosphate (pNPP) (see Fig. 1B, lanes 4,8). This demonstrates that the removal of radioactivity from the proteins was due to phosphatase activity alone and not due to spontaneous hydrolysis or to the presence of contaminating enzymes in the preparation. We conclude from this that most, if not all, of the protein phosphate groups are in the form of phosphoesters.

To determine the effect of phosphoester removal on the electrophoretic mobility of the proteins, a similar experiment was performed using c-*fos* and v-*fos* proteins immunoprecipitated from cells metabolically labeled with L-[^{35}S]methionine. As shown in Figure 1C, hydrolysis of protein phosphoesters results in a dramatic increase in the electrophoretic mobility of the c-*fos* protein as well as a more subtle, but reproducibly observed, shift for the v-*fos* protein. It is thus likely that covalent modification by phosphorylation is solely responsible for the electrophoretic heterogeneity of both proteins in SDS gels.

Sites of phosphorylation of v-*fos* and c-*fos* proteins. Since phosphorylation causes the electrophoretic heterogeneity of *fos* proteins (Fig. 1B) and since v-*fos* protein forms are more homogeneous than the c-*fos* forms, it would appear that c-*fos* is more highly phosphorylated than v-*fos*. However, it is formally possible that both proteins are phosphorylated to the same extent but that phosphorylation of the v-*fos* protein simply does not result in the same unusually large electrophoretic shift in SDS gels. Direct comparisons of metabolic incorporation of [^{32}P]phosphate vs. L-[^{35}S]methionine indicates that the most extensively modified forms of the c-*fos* protein contain 4–5-fold more phosphate than the v-*fos* protein (data not shown).

To determine if the greater degree of phosphorylation of the c-*fos* protein was due to the phosphorylation of additional sites unique to c-*fos*, metabolically ^{32}P-labeled c-*fos* and v-*fos* proteins were trypsinized, and the resultant phosphopeptides compared by two-dimensional analysis. The data in Figure 2A indicate that there are similar or identical phosphopeptides in common between v-*fos* and c-*fos* proteins (compare V and M, peptides 1–3). However, there are at least four major phosphopeptides that are unique to the c-*fos* protein (peptides 5–8). This is the first direct evidence that c-*fos* protein is more highly modified than v-*fos* due to phosphorylation at additional c-*fos* unique sites. A tryptic phosphopeptide that appears to be unique to v-*fos* (Fig. 2A, V spot 4) is not seen reproducibly.

A similar experiment was performed with cells expressing a protein encoded by a chimeric plasmid [LJ40A, ref. 16]. In this construct, the LTR and coding sequences

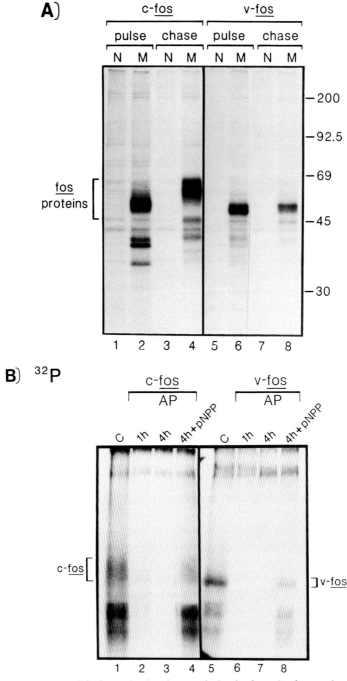

Fig. 1.   A) Immunoprecipitation and pulse-chase analysis of c-*fos* and v-*fos* proteins. Cells were pulse-labeled for 10 minutes with L-[^{35}S]methionine and then either lysed immediately (lanes 2,6) or first "chased" for an additional 20 min by the addition of a 1,000-fold molar excess of unlabeled L-methionine (lanes 4,8). C-*fos* and v-*fos* proteins were then immunoprecipitated and analyzed by SDS gel electrophoresis and autofluorography as described [18]. Odd lanes (N)–normal preimmune serum; even lanes (M)–αM2 *fos* antiserum. Arrows on the side indicate molecular weight size markers. B) Treatment of c-*fos* and v-*fos* proteins with alkaline phosphatase. Cells were metabolically labeled for 4 hr with [^{32}P]phosphate, denatured lysates were prepared, and c-*fos* (left) and v-*fos* (right) proteins were immunoprecipitated as described in A. The proteins were removed from the final Pansorbin pellet by boiling for 2 min in 50 mM tris, 2 mM PMSF, 0.3% SDS, 5 mM DTT, pH 8.0. After removal of the final Pansorbin pellet by centrifugation, concentrated solutions of Non-idet P-40, deoxycholate, and

for the first 316 amino acid residues are contributed by v-*fos*, whereas the remaining c-terminal sequences originate from the c-*fos* gene. The resultant hybrid protein should be identical to v-*fos* except for the carboxy-terminal 48 amino acids, which are unique to the c-*fos* protein [15]. This protein displays c-*fos* protein electrophoretic mobility (not shown) and generates similar or identical tryptic phosphopeptides compared to c-*fos* (Fig. 2A, compare M and VM). It therefore appears that the presence of the c-terminal 48 amino acid residues of c-*fos* are sufficient to lead to the phosphorylation of the c-*fos* unique phosphopeptides (peptides 5–8).

Two-dimensional separation of the phosphoamino acids resulting from partial acid hydrolysis of ^{32}P-labeled c-*fos*, v-*fos*, and hybrid proteins indicates that all are phosphorylated mostly on serine, with trace amounts of phosphothreonine (Fig. 2B). No phosphotyrosine is detectable even when the film is overexposed.

TPA and serum stimulate phosphorylation only of c-*fos*. Because phosphorylation could be involved in regulating the biochemical properties of the proteins, we have investigated the regulation of c-*fos* and v-*fos* phosphorylation. Addition of serum to growth-arrested cells as well as TPA addition to actively growing cells in culture results in a substantial but transient induction of expression of the endogenous c-*fos* proto-oncogene [compare refs. 20–24]. We therefore decided to test whether TPA or serum might also induce changes in the steady-state level of phosphorylation

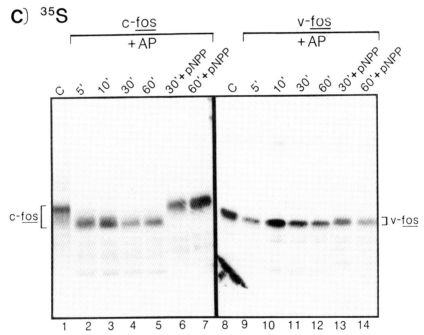

NaCl were added to a final concentration of 1%, 1%, and 150 mM, respectively. The samples were then aliquoted and incubated at 37°C as follows: 1 and 5, no incubation; 2 and 6, 1 hr with alkaline phosphatase (AP); 3 and 7, 4 hr with AP; 4 and 8, 4 hr with AP plus 2 mM P-nitrophenylphosphate (p-NPP). One volume of 2X electrophoresis sample buffer was then added, the samples were analyzed by SDS polyacrylamide gel electrophoresis, and the radioactive bands were visualized by autofluorography. C) The experiment was essentially as described in B, but cells were metabolically labeled with L-[^{35}S]methionine for 1 hr and the resultant immunoprecipitated proteins at 37°C with AP as follows: 1 and 8, no incubation; 2 and 9, 5 min; 3 and 10, 10 min; 4 and 11, 30 min; 5 and 12, 60 min; 6 and 13, 30 min plus 10 mM p-NPP; 7 and 14, 60 min plus 10 mM pNPP.

A

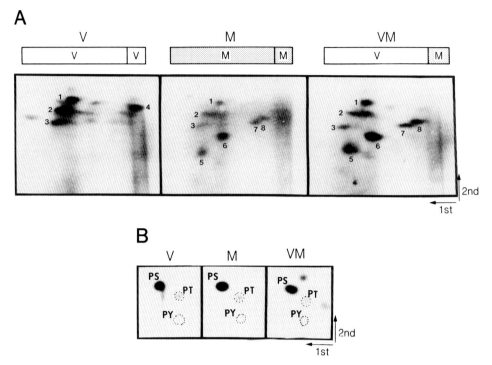

Fig. 2. Two-dimensional separation of tryptic phosphopeptides and phosphoamino acid analysis of c-*fos*, v-*fos*, and a v-*fos*: c-*fos* chimeric protein. Cells were metabolically labeled with [^{32}P]phosphate for 4 hr, (v-*fos*, 4 mCi; c-*fos*, 20 mCi; VM, 10 mCi). Denatured lysates were then prepared and immunoprecipitated c-*fos* and v-*fos* proteins were analyzed by SDS polyacrylamide gel electrophoresis and extracted from the gel slices. A) A fraction was then trypsinized, and the resultant tryptic phosphopeptides were separated (anode, left; cathode, right). B) The remainder of the ^{32}P-labeled proteins was subjected to partial acid hydrolysis and the resultant phosphoamino acids separated. V, v-*fos*; M, c-*fos*; VM, chimeric v-*fos* with the c-*fos* c-terminus. PS, phosphoserine; PT, phosphothreonine; PY, phosphotyrosine.

of the protein. In Figure 3 c-*fos* and v-*fos*-transformed cells were metabolically prelabeled with L-[^{35}S]methionine and then chased with excess unlabeled L-methionine before the addition of TPA. A dramatic and rapid shift to the lower mobility forms of the c-*fos* proteins can be observed (Fig. 3, upper panel, compare lanes 2, 4). This is true even if the radiolabeled cells are "chased" for 45 min before the addition of TPA (lane 6) to allow adequate time for the labeled protein to be completely sequestered within the nucleus [14]. In a similar experiment with cells expressing the v-*fos* protein, however, no detectable shift in electrophoretic mobility of the v-*fos* protein is observed (Fig. 3 lower panel, compare lane 2 with lanes 4,6).

Modulation of c-*fos* Gene Transcription

The rapid and transient induction of the c-*fos* gene transcription lends itself to a search for transcriptional enhancers and inducible sequences in the c-*fos* gene. Several investigators have recently reported the identification and localization of transcriptional enhancer elements of the c-*fos* promoter [25–27]. An element essential for transcriptional activation and inducibility in response to serum is located between nucleotides-276 and -332, relative to the 5'-cap site. The 5' upstream sequences

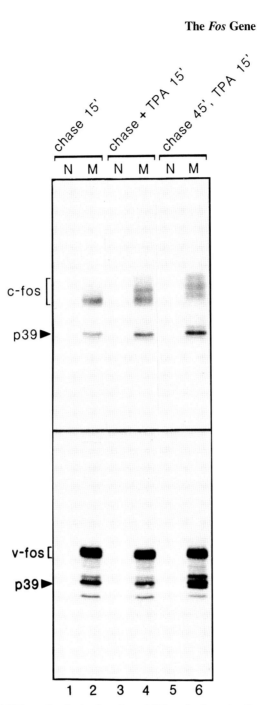

Fig. 3. The effect of TPA on the electrophoretic mobilities of c-*fos* and v-*fos* proteins. A) Cells were pulse-labeled for 15 min with L-[^{35}S]methionine and then "chased" for either an additional 15 min (lanes 1–4) or 60 min (lanes 5,6) by the addition of a 1,000-fold excess of unlabeled L-methionine. Lanes 1 and 2, no additions during the chase; lanes 3 and 4, 140 nM TPA added at the beginning of the chase; lanes 5 and 6, 140 nM TPA added 45 min into the chase. RIPA cell lysates were then prepared and c-*fos* (upper panel) and v-*fos* (lower panel) proteins were then immunoprecipitated and analyzed by SDS polyacrylamide gel electrophoresis and autofluorography as described in Figure 1A. Odd lanes (N) = nonimmune serum; even lanes (M) = αM2 antiserums.

essential for transcriptional activation are conserved between human and mouse c-*fos* genes; these sequences also contain one of the two DNase I hypersensitive sites [26]. The large variety of cell types where *fos* gene expression can be induced shows that, as expected, the *fos* enhancer is not strictly tissue-specific [26].

Induction of c-*fos* expression does not require synthesis of new proteins because addition of protein synthesis inhibitors like cycloheximide prior to induction does not diminish transcription [28,29]. However, the presence of cycloheximide stabilizes c-*fos* mRNA transcripts, presumably by preventing their degradation [29]. In serum-stimulated resting fibroblasts, specific factors bind to the c-*fos* gene enhancer element to induce transcription [30–33]. We hypothesize that in the serum-starved cells, the c-*fos* gene is under negative regulation, either because repressorlike molecules are bound to the promoter-enhancer element or positive factors needed to initiate transcription are in an inactive state (Fig. 4). Upon serum induction, the positive factors are presumably modified to increase its binding affinity to the enhancer, remove the repressor, and initiate transcription. Alternatively the negative factor can also be modified to reduce its binding affinity to the enhancer sequence. This scenario would predict that if excess *fos*-enhancer fragments are added to resting cells prior to serum stimulation, c-*fos* transcription would be inhibited because the positive factors are titrated by excess enhancer sequences. Figure 5 shows one such experiment where growing cells in 10% FCS were transfected with *fos*-CAT construct FC4 [26] or FC4 mixed with pBR322 or enhancer element (*fos*-E) or SV40 enhancer element (SE1) for a 12-hr period. The cells were then serum-starved for 72 hr followed by addition of 15% FCS and CAT enzymatic activity was assayed 30–40 min postinduction. Cells transfected with FC4 construct show conversion to acetylated chloramphenicol. Neither pBR322 sequences nor SV40 enhancer sequences have any effect on the extent of conversion to acetylated chloramphenicol. In contrast, when a fragment containing *fos* enhancer sequences (*fos*-E) is introduced, little or no conversion to acetylated

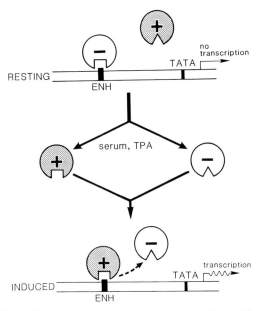

Fig. 4.   Schematic model of c-*fos* transcriptional activation by serum. See text for complete description.

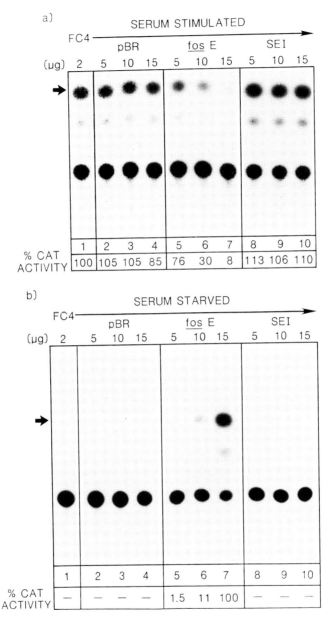

Fig. 5. Competition experiments in 3T3 fibroblasts stimulated or starved by serum. a) CAT activity after transfection of 2 μg of FC4 DNA in serum-stimulated 3T3 fibroblasts is indicated in lane 1. Increasing amounts of pBR322 (lanes 2–4) and SE1 (lanes 8–10) competitor DNAs, as indicated, do not affect the FC4 expression. Increasing amounts of *fos* E (lanes 5 to 7) decreased the CAT activity of the cotransfected FC4. This experiment was repeated three times. b) CAT activity after transfection of 2 μg of FC4 DNA in serum-starved 3T3 fibroblasts. Increasing amounts of pBR322 (lanes 2–4) and SE1 (lanes 8–10) competitor DNA do not affect FC4 experiments. Increasing amounts of *fos* E (lanes 5 to 7) increased the CAT activity of the cotransfected FC4. This experiment was repeated three times. Quantification of the CAT activity, indicated below each lane, was achieved by densitometer scanning of several autoradiograms.

form could be detected. Thus it appears the *fos*-E fragment competes for the positive elements and thus inhibits the serum-dependent stimulation of transcription.

Figure 5B shows the converse experiment. Addition of DNA frgment containing enhancer sequences to serum-starved cells leads to the formation of acetylated chloramphenicol. Presumably, the negatively acting factors can be titrated to allow the binding of positively acting factors to initiate transcription. Thus we conclude that transcription of c-*fos* gene is modulated by negatively and positively acting cellular factors.

DISCUSSION

Fos is a multifaceted gene whose product may play a role during developmment, cellular differentiation, and cell growth [34]. Because products of both the viral and cellular *fos* genes can induce transformation of fibroblasts in vitro, it is puzzling that expression of the *fos* protein in vivo and induced expression of *fos* in vitro do not result in transformation. It is possible that some cell types, such as peritoneal macrophages or macrophages in culture, are refractory to transformation by *fos*, even during sustained expression of *fos* mRNA. Perhaps fibroblasts and other cells that are normally susceptible to c-*fos*-induced transformation are not transformed because the expression of the *fos* protein is only transient.

A common mechanism by which the biochemical properties of a protein can be regulated is by reversible covalent modification. The resultant changes in protein structure, sometimes manifested by anomolous electrophoretic mobility in SDS gels, can have profound effects on the biochemical and biological properties of the protein. Since the *fos* proteins are extensively modified, we have performed a detailed analysis of the nature of this posttranslational modification. The effect of the enzymatic removal of phosphoester groups on the electrophoretic mobility of the c-*fos* and v-*fos* proteins (Fig. 1) strongly supports the notion that their electrophoretic heterogeneity is due largely, if not exclusively, to phosphorylation. We have, however, investigated whether other forms of covalent modification might also contribute to the heterogeneous nature of the *fos* proteins in SDS gels. The proteins are not detectably ubiquitinylated, as judged by protein immunoblots probed with antiubiquitin monoclonal antibodies (V. Fried, J.R.B., I.M.V., unpublished observations). Furthermore, metabolic inhibitor studies failed to reveal any evidence that N-linked glycosylation, poly-ADP-ribosylation, or methylation contributed to the electrophoretic heterogeneity of *fos* proteins. This does not exclude the possibility that the proteins are modified by these or other processes, only that these modifications, if they occur, do not affect the electrophoretic mobility of either protein. However, the fact that essentially all of the metabolically incorporated [^{32}P]phosphate can be removed by alkaline phosphatase treatment (Fig. 1B) essentially excludes the possibility of significant amounts of other phosphorous-containing groups such as ADP-ribosylation, poly-ADP-ribosylation, or adenylylation, since these groups would not normally be removed by this enzyme. The alkaline phosphatase preparation was shown to be free of contaminating phosphodiesterase activity, which could remove groups of this kind, by direct assay using the phosphodiesterase substrate, bis-(p-nitrophenyl) phosphate. The conclusion that phosphorylation results in the electrophoretic shifts observed in Figure 1C for both c-*fos* and v-*fos* protein populations suggests that on the average v-*fos* protein is modified to an extent aproaching one phosphoryl group per protein molecule, whereas the c-*fos* protein probably contains substantially more than one phosphoryl group per molecule. Quantitative comparisons of the relative steady-state degree of phosphorylation of c-*fos* and v-*fos* proteins suggest that the most highly modified forms of the c-*fos* protein may contain an average of 4–5 phosphoryl groups per protein molecule (data not shown). This is consistent with the existence of at least four tryptic phosphopeptides unique to c-*fos* (Fig. 2A). Multiple phosphorylation sites per molecule probably explain the enormous range between the extreme electrophoretic forms of the c-*fos* protein (15,000 daltons difference in apparent molecular mass, Fig. 1) and makes it very likely that phosphorylation will have profound effects on the biological properties of the protein.

Protein kinase C (PK-C) is a cytoplasmic serine/threonine kinase that requires phospholipid, Ca^{++}, and diacylglycerol for optimal activity [35]. Many of the biological effects of TPA are apparently a result of its ability to directly substitute for cellular diacylglycerol, activating PK-C [36,37]. Intracellular diacylglycerol can otherwise be released as a biological response to various stimuli. The stimulation of in vivo phosphorylation of c-*fos* protein by TPA and serum (Fig. 3) could thus conceivably be mediated through PK-C. However, several observations make it unlikely that PK-C is involved in this stimulation of c-*fos* phosphorylation: 1) c-*fos* protein is phosphorylated in the nucleus and only cytoplasmic and plasma membrane forms of PK-C have as yet been identified, 2) the phosphorylation of c-*fos* protein is not stimulated by Ca^{++} or diacylglycerol even though PK-C has presumably been activated as judged by stimulation of phosphorylation of several cellular proteins (data not shown); addition of the enzyme, phospholipase C, which activates PK-C by directly producing intracellular diacylglycerol [38], also has no effect on c-*fos* phosphorylation (data not shown), and 3) prior removal of intracellular free Ca^{++} by the addition of A23187 and EGTA does not prevent the stimulation of c-*fos* phosphorylation by TPA. These data taken together suggest that PK-C activation is neither sufficient nor necessary for the observed effect of TPA on c-*fos* phosphorylation. Phosphorylation of the c-*fos* protein thus appears to fall into the same category as other recently characterized phenomena for which PK-C activation alone is insufficient to account for the observed biological effect of TPA.

Histones are the only other nuclear protein whose phosphorylation has been reported to be stimulated by TPA [39,40]. However, a number of other nuclear oncogene proteins like *myc* [14,40], *myb* (W. Boyle, T. Hunter, personal communication), *p53* cellular tumor antigen, SV40 large T antigen, polyoma large T antigen, and adenovirus E1A are phosphorylated on serine residues. it is tempting to speculate that they may all be phosphorylated, and perhaps regulated, by a mechanism similar to that observed here for the *fos* protein. Recently, a family of protein kinase genes related to PK-C has been reported [41]. Perhaps one of these gene products is responsible for the nuclear, TPA-dependent phosphorylation of the c-*fos* protein. Alternatively, this unusual effect of TPA may be due to alteration of protein phosphoesterase activity.

The predicted amino acid sequences of the c-*fos* and v-*fos* proteins are identical throughout the first 332 residues with the exception of five scattered amino acid substitutions [13]. The major difference in the primary structure between the proteins is in the c-termini, where the last 48 amino acid residues of c-*fos* are entirely unrelated in sequence to the c-terminal 49 amino acid residues of the v-*fos* protein [13] (Fig. 6). To help us identify the amino acid sequences in c-*fos* that are responsible for its

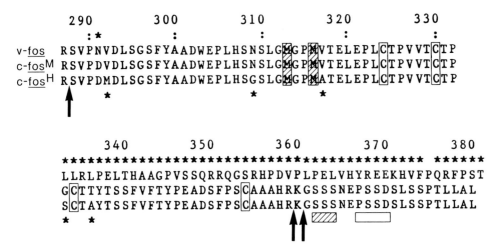

Fig. 6. C-terminal amino acid sequences of *fos* proteins. (Amino acid sequences were obtained from ref. 13.) Arrows indicate preferential sites of trypsin cleavage. Asterisks above the sequence denote differences between murine c-*fos* (c-*fos*[M]) and v-*fos*; asterisks below the sequence denote amino acid differences between c-*fos*[M] and human c-*fos* (c-*fos*[H]). Cysteine residues are enclosed in open boxes; methionine residues are enclosed in hatched boxes. The three serine residues underscored with a hatched box match protein kinase consensus sequences, whereas the sequence homology underscored by the open box is phosphorylated in SV40 large T antigen (see text).

unique sites of phosphorylation relative to v-*fos*, we investigated the sites of phosphorylation in the protein encoded by a chimeric *fos* DNA construct. The resultant protein ("VM") should be identical in amino acid sequence with the v-*fos* protein except that it contains the c-terminal 48 residues unique to c-*fos*. The tryptic phosophopeptides of this protein are similar or identical to those obtained from the c-*fos* protein (Fig. 2A, compare "M" and "VM"). Furthermore, the phosphorylation of the protein is stimulated by TPA (data not shown). It is therefore the 48 c-terminal amino acid residues of c-*fos* that confer upon the protein the ability to be phosphorylated at the c-*fos*-unique sites in a TPA-dependent manner. Because the c-terminus of the c-*fos* protein is high in serine and threonine (17 out of the last 48 amino acids; see Fig. 6), the simplest interpretation of these data is that this region contains the c-*fos* unique sites of phosphorylation. However, we cannot rule out the possibility that conformational differences conferred upon the protein by the c-terminus might allow residues in another region of the molecule to become phosphorylated.

Determination of the effect of phosphorylation on the functional properties of the c-*fos* and v-*fos* proteins will require the ability to specifically prevent the phosphorylation of these proteins. To this end we are currently attempting more precisely to identify the sites of phosphorylation to determine the effect of mutagenesis of these serine and threonine residues on the biological properties of the proteins.

The results presented here indicate that the c-*fos* gene expression is regulated by both positive and negative trans-acting cellular factors. We show that the positive cellular factor(s) are present in fibroblasts, both when they are starved or stimulated with serum. The negative factor(s) is responsible for the c-*fos* transcriptional block in serum-starved fibroblasts, which is perhaps modified upon serum stimulation to allow efficient expression. The modification(s) that occur after serum treatment may involve variations in the factor's affinity to specific sites on the promoter. We cannot exclude the possibility that positive and negative cellular components may be associated and that serum stimulation could change the properties of this complex. However, the ability to titrate out the negative factor in serum-starved fibroblasts, using an excess of the upstream c-*fos* promoter element, is indicative of specific binding properties to promoter sequences. We propose that in serum-starved cells the negative factor(s) are associated with the c-*fos* promoter (or to the promoter transcriptional complex), which results in the "shut-off" of transcription. Upon serum stimulation, this factor or factors are modified and affinity to the regulatory sequences decreases. Alternatively, the positive factor is modified and its affinity to the regulatory sequences increases. In this scenario, the intracellular balance of the two classes of factors is crucial, since their affinity to c-*fos* regulatory sequences changes upon serum treatment. The model in Figure 4 is compatible with the results.

Other examples of negative regulation by trans-acting factors have been described, especially in viral systems. In undifferentiated embryonal carcinoma cells, both MSV and polyoma enhancers are under negative regulation [42]. The Adenovirus-2 E1A products are the prototype of transrepressors of transcriptional activity of enhancer sequences [43,44]. We do not know if the repressor molecule described here has any similarity to the E1A-like proteins described in F9 cells [45]. This is, however, not a general feature of enhancers because SV40 and RSV promoter-enhancer activity does not appear to be reduced in serum-starved fibroblasts (our unpublished observations). At present, examples of cellular regulatory regions that undergo a negative transregulation include the mouse immunoglobulin heavy chain enhancer [46], the rat insulin 1 promoter [47], and the interferon gene [48]. The negative transregulation reported here is the first described for a proto-oncogene. A detailed understanding of the transcriptional regulation of cellular oncogenes is of great interest because of their possible role in differentiation and normal cell growth.

REFERENCES

1. Bishop JM: Ann Rev Biochem 52:301–354, 1983.
2. Hunter T: Sci Amer 251:70, 1984.
3. Cooper GM: Science 217:801–806, 1982.
4. Weinberg RA: Sci Amer 249:126–142, 1983.
5. Bishop JM: Trends Genet 1:245–249, 1985.
6. Sherr CJ, Rettenmier CW, Sacca R, Roussel MF, Look AT, Stanley ER: Cell 41:665–676, 1985.
7. Doolittle RF, Hunkapiller MW, Hood LE, Devare SG, Robbins KC, Aaronson SA, Antoniades HW: Science 221:275, 1983.
8. Waterfield MD, Scrace GT, Whittle N, Stroobant P, Johnsson A, Wasteson A, Westermark B, Heiden CH, Huang JS, Duel TF: Nature 304:35, 1983.
9. Ross R, Raines EW, Bowen-Pope DF: Cell 46:155–169, 1986.
10. Finkel MP, Biskis BO, Jinkins PB: Science 151:598–701, 1966.
11. Curran T, Peters G, Van Beveren C, Teich NM, Verma IM: J Virol 44:674–682, 1982.
12. Levy JA, Hartley JW, Rowe WP, Huebner RJ: J Natl Cancer Inst 51:529–539, 1973.
13. Van Beveren C, van Straaten F, Curran T, Muller R, Verma IM: Cell 32:1241–1255, 1983.
14. Curran T, Miller AD, Zokas L, Verma IM: Cell 36:259–268, 1984.
15. Miller AD, Curran T, Verma IM: Cell 36:51–60, 1984.
16. Meijlink F, Curran T, Miller AD, Verma IM: Proc Natl Acad Sci USA 82:4987–4991, 1985.
17. Curran T, Van Beveren C, Ling N, Verma IM: Mol Cell Biol 5:167–172, 1985.
18. Barber J, Verma IM: Mol Cell Biol 1987.
19. Curran T, Teich NM: J Virol 42:114–122, 1982.
20. Greenberg ME, Ziff EB: Nature 311:433–438, 1984.
21. Kruijer W, Cooper JA, Hunter T, Verma IM: Nature 312:711–716, 1984.

22. Kruijer W, Schubert D, Verma IM: Proc Natl Acad Sci USA 82:7330–7334, 1985.
23. Mitchell RL, Zokas L, Schreiber RD, Verma IM: Cell 40:209–217, 1986.
24. Muller R, Bravo R, Burckhardt J, Curran T: Nature 312:716–720, 1984.
25. Treisman R: Cell 42:889–902, 1985.
26. Deschamps J, Meijlink F, Verma IM: Science 230: 1174–1177, 1985.
27. Renz M, Neuberg M, Kurz C, Bravo R, Muller R: EMBO J 4:3711–3716, 1985.
28. Greenberg ME, Hermanowski AL, Ziff EB: Mol Cell Biol 6:1050–1057, 1986.
29. Mitchell RL, Henning-Chubb C, Huberman E, Verma IM: Cell 45:497–504, 1986.
30. Treisman R: Cell 46:567–574, 1986.
31. Gilman MZ, Wilson RN, Weinberg RA: Mol Cell Biol 6:4305, 1986.
32. Greenberg ME, Siegfried Z, Ziff EB: Mol Cell Biol 7:1217–1225, 1987.
33. Sassone-Corsi P, Verma IM: Nature 1987.
34. Verma IM: Trends Genet 2:93–96, 1986.
35. Nishizuka Y: Science 233:305–312, 1986.
36. Castagna M, Takai Y, Kalbuchi K, Sano K, Kikkawa U, Nishizuka Y: Biol Chem 257:7847–7851.
37. Nishizuka Y: Nature 308:693–698, 1984.
38. Rozengurt E, Rodriguez-Pena M, Smith KA: Proc Natl Acad Sci USA 80:7244–7248, 1983.
39. Patskan GJ, Baxter CS: J Biol Chem 260:12899–12903, 1985.
40. Butler AP, Byus CV, Siaga TJ: J Biol Chem 261:9421–9425, 1986.
41. Knopf JL, Lee M, Suitzman LA, Kriz RW, Loomis CR, Hewick RM, Bell RM: Cell 46:491–502, 1986.
42. Gorman CM, Rigby PWJ, Lane DP: Cell 42:519, 1985.
43. Borrelli E, Hen R, Chambon P: Nature 312:608, 1984.
44. Velcich A, Ziff E: Cell 40:705–716, 1985.
45. Imperiale MJ, Kas HT, Feldman LT, Nevins JR, Strickland S: Mol Cell Biol 4:867, 1984.
46. Borrelli E, Hen R, Wasylyk B, Wasylyk C, Chambon P: Proc Natl Acad Sci USA 83:2846, 1986.
47. Nir U, Walkeeer MD, Rutter WJ: Proc Natl Acad Sci USA 83:3180, 1986.
48. Goodbourn S, Burstein H, Maniatis T: Cell 45:601, 1986.

Growth Regulation of Cancer
189–199 (1988)

Oncogenic Potential of the *erb*B-2 Gene: Frequent Overexpression in Human Mammary Adenocarcinomas and Induction of Transformation In Vitro

C. R. King, P. P. Di Fiore, J. H. Pierce, O. Segatto, M. H. Kraus, and S. A. Aaronson

Laboratory of Cellular and Molecular Biology, National Cancer Institute, Bethesda, Maryland 20892

The oncogenes of acute transforming retroviruses have counterparts, designated proto-oncogenes, that are conserved within the human genome [1]. The human *sis* proto-oncogene encodes one major polypeptide chain of platelet-derived growth factor (PDGF) [2,3], and the *erb*B proto-oncogene encodes a truncated receptor for epidermal growth factor (EGF) [4]. A number of other proto-oncogenes, like *erb*B, share nucleotide sequence homology with the tyrosine kinase-encoding *src* gene [5–8]. The fact that cellular receptors for several growth factors or hormones, including the EGF receptor, possess this enzymatic activity suggests that other proto-oncogenes may encode growth factor receptors as well. Genetic alterations affecting proto-oncogenes of the tyrosine kinase family can play a role in spontaneous tumor development. A specific translocation affecting the c-*abl* locus, for example, is associated with chronic myelogenous leukemia [9,10]. Several recent studies have also documented amplification or rearrangement of the gene for the EGF receptor in certain human tumors [11] or tumor cell lines [12–14].

The identification of additional members of some proto-oncogene families has emerged from findings of related sequences amplified sufficiently in a particular tumor to allow detection [15–16]. Because of our interest in genes coding for growth factor receptors, we used the v-*erb*B gene to probe for related genes that might be candidates for other receptor coding sequences. The present report summarizes investigations that have led to the discovery of a novel EGF receptor-related gene. This gene, designated *erb*B-2, was found amplified and/or overexpressed in a significant fraction of human mammary adenocarcinomas, and its direct oncogenic potential in vitro was demonstrated.

Received June 11, 1987.

A Novel EGF Receptor-Related Gene in a Human Mammary Adenocarcinoma

In an initial attempt to identify genes that might be candidates for new receptor coding sequences with oncogenic potential, we analyzed DNAs from primary tumors and carcinoma cell lines by Southern blot analysis using nick translated v-*erb*B DNA as a probe [17]. For these experiments, we selected moderate stringency hybridization conditions under which different oncogenes of the tyrosine family did not cross-hybridize (data not shown). Thus, any gene detected might be expected to have a closer relationship to v-*erb*B than to other members of the tyrosine kinase family.

DNA prepared from tissue of a human mammary carcinoma, MAC117, showed a pattern of hybridization (Fig. 1A) differing both from that observed with DNA of normal human placenta and the A431 squamous-cell carcinoma line, which contains amplified EGF receptor genes [12–14]. In A431 DNA, we observed four EcoR I fragments that had increased signal intensities compared to those of corresponding fragments in placenta DNA (Fig. 1A). In contrast, MAC117 DNA contained a 6-kilobase pair (kdp) filament, which appeared to be amplified compared to corresponding fragments observed in both A431 and placenta DNA's (Fig. 1A). These findings were consistent with the possibility that the MAC117 tumor contained an amplified DNA sequence related to, but distinct from, the cellular *erb*B proto-oncogene [17].

To define its nature, we undertook the molecular cloning of the 6-kbp EcoR I fragment. We determined its nucleotide sequence in the region most homologous to v-*erb*B. This sequence contained two regions of nucleotide sequence homology to v-*erb*B separated by 122 nucleotides (Fig. 2). These regions shared 69% nucleotide

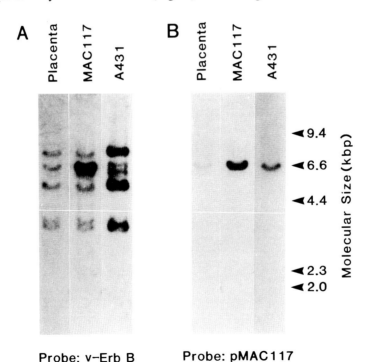

Fig. 1.   Detection of v-*erb*B- and pMAC117-specific gene fragments in normal human placenta, A431 cells, or human mammary carcinoma MC117.

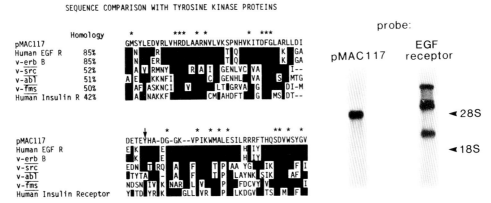

Fig. 2. Left: Comparison of the putative encoded amino acid sequence in pMAC117 with known tyrosine kinase sequence. Black regions represent homologous amino acids. Differing amino acid residues are shown in one letter code. Amino acid positions conserved in all sequences are denoted by *. The tyrosine homologous to that autophosphorylated by the v-*src* protein is shown by an arrow. The v-*abl* sequence contains a tyrosine residue in this region displaced by two positions. The amino acid sequences of human EGF receptor, v-*erb*B, v-*src*, v-*abl*, v-*fms*, and human insulin receptor were aligned by the computer program described [43]. The homology observed with the predicted amino acid sequences of v-*yes* and v-*fes* was 51% and 48%, respectively. Right: Detection of distinct messenger RNA species derived from the pMAC117 gene and the human EGF receptor gene.

sequence identity with both the v-*erb*B and the human EGF receptor gene. The predicted amino acid sequence was 85% homologous to two regions that are contiguous in the EGF receptor sequence [12]. Furthermore, the two putative coding regions were each flanked by the AG and GT dinucleotides, which are known to border the exons of eukaryotic genes. All of these findings argue strongly that the sequence represents two exons, separated by an intron, of a gene related to but distinct from the v-*erb* B/EGF receptor gene.

By comparison of the predicted amino acid sequence of the clone designated pMAC117 with corresponding sequences of several members of the tyrosine kinase family, the most striking homology was observed with the human EGF receptor and v-*erb*B. However, we observed 42% to 52% homology with the predicted amino acid sequences of other tyrosine kinase encoding genes as well. In fact, at 25% of the positions, there was identity among each of the sequences analyzed. All of these findings placed the pMAC117 encoding sequence within the tyrosine kinase gene family.

The availability of cloned probes of the gene made it possible to investigates its expression in a variety of cell types. The probe detected a single 5-kb transcript in A431 cells (Fig. 2). Under the stringent conditions of hybridization utilized, this probe did not detect any of the three RNA species recognized by EGF receptor complementary DNA. Thus, the gene, designated *erb*B-2, represented a new functional gene within the tyrosine kinase family, closely related to but distinct from the gene encoding the EGF receptor [17].

Overexpression of the *erb*B-2 Gene in Human Mammary Tumor Cell Lines by Different Molecular Mechanism

To assess the role of *erb*B-2 in human mammary neoplasia, we compared mRNAs of 16 mammary tumor cell lines to normal human fibroblasts, M413, and a human mammary epithelial cell line, HBL100 [18]. Increased expression of an apparently normal size 5-kb transcript was detected in 8 of 16 tumor cell lines, when total cellular RNA was subjected to Northern blot analysis. An aberrantly sized erbB-2 mRNA was not detected in any of the cell lines analyzed.

To quantitate more precisely the amount of erbB-2 transcript in eight mammary tumor cell lines that overexpress erbB-2, serial twofold dilutions of total cellular RNA were subjected to dot blot analysis using human β actin as a control for the amount of RNA applied to the nitrocellulose filters. The highest levels of erbB-2 mRNA, which ranged from 64- to 128-fold over that of our controls, were observed in the cell lines MDA-MB453, SK-BR-3, MDA-MB361, and BT474. Moreover, erbB-2 mRNA levels were increased 4- to 8-fold in four cell lines including BT483, MDA-MB175, ZR-75-30, and ZR-75-1 (Table I).

To investigate alterations of the erbB-2 gene associated with its overexpression, we examined the erbB-2 gene locus by Southern blot analysis in these cell lines. The normal restriction pattern was detected in all DNA samples tested, indicating that gross rearrangements in the proximity of the erbB-2 coding region did not occur in these cell lines. When compared with normal human fibroblast DNA, the erbB-2 specific restriction fragments appeared amplified in several cell lines including SK-BR-3, BT474, and MDA-MB361.

Quantitation of erbB-2 gene copy number was accomplished using DNA dot-blot analysis. These studies revealed a 4- to 8-fold erbB-2 gene amplification in SK-BR-3 and BT474 relative to normal human DNA, and a 2- to 4-fold erbB-2 gene amplification in the MDA-MB453 and MDA-MB361 cell lines. Thus, gene amplification was associated with overexpression in the four tumor cell lines with the highest levels of erbB-2 mRNA (Table 1). In contrast, gene amplification could not be detected by Southern blot analysis or DNA dot-blot analysis in four tumor cell lines in which the erbB-2 transcript was increased to intermediate levels [18].

Mammary Tumor Cell Lines Overexpressing erbB-2: No Transforming Genes Detectable by DNA Transfection

In chemically induced rat neuroblastomas, a point mutation within the transmembrane domain activates neu, the rat homologue of erbB-2, to acquire transform-

TABLE I. Overexpression of erbB-2 in Human Mammary Neoplasia

	erbB-2	
	Overexpression of mRNA[a]	Gene amplification
M413	1	1
HBL100	1	1
MCF-7	1	1
SK-BR-3	128	4–8
BT474	128	4–8
MDA-MB361	64	2–4
MDA-MB453	64	2
ZR-75-1	8	1
ZR-75-30	4	<1
MDA-MB175	8	1
BT483	8	<1

[a]Overexpression above normal fibroblast and HBL100.

ing activity in the NIH/3T3 transfection assay [19]. Previous transfection analysis of a large series of mammary tumors and tumor cell lines did not reveal activation of *erb*B-2 as a transforming gene in human mammary tumors [20]. To investigate whether an activating lesion similar to that observed in rat *neu* was associated with *erb*B-2 overexpressed in human mammary tumor cell lines, we transfected genomic DNAs of such cell lines on NIH/3T3 cells [18]. Under conditions where high mw DNA from the T24 bladder carcinoma cell line, which contains an activated H-*ras* oncogene, induced 4–8 foci/plate, genomic DNA from eight mammary tumor cell lines that overexpressed *erb*B-2 did not induce detectable morphological transformation (Table II). The above findings along with evidence of frequent *erb*B-2 amplification in the absence of aberrant transcript suggested that a structurally normal *erb*B-2 coding sequence was overexpressed as mRNA in some human mammary tumor cell lines. Furthermore, protein analysis of representative samples established that the elevated *erb*B-2 transcript levels are translated into *erb*B-2 protein (data not shown).

It is not yet clear exactly how *erb*B-2 overexpression and gene amplification are involved in the transition of cells from the normal to the neoplastic state. However, the identification of overexpression without gene amplification raises the possibility of a multistep mechanisms. Overexpression of *erb*B-2 might confer an initial selective growth advantage to the tumor cell. As a further step, gene amplification might enhance and stabilize this selective growth advantage. *erb*B-2 overexpression was consistently higher in those tumors with gene amplification compared to those lacking gene amplification [18]. However, the amount of overexpression per gene copy was approximately constant in the different cell lines (Table I).

The *erb*B-2 Gene: Potent Oncogene When Overexpressed in NIH/3T3 Cells

To directly assess the effects of *erb*B-2 overexpression on cell growth properties, we undertook the isolation of cDNA clones comprising the entire human *erb*B-2 coding sequence [18]. A series of overlapping cDNA clones were isolated from normal human fibroblast and MCF-7 cDNA libraries utilizing fragments from the previously described human genomic *erb*B-2 clones as probes. A full-length normal human *erb*B-2 clone was assembled from overlapping clones [21]. By sequence analysis the coding sequence was found to be identical to previously published normal *erb*-2 coding sequences except for a few conservative substitutions [21–23].

TABLE II. DNA Transfection of Human Mammary Tumor Cell Lines

Source of genomic DNA	FFU/plate[a]
T24 prep 1	32/4
T24 prep 2	19/4
T24 prep 3	16/4
SK-BR-3	0/12
BT474	0/12
MDA-MB361	0/2
MDA-MB453	0/4
ZR-75-30	0/4
BT483	0/4
MDA-MB175	0/8

[a]Focus-forming units/number of transfected plates.

Expression vectors based on the transcriptional initiation sequences of either the Moloney murine leukemia virus long terminal repeat (MuLV LTR) or the SV40 early promoter were constructed in an attempt to express the *erb*B-2 cDNA at different levels in NIH/3T3 cells (Fig. 3) [21]. Previous studies have indicated different strengths of LTR and the SV40 promoters in these cells [24]. Because of the presence of the MuLV donor splice site close to the 5' LTR [25], we engineered one of the LTR-based vector (LTR-1/*erb*B-2) to contain an acceptor splice site immediately upstream of the translation initiation codon of the *erb*B-2 coding sequence (Fig. 3). This vector was constructed to ensure correct splicing of the message even if a cryptic splice acceptor site were present within the *erb*B-2 open reading frame. In the SV40-based expression vector (SV40/*erb*B-2), the *erb*B-2 coding sequence replaced the neomycin-resistance gene of pSV2/neo (26)(Fig. 3).

To assess the biologic activity of our human *erb*B-2 vectors, we transfected NIH/3T3 cells with serial dilutions of each DNA. As shown in Table III, both LTR-1/*erb*B-2 and LTR-2/*erb*B-2 DNAs induced transformed foci at high efficiencies of 4.1×10^4 and 2.0×10^4 focus-forming units per picomole of DNA (ffu/pM), respectively. In striking contrast, the SV40/*erb*B-2 construct failed to induce any detectable morphological alteration of NIH/3T3 cells transfected under identical assay conditions (Table III). Since the SV40/*erb*B-2 construct lacked transforming activity, these results demonstrated that the higher levels of *erb*B-2 expression under LTR influence correlated with this ability to exert transforming activity.

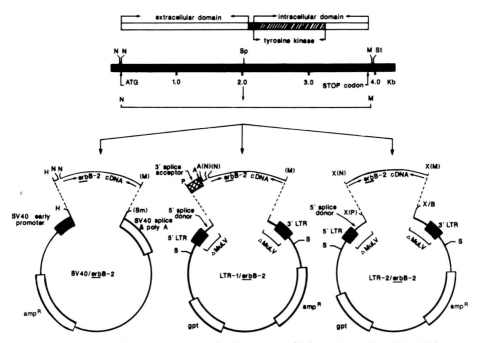

Fig. 3. Construction of expression vectors for the human *erb*B-2 cDNA. A Nco I-Mst II fragment encompassing the entire *erb*B-2 open reading frame was cloned under the transcriptional control of either the SV40 early promoter on MuLV LTR. Symbols: Cross-hatching represents *erb*A-*erb*B intergenic region of pAEV11 containing the 3' splice acceptor site; N, Nco I; Sp, Sph I; M, Mst II; St, Stu I; H, Hind III; Sm, Sma I; P, Pst I; B, BamH I; X, Xho I. Sites indicated in parentheses were not reconstituted after the cloning procedure.

TABLE III. Transformed Phenotype of *erb*B-2 Transfectants

DNA transfectant[a]	Specific transforming activity[b] (ffu/pM)	Colony-forming efficiency in agar (%)[c]	Cell number required for 50% tumor incidence[d]
LTR-1/*erb*B-2	4.1×10^4	45	10^3
SV40/*erb*B-2	$< 10^0$	<0.01	$> 10^6$
LTR/v-*erb*B	5.0×10^2	20	5×10^4
LTR/*ras*	3.6×10^4	35	10^3
pSV2/gpt	$< 10^0$	<0.01	$> 10^6$

[a]All transfectants were isolated from plates that received 1 μg cloned DNA and were selected by their ability to grow in the presence of killer HAT medium [44].
[b]Focus-forming units were adjusted to ffu/pM of cloned DNA added based on the relative molecular weights of the respective plasmids.
[c]Cells were plated at 10-fold serial dilutions in 0.33% soft agar medium containing 10% calf serum. Visible colonies comprising > 100 cells were scored at 14 days.
[d]NFR nude mice were inoculated subcutaneously with each cell line. Ten mice were tested at cell concentrations ranging from 10^6 to 10^3 cells/mouse. Tumor formation was monitored at least twice weekly for up to 30 days.

To compare the growth properties of NIH/3T3 cells transfected by these genes, we analyzed the transfectants for anchorage-independent growth in culture, a property of many transformed cells. The colony-forming efficiency of a LTR-1/*erb*B-2 transformant was very high and comparable to that of cells transformed by LTR-driven v-H-*ras* and v-*erb*B (Table III). Moreover, the LTR-1/*erb*B-2 transfectants were as malignant in vivo as cells transformed by the highly potent v-H-*ras* oncogene, and 50-fold more tumorigenic than cells transfected with v-*erb*B. In contrast, SV40/*erb*B-2 transfectants failed to display anchorage-independent growth in vitro and did not grow as tumors in nude mice even when 10^6 cells were injected (Table III).

Whereas the predicted *erb*B-2 protein bears structural similarity to the EGF receptor, there is evidence that EGF is not the ligand for the *erb*B-2 product [27, 28]. In fact, the normal ligand for this receptorlike protein has yet to be identified. If present in serum, this ligand might be responsible for stimulating the overexpressed *erb*B-2 product and triggering its transforming ability. To address this possibility, we investigated whether *erb*B-2 transformed cells maintained their altered phenotype when cultured in medium lacking serum [21]. NIH/3T3 cells grow as a contact-inhibited monolayer in a chemically defined medium that contains EGF, fibroblast growth factor (FGF), and insulin [29]. These growth factors have been excluded as possible exogenous ligand for the *erb*B-2 gene product [27, 28]. In this medium, LTR-1/*erb*B-2-transfected cells continued to exhibit a stable transformed phenotype by growing as foci of densely packed cells (Fig. 4). These findings demonstrated that neither EGF nor any factors present in serum are required for maintaining the transformed phenotype of NIH/3T3 cells overexpressing *erb*B-2.

Human Tumors With Amplified *erb*B-2 Genes Express the *erb*B-2 Protein at High Levels Comparable to LTR/*erb*B-2 NIH/3T3 Transformants

Since we and others detected amplification and/or overexpression of the *erb*B-2 gene in a wide variety of human malignancies [17,18,30–33], we sought to compare the level of overexpression of the *erb*B-2-encoded 185 kd protein in human mammary tumor cell lines possessing amplified *erb*B-2 genes with that of NIH/3T3 cells

+EIF   LTR-1/erbB-2   +IF

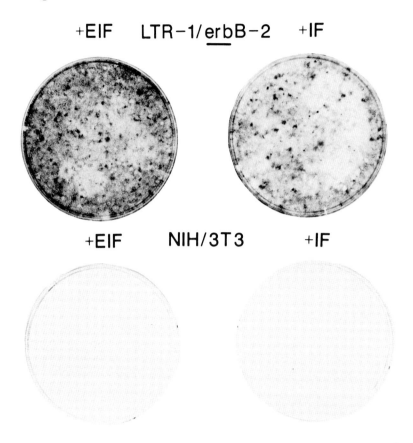

+EIF   NIH/3T3   +IF

Fig. 4.   Growth of LTR-1/erbB-2-transformed cells in chemically defined medium. Around 10^4 LTR-1/ erbB-2-transfected or control NIH/3T3 cells were plated in chemically defined medium (1:1:1 mixture of Ham's F12, Leibowitz's L-15, and MCDB401), supplemented with 10 µg/ml transferrin, and 10^{-8} M Na_2SeO_3 [23]. This medium was supplemented with either the mixture designated EIF, 10 ng/ml EGF, 10 ng/ml insulin, and 10 ng/ml FGF, or the mixture designated IF; 10 µg/ml insulin and 10 ng/ml FGF.

transformed by the erbB-2 coding sequence [21]. An antierbB-2 peptide serum detected several discrete protein species ranging in size from 150 to 185 kd in extracts of MDA-MB361 and SK-BR-3 mammary tumor cell lines, as well as LTR/erbB-2 NIH/3T3 transformants (Fig. 5). The relative levels of the 185 kd erbB-2 product were similar in each of the cell lines and markedly elevated over that expressed by MCF-7 cells, where the 185 kd erbB-2 protein was not detectable under these assay conditions (Fig. 5). Thus, human mammary tumor cells that overexpressed the erbB-2 gene demonstrated levels of the erbB-2 gene product capable of inducing malignant transformation in a model system.

Role of Growth Factor Receptor Overexpression in Neoplasia

The profound cellular alterations induced by the activated cellular transforming genes have similarities to the growth promoting actions of hormones and growth factors. Each exerts pleiotropic effect on cellular metabolism, including the induction of sustained cell replication. There is considerable evidence that genes encoding

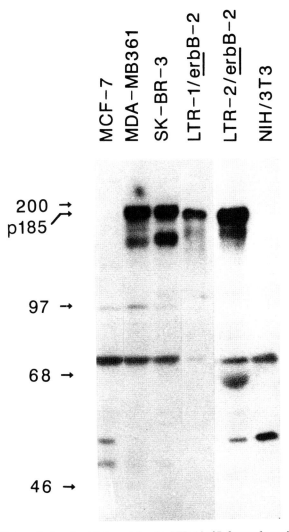

Fig. 5. Immunoblot analysis of *erb*B-2 proteins in LTR-1/*erb*B-2-transformed NIH/3T3 cells and human tumor cell lines.

growth factor receptors can be activated as transforming genes by structural alterations in their coding sequences [8,12,19,34–40]. For example, the chemically activated *neu* gene, activated by a point mutation in its transmembrane domain [19], was initially detected by its ability to induce foci upon DNA transfection of NIH/3T3 cells [41]. To date, transforming genes encoding growth factor receptors have not been detected in human tumors by this approach. Instead, abnormalities involving growth factor receptors in human malignancies appear most commonly to involve their overexpression as reported for EGF receptor or *erb*B-2 genes in a significant fraction of human epithelial malignancies [11,13,17,18,30–33,43].

Our studies show that the human *erb*B-2 gene can be activated as an oncogene by its overexpression in NIH/3T3 cells. The level of the *erb*B-2 product was shown to be critical in determining its transforming ability. This in vitro observation is paralleled by in vivo findings that a number of human tumors, which include a significant percentage of human mammary adenocarcinomas, display overexpression of the *erb*B-2 gene. In addition, we demonstrated that the levels at which the *erb*B-2 protein is capable of inducing in vitro transformation are comparable to those detected in naturally occurring tumors exhibiting *erb*B-2 overexpression. Taken together, all these observations establish a mechanistic basis for growth factor receptor gene amplification as representing a causal driving force in the clonal evolution of a tumor cell rather than being an incidental consequence of tumorigenesis.

Our results indicate that a ligand in serum is not required for transforming activity of the overexpressed *erb*B-2 product. In fact, transfected NIH/3T3 cells overexpressing the *erb*B-2 product were still capable of altered growth in chemically defined medium supplemented with EGF, FGF, and insulin, which have been excluded as exogenous ligands for this receptorlike protein. As the ligand for the *erb*B-2 protein has yet to be identified, it is not possible to exclude that *erb*B-2 transformed cells themselves might produce the ligand for the *erb*B-2 receptor protein. Alternatively, an increased number of receptors may cause transformation either by raising the level of constitutive tyrosine kinase activity to a threshold required for growth stimulation or by facilitating receptor–receptor interactions that may be a prerequisite for their activation.

REFERENCES

1. Bishop JM: Annu Rev Biochem 52:301–354, 1983.
2. Doolittle RF, Hunkapiller MW, Hood LE, Devare SG, Robbins KC, Aaronson SA, Antoniades HN: Science 221:275–277, 1983.
3. Waterfield MD, Scrace GT, Whittle N, Stroobant P, Johnsson A, Wasteson A, Westermark B, Heldin CH, Huang JS, Deuel TF: Nature 304:35–39, 1983.
4. Downward J, Yarden Y, Mayes E, Scrace G, Totty N, Stockwell P, Ullrich A, Schlessinger J, Waterfield MD: Nature 307:521–527, 1984.
5. Hampe A, Paprevotte I, Galibert F, Fedele LA, Sherr CJ: Cell 30:775–785, 1982.
6. Kitamura N, Kitamura A, Toyoshima K, Hirayama Y, Yoshida M: Nature 297:205–208, 1982.
7. Shibuya M, Hanfafusa H: Cell 30:787–795, 1982.
8. Yamamoto T, Nishida T, Miyajima N, Kawai S, Ooi T, Toyoshima K: Cell 35:71–78, 1983.
9. de Klein A, van Kessel AG, Grosveld G, Bartram CR, Hagemeijer A, Bootsma D, Spurr NK, Heisterkamp N, Groffen J, Stephenson JR: Nature 300:765–767, 1982.
10. Collins SJ, Groudine MT: Proc Natl Acad Sci USA 80:4813–4817, 1983.
11. Libermann TA, Nusbaum HR, Razon N, Kris R, Lax I, Soreq H, Whittle N, Waterfield MD, Ullrich A, Schlessinger J: Nature 313:144–147, 1985.
12. Ullrich A, Coussens L, Hayflick JS, Dull TJ, Gray A, Tam AW, Lee J, Yarden Y, Libermann TA, Schlessinger J, et al.: Nature 309:418–425, 1984.
13. Xu Y, Richert N, Ito S, Merlino ST, Pastan I: Proc Natl Acad Sci USA 81:7308–7312, 1984.
14. Lin CR, Chen WS, Kruiger W, Stolarsky LS, Weber W, Evans RM, Verma IM, Gill GN, Rosenfeld MG: Science 224:843–848, 1984.
15. Schwab N, Alitalo K, Klempnauer KH, Varmus HE, Bishop JM, Gilbert F, Brodeur G, Goldstein M, Trent J: Nature 305:245–248, 1983.
16. Kohl NE, Kanda N, Schreck RR, Bruns G, Latt SA, Gilbert F, Alt FW: Cell 35:359–367, 1983.
17. King CR, Kraus MH, Aarsonson SA: Science 229:974–976, 1985.
18. Kraus MH, Popescu NC, Amsbough SC, King CR: EMBO J 6:605–610, 1987.
19. Bargmann CI, Hung MC, Weinberg RA: Cell 45:649–657, 1986.
20. Kraus MH, Yuasa Y, Aaronson SA: Proc Natl Acad Sci USA 81:5384–5388, 1984.
21. DiFiore PP, Pierce JH, Kraus MH, Segetto O, King CR, Aaronson SA: Science 237:178–182 (1987).

22. Yamamoto T, Ikawa S, Akiyama T, Semba K, Nomura N, Miyajima N, Saito T, Toyoshima K: Nature 319:230–234, 1986.
23. Coussens L, Yang-Feng TL, Liao YC, Chen E, Gray A, McGrath J, Seeberg PH, Libermann TA, Schlessinger J, Francke U, et al: Science 230:1132–1139, 1985.
24. Gorman CM, Merlino GT, Willingham MC, Pastan I, Howard BH: Proc Natl Acad Sci USA 79:6777–6781, 1982.
25. Shinnick TM, Lerner RA, Sutcliffe JG: Nature 293:543–548, 1981.
26. Southern PJ, Berg P: J Mol Appl Genet 1:327–341, 1982.
27. Akiyama T, Sudo C, Ogawara H, Toyoshima K, Yamamoto T: Science 232:1644–1646, 1986.
28. Stern DF, Heffernan PA, Weinberg RA: Mol Cell Biol 6:1729–1740, 1986.
29. Taylor W, Segatto O, Aaronson SA (unpublished observations).
30. Fukushige S, Matsubara K, Yoshida M, Sasaki M, Suzuki T, Semba K, Toyoshima K, Yamamoto T: Mol Cell Biol 6:955–958, 1986.
31. Semba K, Kamata N, Toyoshima K, Yamamoto T: Proc Natl Acad Sci USA 82:6497–6501, 1985.
32. Yokota J, Yamamoto T, Toyoshima K, Terada M, Sugimura T, Battifora H, Cline MJ: The Lancet 765–767, 1986.
33. Slamon D, Clark GM, Wong SG, Levin WJ, Ullrich A, McGuire WL: Science 235:177–182, 1987.
34. Sherr CJ, Rettenmier CW, Sacca R, Roussel MF, Look AT, Stanley ER: Cell 41:665–676, 1985.
35. Weber W, Gill GN, Spiess J: Science 224:294–297, 1984.
36. Merlino GT, Xu YH, Ishii S, Clark AJ, Semba K, Toyoshima K, Yamamoto T, Pastan I: Science 224:417–419, 1984.
37. Lax I, Kris R, Sasson I, Ullrich A, Hayman MJ, Beug H, Schlessinger J: EMBO J 4:3179–3182, 1985.
38. Nielsen TW, Maroney PA, Goodwin RG, Rottman FM, Crittenden LB, Raines MA, Kung HJ: Cell 41:719–726, 1985.
39. Hampe A, Gobet M, Sherr CJ, Galibert F: Proc Natl Acad Sci USA 81:85–89, 1984.
40. Coussens L, Van Beveran C, Smith D, Chen E, Mitchell RL, Isacke CM, Verma IM, Ullrich A: Nature 320:277–280, 1986.
41. Shih C, Padhy LC, Murray M, Weinberg RA: Nature 290:261–264, 1981.
42. King CR, Kraus MH, Williams LT, Merlino GT, Pastan IH, Aaronson SA: Nucleic Acid Res 13:8477–8486, 1985.
43. Ullrich A, Bell JR, Chen EY, Herrera R, Petruzzelli LM, Dull TJ, Gray A, Coussens L, Liao YC, Tsubokawa M, et al: Nature 313:756–761, 1985.
44. Mulligan RC, Berg P: Proc Natl Acad Sci USA 78:2072–2076, 1981.

Growth Regulation of Cancer
201–204 (1988)

Proto-Oncogenes as Mediators of Growth and Development: Discussion Summary

Mark A. Israel

Molecular Genetics Section, Pediatric Branch, National Cancer Institute, National Institutes of Health, Bethesda, Maryland 20892

Experimental evidence from various animal species indicates that the expression of some proto-oncogenes is differentially regulated in a tissue- and stage-specific manner. In some instances, it appears that proto-oncogenes play important roles in regulating the molecular processes by which differentiation is mediated. Such findings complement other lines of investigation demonstrating that the altered expression of some proto-oncogenes, as well as the pathologic expression of their corresponding oncogenes, can perturb normal cellular differentiation and the growth properties of many different cell types. Given the paucity of genes known to play regulatory roles in the differentiation of mammalian tissues, it is remarkable that even at this time we know relatively little about the tissue-specific expression of most proto-oncogenes during the maturation of normal animal cells and tissues. For this reason, the workshop focused on: 1) the distribution of proto-oncogene expression in selected tissues during maturation, and 2) experimental approaches to the study of the regulatory roles that the proteins encoded by these genes may have during the maturation of such tissues.

In particular, data describing proto-oncogene expression during muscle cell differentiation was of interest to workshop participants. Several experimental model systems were described. Molecular probes for the specific analysis of skeletal, smooth, and cardiac muscles were discussed and may provide insights into the regulation of tissue subsets not as easily examined in other settings. In vitro, rodent cell lines of myoblasts whose differentiation into myotubes can be marked by morphologic, biochemical, and molecular changes provide particularly powerful models in which to examine the regulatory role of proto-oncogenes in tissue maturation.

Much of the discussion about the use of such model systems was based on data reported by two of the meeting's participants, J. Harel (Institute Gustave Roussy,

Received September 22, 1987.

Villejuif, France) and M.D. Schneider (Baylor University, Houston, TX). Dr. Harel reviewed time-course studies evaluating the expression of a large number of different proto-oncogenes during the maturation in vitro of the rat myoblast cell line, L6 1 [1]. In 10% serum these cells become growth arrested upon reaching confluence, and genes encoding muscle-specific products are turned on. For morphologic differentiation and myoblast fusion to take place, however, the cells require several additional days of incubation in media containing very low amounts of serum. In growing L6 1 cells, the expression of *abl*, *erb*A, *erb*B, *fes*, *fgr*, *fms*, *fos*, Ha-*ras*, Ki-*ras*, N-*ras*, *myb*, *myc*, *sis*, and *src* can be detected by Northern blot analysis. C-mos expression could not be detected in these cells. As growing L6 1 cells approach confluency, the level of c-*fos* expression increases, whereas the level of expression of other proto-oncogenes does not change until the induction of myotube formation. At that time, *fos*, *myc*, and Ki-*ras* expression becomes undetectable and N-*ras* expression increases.

These findings were of particular interest to the discussion group in light of data presented by Dr. Schneider describing selected effects of several activated oncogenes transfected into another rodent cell line that can also be induced to develop muscle-specific properties after mitogen withdrawal [2]. The experiments discussed focused on the development of several different voltage-gated ion channels that were monitored in the BC3H1 rodent myocyte cell line transfected with various combinations of the v-*erb*B, c-*myc* (under the control of an SV40 promoter), and Ha(va1-12)-*ras* oncogenes. Although the development of ion channels was not blocked by either *myc* or *erb*B alone, a combination of these two oncogenes or the activated Ha-*ras* alone did suppress the development of both Na$^+$ and Ca^{2+} channels. The development of K$^+$ channels was not blocked in any of the transfected cells examined.

Participants speculated that during physiologic muscle differentiation the transient enhancement of *fos* expression and the decreased expression of Ki-*ras* genes may foster the progress of muscle-specific maturation, whereas *myc* and *erb*B may have the potential to block such progression in either a physiologic setting or during oncogenesis. In this regard, Dr. Harel's data indicating that *ras* and *myc* oncogenes were expressed at high levels in two malignant cell lines, M4 and RMS4 (both derived from the L6 1 cell line), were of considerable interest, and the implications of altered expression of these proto-oncogenes in the pathogenesis of muscle tumors in general and rhabdomyosarcoma in particular were discussed.

Since many of the session participants had a special interest in mitogen-stimulated growth, there was considerable discussion about the similarities between the suppression of muscle cell differentiation by media that supported rapid cell growth and the effects of transfected oncogenes. In particular, there was interest in the possibility that the apparent regulatory action of oncogenes important for the induction of muscle-specific gene programs is mediated directly through alterations in the molecular pathways by which the growth of myoblasts is mediated.

Similar approaches to the study of peripheral nervous system differentiation were also reported, and data describing changes in the expression of several of these same proto-oncogenes during the retinoic acid-induced differentiation of human neuroblastoma tumor cells were presented by M.A. Israel [4]. Of particular interest, in light of the pathologic potential of N-*myc* in the development of this childhood tumor, was the observation that, although morphologic and biochemical differentiation of neuroblastoma tumor cells cannot be detected for several days after the initiation of retinoic acid treatment, N-*myc* expression drops to 50% of basal levels in about 6 hr after the initiation of treatment, and to less than 10% in 36 hr. This decrease in N-*myc* expression is seen not only in association with retinoic acid-induced differentiation of these cells, but also when differentiation is induced by other agents, such as cyclic AMP and bromodeoxyuridine.

In neuroblastoma cells it has been possible to design experiments that permit changes in gene expression closely associated with the induction of differentiation to be distinguished from those associated with the growth arrest that almost invariably accompanies the differentiation of cells both in culture and in vivo. Whereas N-*myc* decreases in association with differentiation as described above, it is possible to growth arrest neuroblastoma cells in culture either by nutriment deprivation or by the use of a thymidine blockade. Experiments described during the workshop indicated that, although growth arrest was very effectively achieved by these manipulations in vitro, N-*myc* expression was not detectably altered. These findings were interpreted as indicating that the decreased expression of N-*myc* described above is associated with the differentiation of these neuronal cells and not with their altered growth potential.

In related experiments, P. Maness (University of North Carolina, Chapel Hill) described the developmentally regulated expression of c-*src* [3].These studies were unique in that they utilized an in vivo-based approach and highlighted immunocyto-chemical analysis of embryonic tissue specimens as a complement to biochemical studies of excised embryonal tissues. Dr. Maness demonstrated the expression of c-*src* in a diversity of chick embryonic tissues, although it was especially high in the nervous system. Earlier studies describing very high levels of pp60c-*src* tyrosine kinase activity in nervous system tissues were discussed, but participants were especially interested in Dr. Maness's description of the dramatic increase in c-*src* expression that occurs during early development of the retina and diminishes just before birth. Interestingly, this burst of c-*src* expression occurs about the time at which growth is arrested. Together with the observation that fetal tissues invariably have a higher level of c-*src* than corresponding adult tissues, although even adult nervous system tissues express high levels of c-*src*, these data were interpreted as suggesting a developmental role for c-*src*.

Other studies by Dr. Maness focusing on the expression of c-*src* very early in avian development extended these findings and stimulated discussion among the workshop's participants. By means of immunohistochemical analysis of tissue specimens from embryos during the first 2 days after fertilization, it was possible to observe c-*src* expression during gastrulation and formation of the neural tube. At this time expression appeared to be localized to neural ectoderm, with only the suggestion of limited expression in tissues of the other embryonic layers. Although c-*src* was expressed in neural ectoderm throughout the course of development, the highest levels were noted in very early specimens before neural tube closure. These findings were appreciated as important evidence for a developmental role for c-*src* at very early times that might be distinct from the role it plays late in development.

The workshop ended with a discussion of how investigators might utilize available reagents and techniques to evaluate more efficaciously the distribution of proto-oncogene expression in embryonic tissues. The importance of new techniques to prepare antipeptide as well as conventional antibodies for immunohistochemical studies was stressed. The hope that such reagents would become commercially available and thereby increase the number of investigators who would have access to them was a clearly expressed sentiment. The advantages and pitfalls of using in situ hybridization to molecular probes for similar experiments were also discussed. Most investigators seemed to believe that the difficulty of establishing this procedure in their laboratories, and the apparent insensitivity of currently available experimental techniques, would greatly limit its usefulness.

Participants in this workshop indicated clearly their enthusiasm for the evaluation of proto-oncogenes as mediators of the molecular processes by which cells progress along lineage-specific differentiation pathways. No consensus was reached on whether these same genes were likely to play a role in the commitment process. Several investigators suggested that future research would not only broaden our knowledge of the distribution of proto-oncogene expression during development, but also would be directed at more mechanistic questions. Eukaryotic systems, other than mammalian cells, were considered to be settings in which to gain initial insights into the mechanisms by which the effects of such regulatory genes are mediated. On the other hand, there was considerable interest in the use of gene transfer techniques in mammalian cells to pursue functional studies. Participants agreed that study of the aberrations in differentiation and growth control found in malignant tissues might provide opportunities to identify developmental functions for these genes that would not otherwise be evaluable [5].

REFERENCES

1. Leibovitch MP, Leibovitch SA, Hillion J, Guillier M, Schmitz A, Harel J: Exp Cell Res 170:80–92, 1987.
2. Caffrey JM, Brown AM, Schneider MD: Science 236:570–573, 1987.
3. Maness PF, Sorge LK, Fults DW: Dev Bio 117:83–89, 1986.
4. Thiele CJ, Reynolds CP, Israel MA, Nature 313(6001):404–406, 1985.
5. Israel MA, Helman LJ, Miser J: In DeVita VT, Hellman S, Rosenberg SA (eds): "Important Advances in Oncology 1987." Philadelphia: J.B. Lippincott, 1987, pp 87–104.

Growth Regulation of Cancer
205–211 (1988)

Host Microenvironment Determinants in Cancer Metastasis

Isaiah J. Fidler and Janet E. Price

Department of Cell Biology, The University of Texas, M.D. Anderson Hospital and Tumor Institute at Houston, Houston, Texas 77030

The process of metastasis consists of a sequence of events during which tumor cells disseminate from a primary site to distant organs. It is generally regarded as a selective process, as only the tumor cells possessing multiple properties will survive interactions with host factors and produce metastases; these cells represent only a minor subset of the heterogeneous neoplastic population. These findings agree with the concept forwarded by Paget that metastasis results only when certain tumor cells ("seeds") can favorably interact with certain organs ("soil"). Metastasis, therefore, can be regarded as a selective biological process whose outcome is regulated by the interaction of tumor cells with the host. As such, the process must be governed by mechanisms that can be studied and ultimately understood in sufficient detail to allow rational therapeutic interaction.

Key words: metastasis, organ environment, selection, growth factors

Recently, well-deserving emphasis has been given to the effect(s) that various host-derived and tumor-derived growth factors have on the development and growth of neoplasms. It is therefore most appropriate that in this review on the pathogenesis of metastasis, we emphasize the unique interactions of tumor cells with host organ microenvironment.

The most devastating aspect of cancer is the propensity of malignant cells to spread from a primary site to distant organs where new lesions develop. Indeed, the majority of deaths from cancer are attributed to the continued proliferation of metastases that are resistant to conventional therapeutics. There are several reasons for the failure of treatment for established metastases. First, by the time of diagnosis of primary tumors, metastasis may have already occurred, although the lesions are often too small to be detected. Second, the anatomic location of many metastases may limit the effective dose of therapeutic agents that can be delivered to the lesions without being toxic to normal tissues. Third, and the most formidable problem, is the heterogeneous nature of malignant neoplasms, which leads to the rapid biological diversification of tumor cells and to the development of resistance to conventional therapy [1–5].

Received February 19, 1987.

By the time of diagnosis, malignant neoplasms contain multiple cell populations that exhibit almost limitless biological heterogeneity. Cells obtained from individual tumors can be different with respect to cell surface properties, immunogenicity, antigenicity, growth rate, karyotype, sensitivity to various cytotoxic drugs, and the ability to invade and metastasize [1–7]. Biological heterogeneity is not confined to cells in primary tumors and is equally prominent among the cells populating metastases [1,3]. Many clinical observations reveal that multiple metastases proliferating in different organs or even in the same organ are heterogeneous in many biological characteristics such as hormone receptors, antigenicity-immunogenicity, and sensitivity to various chemotherapeutic drugs. This biological diversity may be due to the nature of the metastatic process, or to the process of tumor evolution and progression, or to both.

THE PROCESS OF CANCER METASTASIS

The process of metastasis begins with the local invasion of the surrounding host stroma by either single cells or clumps of cells from the primary tumors. Once the invading tumor cells have gained entrance into the vascular channels, they may grow at the site of penetration, or detach as single cells or aggregates to be carried in the circulatory system where they are susceptible to various host immune and nonimmune defenses, such as blood turbulence, lymphocytes, natural killer cells, and monocytes. Tumor cells that survive in the circulation can arrest in the capillary beds of distant organs and then extravasate into the organ parenchyma. To proliferate in the organ parenchyma, the tumor cells first respond to local growth factors, and then develop a vascular network. When the micrometastases have attained a certain size, they may give rise to additional metastases. Thus, in a short time, a small primary tumor can produce a multitude of distant metastases [5,6,8,9].

To produce a clinically relevant metastasis, malignant tumor cells must complete a number of sequential and potentially lethal interactions with host homeostatic mechanisms, which include various host defenses. Failure to complete any of the steps in metastasis leads to the elimination of the disseminating tumor cell. The complexity of the metastatic process explains, in part, why the presence of tumor cells in the circulation does not predict that metastasis will occur. In fact, most tumor cells that enter the bloodstream are rapidly eliminated [10]. Using radiolabeled tumor cells, we have observed that after entry into the circulation, < 0.1% of tumor cells survived to produce metastases [10]. This observation prompted us to question whether the 0.1% of the circulating cells that were responsible for the development of metastases survived at random, or whether the cells represented the selective survival and growth of pre-existent subpopulations of cells endowed with special properties [11]. In other words, do neoplasms exhibit metastatic heterogeneity? Can all cells growing in a malignant neoplasm produce metastases, or can only unique cells produce secondary lesions? The first experimental proof for metastatic heterogeneity in neoplasms was provided by Fidler and Kripke in 1977 working with the murine B16 melanoma [12]. Based on the modified fluctuation assay of Luria and Delbruck [13], we demonstrated that different tumor cell clones isolated from the parent tumor varied dramatically in their potential to form pulmonary tumor colonies following i.v. inoculation into syngeneic mice. Control subcloning procedures demonstrated that the observed diversity was not a consequence of the cloning procedure

[12]. The finding that pre-existing tumor cell subpopulations growing in the same tumor exhibit heterogeneous metastatic potential has since been confirmed in numerous laboratories using a wide range of experimental animal tumors of different histories and histological origins [1–7,14]. Similar data have recently been documented for human neoplasms implanted into nude mice [15].

PAGET'S "SEED AND SOIL" HYPOTHESIS

Clinical observations of cancer patients have concluded that certain tumors have a marked predilection for metastasis to specific organs, and that these metastatic patterns are not merely determined by vascular anatomy, rate of blood flow, and number of tumor cells reaching an organ. Interest in factors that affect metastatic patterns is not new. In 1889, the pathologist Paget analyzed 735 autopsies of women with breast cancer and concluded that the nonrandom pattern of breast cancer metastases was not due to chance; rather, some tumor cells ("seeds") traveling by vascular routes had affinity for growth in the environment provided by certain organs ("soil"). The development of metastases occurred only when the "seed and soil" were matched [16]. Recent experiments have shown that site-specific metastasis occurs with many transplantable experimental tumors [1–7,17] and has been reported recently in autochthonous human tumors in patients with peritoneovenous shunts [18–20]. A present definition of the "seed and soil" hypothesis could consist of three important principles. First, the process of metastasis is not random. Second, neoplasms are not uniform entities but contain cells exhibiting heterogeneous metastatic capabilities. Third, the outcome of metastasis depends on the properties of tumor cells and host factors, and the balance of their contributions varies among tumors arising in different tissues, and even among tumors of similar histologic origin in different patients.

THE INFLUENCE OF ORGAN MICROENVIRONMENT ON THE GROWTH OF METASTASES

Studies using experimental animal tumor systems have demonstrated that the formation and anatomical location of metastases are determined by host factors and tumor cell properties [1]. The distribution and fate of hematogenously disseminated radiolabeled tumor cells in rodent systems demonstrate that tumor cells reach and arrest in the microvasculature of many organs. Tumor cell proliferation that results in visible metastases occurs in only some of the organs tumor cells reach. Thus, the arrest of viable tumor cells in an organ does not guarantee that metastases will develop [1].

Experimental data derived in mouse tumor systems supporting the "seed and soil" hypothesis of Paget were first reported by Kinsey [21] and then by Sugarbaker et al. [22]. We carried out experiments to determine whether metastatic tumor cells arrest specifically in some organs where metastases develop, or whether metastatic tumor cells distribute to many organs but proliferate in only particular sites. We also questioned whether the mechanical arrest of circulating tumor emboli can explain the unique patterns of metastasis of B16 melanoma, or whether tumor cell and organ affinities were responsible for the growth of metastatic foci [23].

The preferential growth of B16 melanoma metastases in specific organs was therefore studied. Following the i.v. injection of B16 melanoma cells into syngeneic

C57BL/6 mice, tumor growths developed in the in situ lungs and in fragments of lung or ovary implanted either subcutaneously or intramuscularly into the quadriceps femoris. Melanoma lesions did not develop in control implanted kidney tissue or at the site of surgical trauma. Parabiosis experiments suggested that the formation of tumors at the transplanted organ was due to the arrest and growth of tumor cells immediately following intravenous injection and not to shedding of malignant cells from foci growing in the in situ lungs. Two weeks after normal, tumor-free mice were joined parabiotically to tumor-bearing animals, there was no evidence of any tumor growth in the "guest" animals. However, when the parabiont animals were allowed to survive for 4 weeks after separation from the tumor-bearing animals, 40% developed lung metastases [23].

To determine whether tumor growth in ectopically implanted organs was due to organ-specific arrest of intravenously injected cells, we monitored the organ distribution of radiolabeled melanoma cells. By 10 min after injection of $[^{125}I]$ IdUrd-labeled cells, no more than 0.8% of the total number of injected cells was found in the hind legs where lung or kidney fragments were implanted. No significant differences were detected between the number of cells lodged in limbs bearing kidney (tumor negative) or lung (tumor positive); between transplant-bearing limbs and the opposite, nonoperated limb, which served as a control; or among the different implanted organs [23].

These data clearly demonstrate the organ-specific growth of the mouse B16 melanoma and illustrate the difficulty encountered in past studies in defining tumor cell "homing." Although B16 melanoma cells do indeed produce gross metastases in the lungs and gonads, it is not apparent that the distribution of metastases can be explained merely by the initial lodgment of tumor cells in these organs. Rather, the lung and gonads provide a receptive organ ("soil") for the multiplication of a few surviving tumor cells.

The patterns of metastasis formation in human patients cannot be explained by blood flow alone [24,25]. For example, a study of the distribution of melanoma metastases in 56 patients concluded that the patterns of metastasis may be related to the embryological derivation or functional properties of the organ tissues affected [26]. That the role of organs as the "soil" is not totally passive has been suggested by studies showing that damage elicited by injury or radiation can enhance metastasis formation, a phenomenon termed "inflammatory oncotaxis" [27].

For obvious reasons, experimental analysis of human tumor dissemination in the ways it has been investigated in animal systems cannot be approved. The introduction of peritoneovenous (p.v.) shunts for palliation of malignant ascites in patients with terminal cancer provided an opportunity to study some of the factors affecting metastatic spread in humans. In a series of elegant studies, Tarin and colleagues [18–20,28] followed the pathology of the disease in patients with different primary tumors. The autopsy findings from 15 patients reflected the clinical observations that the p.v. shunts do not carry the risk of promoting significant metastasis. In eight patients, small metastases were found in extra-abdominal organs (most commonly lungs), possibly seeded since the p.v. shunts were inserted, but these tumor foci were not clinically detectable. In the other seven patients there was no evidence of tumor foci outside the abdomen, even in cases where the p.v. shunt had functioned for several months, and in one case longer than 2 years [18].

Malignant neoplasms do not need the intervention of p.v. shunts to disseminate cells; however, the negative findings in half of these patients are of importance. The identification of cytological markers (psammoma bodies) in the tumors of two patients confirmed the widespread distribution of cells to many organs, but resulting tumor proliferation was seen in only few organ sites or none at all [18,20]. The p.v. shunt findings are directly comparable with those from animal tumor studies, confirming that although viable tumorigenic cells may be distributed to many organs, proliferation into metastases only occurs in few sites, often characteristics for the particular neoplasm. The studies, therefore, provide verification of the near century-old, "seed and soil" hypothesis [16]. Laboratory investigation of properties of the ascites tumor cells and correlation with the metastatic behavior affords opportunities to find markers of metastatic potential and for further research into why tumor cells grow in some organ sites and not others.

THE INFLUENCE OF HOST MICROENVIRONMENT ON THE BIOLOGIC BEHAVIOR OF METASTATIC CELLS

The growth of tumor cells in a given organ is not a random event. Although the mechanisms responsible for organ specific metastasis are not well understood, it is certain that they depend on the interaction of specific tumor cells with organ microenvironment [1].

The response of metastases to therapeutic agents could well depend on the organ site for growth. For example, clinical observations have suggested that the response of metastases in women with breast cancer is influenced by the anatomical location of the lesions. With few exceptions, the metastases in lymph nodes and skin have a better prognosis and treatment response than skeletal or pulmonary metastases [29–31]. The viability and growth of tumor cells depend on an adequate source of nutrients. The degree of tumor vascularity can control the delivery of nutrients, clearance of metabolites, and the delivery of cytotoxic drugs to the lesion. Measurements of blood flow in subcutaneous tumors of rats revealed a lack of autoregulation in response to infusions of angiotensin II. The selective increase in tumor blood flow, with no increase in normal tissues, could therefore enhance chemotherapeutic drug delivery [32]. Moreover, the extent of tumor angiogenesis [33], a host response to a growing neoplasm, can differ among different organs and thus contribute to differential growth of some metastases.

Another example for the ability of an organ environment to influence a biological property of tumor cells comes from our recent studies with a murine melanoma. The K-1735 melanoma is a transplantable UV light induced tumor [34] that produces both pigmented and unpigmented metastases in syngeneic C_3H/HeN mice. The metastases are primarily found in the lungs, but extrapulmonary tumor foci are common. The tumor is heterogeneous and contains cells with different metastatic properties, as well as pigmentation [35]. Clonal analysis of the tumor revealed that many clones were tumorigenic but not metastatic. Other clones were metastatic, and the metastases varied in their size and pigmentation. Some clones produced melanotic lesions, whereas others produced amelanotic lesions [35].

The variant line K-1735 SW-1 was isolated from a small amelanotic lung metastasis produced in a C3H/HeN mouse by parent K-1735 melanoma cells growing subcutaneously [36]. The lesion was enzymatically dissociated and cells established as a monolayer culture. Under culture conditions the cells did not produce melanin. When reinjected intravenously, the SW-1 cells produced numerous amelanotic deposits in the lungs and other organs, and melanin was seen only in tumors growing in the brain in two mice, suggesting a possible relationship between melanin synthesis and site of tumor growth.

We carried out detailed studies to investigate the relationship of the host microenvironment to the metastatic and pigmented phenotypes. Cells of K-1735 SW-1 line were highly metastatic and produced lesions in many organs. In all organs except the brain, the lesions were predominantly amelanotic. K1735 SW-1 cells were isolated from different organ metastases and subsequently reinoculated into normal syngeneic recipients. Whereas the metastatic phenotype was stably expressed, and thus heritable, pigmentation was not and appeared to be modulated by the site of tumor growth.

The findings that tumor cells can produce a product when growing in some organ sites but not others, and certainly not when growing in culture, recommend the need for caution in extrapolating the results of biochemical assays performed on tumor cells in vitro to the behavior of these cells in vivo. For example, it is possible that in addition to melanin synthesis, the production of proteolytic enzymes or expression of hormone receptors occurs in K-1735 SW-1 cells growing in one organ site and not another. Similar to the example of tyrosinase activity in K-1735 SW-1 cells, the production of a given enzyme may not be detected when the tumor cells are cultured in vitro. Thus, the biochemical analyses of the cultured cells might erroneously lead to the conclusion that this enzyme is not produced by the tumor cells in vivo.

CONCLUSIONS

The process of cancer metastasis is not random. Metastatic tumor cells must complete a series of steps to reach an organ parenchyma, and then proliferate to produce clinically relevant metastases. The proliferation of cells in an organ environment is dependent on the favorable interaction of metastatic cells with organ growth factors. It is conceivable that specific organ factors can either directly stimulate the growth of tumor cells or act as signals for the production of growth factors from the tumor cells. In either case, it is the interaction of the "seed" with the favorable "soil" that determines whether metastases will be produced. For this reason, it is important that organ-derived growth factors receive their due attention.

ACKNOWLEDGMENTS

This work was supported by the R.E. "Bob" Smith Chair in Cell Biology.

REFERENCES

1. Fidler IJ: In Nicolson GL (ed): "Cancer Invasion and Metastasis: Biologic and Therapeutic Aspects." New York: Raven Press, 1984, pp 5–30.
2. Hart IR, Fidler IJ: Biochem Biophys Acta 651:37, 1981.
3. Fidler IJ, Poste G: Semin Oncol 12:207, 1985.
4. Fidler IJ, Hart IR: Science 217:998, 1982.
5. Heppner G: Cancer Res 44:2259, 1984.
6. Poste G, Fidler IJ: Nature 283:139, 1979.
7. Nicolson GL, Poste G: Curr Probl Cancer 7:4, 1982.
8. Fidler IJ, Gersten DM, Hart IR: Adv Cancer Res 28:149, 1978.

9. Weiss L: "Principles of Metastasis." New York: Academic Press, 1985.
10. Fidler IJ: JNCI 45:773, 1970.
11. Fidler IJ: Nature (New Biol) 242:148, 1973.
12. Fidler IJ, Kripke ML: Science 197:893, 1977.
13. Luria SE, Delbruck M: Genetics 28:491, 1943.
14. Nicolson GL: Clin Expl Met 2:85, 1984.
15. Fidler IJ: Cancer Metastasis Rev 5:29, 1986.
16. Paget S: Lancet 1:571, 1889.
17. Nicolson GL: Cancer Met Rev 3:25, 1984.
18. Tarin D, Vass ACR, Kettlewell MGW, Price JE: Invasion Metastasis 4:1, 1984.
19. Tarin D, Price JE, Kettlewell MGW, Souter RG, Vass ACR, Crossley B: Br Med J 288:749, 1984.
20. Tarin D, Price JE, Kettlewell MGW, Souter RG, Vass ACR, Crossley B: Cancer Res 44:3584, 1984.
21. Kinsey DL: Cancer 13:874, 1960.
22. Sugarbaker EV, Cohen AM, Ketcham AS: Ann Surg 174:161, 1971.
23. Hart IR, Fidler IJ: Cancer Res 40:2281, 1980.
24. Willis RA: "The Spread of Tumors in the Human Body," 3rd ed. London: Butterworth, 1972.
25. Tarin D: In Weiss L (ed): "Fundamental Aspects of Metastasis." Amsterdam: North-Holland Publishing Co., 1976, pp 151–170.
26. dela Monte SM, Moore GW, Hutchins GM: Cancer Res 43:3427, 1983.
27. DerHagopian RP, Sugarbaker EV, Ketcham A: JAMA 240:374, 1978.
28. Souter RG, Tarin D, Kettlewell MGW: Br J Surg 70:478, 1983.
29. Brambilla C, Delena M, Rossi A, Valagussa P, Bonadonna G: Br Med J 1:801, 1976.
30. Canellos GP, Devita VT, Gold GL, Chabner BA, Schein PS, Young RC: Br Med J 1:218, 1974.
31. Slack NH, Bross JBJ: Br J Cancer 32:78, 1975.
32. Suzuki M, Hori K, Abe I, Saito S, Sato H: JNCI 67:663, 1981.
33. Folkman J: Cancer Res 46:467, 1986.
34. Kripke ML: JNCI 63:541, 1979.
35. Fidler IJ, Gruys E, Cifone MA, Barnes Z, Bucana C: JNCI 67:947, 1981.
36. Talmadge JE, Fidler IJ: JNCI 69:975, 1982.

Growth Regulation of Cancer
213–220 (1988)

Repression of Glucocorticoid Hormone-Dependent Transcription of the Mouse Mammary Tumor Virus LTR by the P37 V-MOS Oncogene Product

Bernd Groner, Robert R. Friis, Alexandra Schläfli, and Rolf Jaggi

Ludwig Institute for Cancer Research, Inselspital, CH-3010 Bern, Switzerland

Transcriptional regulation by oncogenes has been studied in transfected NIH 3T3 mouse fibroblasts. For this purpose the v-mos oncogene coding region was subjected to the control of the hormone-dependent promotor of the mouse mammary tumor virus LTR. The LTR v-mos gene was introduced into NIH 3T3 cells and its transcription and phenotypic effects were studied in the absence and presence of glucocorticoid hormone in the growth medium. No transcription was observed in the absence of hormone and the cells were phenotypically normal. Addition of hormone to the medium results in LTR transcription and a morphologically transformed phenotype. Accumulation of the p37 v-mos oncogene product reduces the efficiency of LTR transcription to about 5% of the maximal level observed shortly after hormone addition. The hormonally regulated MMTV LTR transcription provides a model for oncogene-mediated interference with gene expression.

Key words: inducible oncogene expression, hormone response element, transcriptional regulation

The concept of oncogenes [1] promises the introduction of some order in the description of the large number of naturally occurring tumors affecting different cell types and organs. This promise is based on the assumption that only a relatively small number of genes may classify as oncogenes, i.e., contribute to the primary event in the transformation process [2,3]. This contribution is caused by mutation of the protooncogene form of recessive or dominantly acting oncogenes and results in an alteration of the expression levels or biochemical functions of these genes. Research has focused on 1) the identification of oncogenes and the genetic basis of their activation, 2) the biochemical function of oncogene products, and 3) the consequences of oncogene activation on cellular gene expression. The consequences of oncogene expression may be the most complex of these aspects and little molecular information on the pathways involved is available. The transformed phenotype is likely to be a

Received March 24, 1987.

consequence of altered cellular gene expression. Potentially a large number of cellular genes might be qualitatively or quantitatively deregulated in oncogene expression cells [4]. The signals generated by the oncogene products, the identification of their cellular target sequences, and the mechanisms by which they effect target genes is therefore an important step in the molecular description of the transformation process.

We have used the conditional transformation of NIH 3T3 cells to address the question of transcriptional regulation by oncogenes. For this purpose we have introduced a v-mos oncogene under the control of the MMTV LTR into cultured cells. We selected transfectants strictly dependent in their morphological phenotype on the glucocorticoid regulated oncogene expression. Our experiments show that the MMTV LTR itself is an oncogene target, i.e., the accumulation of p37 v-mos causes a repression of the hormone-dependent transcription [5]. A model is proposed in which the activation of a latent transcriptional regulator (TR) by p37 v-mos leads to a functional interference with the DNA-protein complex comprising the glucocorticoid receptor, the hormone response element (HRE), and possibly other transcription factors.

NIH 3T3 CELLS REVERSIBLY TRANSFORMED BY AN MMTV LTR V-MOS GENE CONSTRUCT

Conditional transformation can be obtained by a temperature shift of cells harboring temperature-sensitive oncogene products or by the introduction into cells of oncogenes transcriptionally controlled by an inducible promoter. The first strategy was successfully applied, e.g., in the case of the v-src gene [6]. It necessitates, however, the availability of rarely occurring spontaneous mutants. The second strategy allows a more systematic approach making use of the well-defined properties of the promoter contained in the mouse mammary tumor virus LTR. This proviral promotor is transcriptionally silent when introduced as a chimeric gene construct into cultured fibroblasts. It can be induced to a high transcriptional activity by addition of glucocorticoid hormone to the culture medium [7]. We have combined the viral mos gene [8], encoding a 374 amino acid protein (p37 v-mos), with the MMTV LTR (Fig. 1). This construct contains the entire U3 region of the MMTV LTR, which harbors the hormone response element (HRE), the R region, and 106 nucleotides of the U5 region. The transcriptional start is located at the 5′ border of R as indicated in Figure 1. The translational intiation condon and the entire protein coding region are contributed by the v-mos fragment. A polyadenylation signal has been added at the 3′ side of the v-mos coding fragment [5].

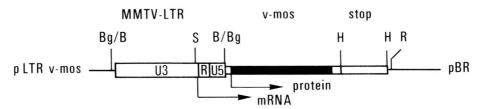

Fig. 1.   Diagram of the MMTV LTR v-mos chimeric gene construct [5]. The LTR of MMTV provides the transcriptional regulation to the gene. A promoter element and a hormone response element are contained in the U3 region [7,9]. RNA synthesis is initiated at the 5′ side of the R region (indicated by an arrow). The protein coding sequence is contributed the v-mos fragment (indicated by an arrow) [8].

DNA mediated gene transfer was used to introduce the LTR v-mos construct into NIH 3T3 cells. Transfected cells grown in the absence of glucocorticoid hormone are phenotypically not distinguishable from untransfected control cells. The addition of hormone to the growth medium resulted in a morphological transformation within 24 hrs. The transformed phenotype could also be observed in cells grown in soft agar. Only transfected cells grown in the presence of glucocorticoid hormone were able to grow anchorage independently and form soft agar colonies. Transfected cells injected into nude mice formed tumors with a short latency. Nontransfected NIH 3T3 cells did not form tumors [5]. The circulating levels of glucocorticoids in the animals are probably sufficient to induce the LTR v-mos oncogene construct and are thus responsible for the oncogene activation. The transformation parameters tested in vitro, soft agar growth and morphological appearance, were reversed when the hormone was removed from the culture medium. This shows that the continous presence of p37 v-mos is required to maintain the transformed phenotype and that the MMTV LTR transcription returns to an undetectable level in the absence of hormone.

MMTV LTR TRANSCRIPTION REPRESSED BY V-MOS ONCOGENE EXPRESSION

The MMTV LTR contains a hormone response element located at position − 59 to − 202 with respect to the RNA initiation site [9]. This sequence is required for the hormonal induction of transcription in vivo and is able to preferentially interact with the glucocorticoid receptor in vitro [10]. The hormonal effect on transcription is thought to be mediated through the association of the hormone receptor complex with target sequences adjacent to a regulated gene and results in an increase in the rate of initiation of RNA synthesis [11]. The effect of glucocorticoid hormone on the rate of RNA transcription can be visualized. For this purpose nuclei were prepared from LTR v-mos transfected cells incubated with glucocorticoid hormone for 0, 1, and 5 hr in vivo. The nuclei were incubated in vitro under conditions that allow elongation of RNA molecules initiated in vivo and the incorporation of radioactive precursors offered in vitro. Only in vitro synthesized RNA becomes radioactive. Nuclear RNA is then hybridized to specific filter-bound DNA sequences and the hybridization signals obtained can be considered proportional to the transcription rate. Figure 2, lane 1 shows the transcriptional activity of the LTR v-mos gene in the absence of hormone. A signal for v-mos transcription is observed that is very similar to the background signal. The transcription rate is induced to a maximal level within 1 hr after hormone addition (lane 3). A signal similar to the one observed at 0 time is obtained from nuclei of cells stimulated for 5 hr with glucocorticoid hormone (lane 7). The decrease in the LTR v-mos transcriptional rate is due to the expression of the v-mos oncogene. We have shown previously that a similar effect of oncogene accumulation can be observed when the activated human H-ras oncogene is induced in NIH 3T3 cells. The nonactivated protooncogene form of the human H-ras gene does not repress MMTV LTR transcription [5].

Additional evidence for the involvement of the p37 v-mos oncogene product was obtained in protein synthesis inhibition experiments. Simultaneous protein synthesis is not required for the induction of the MMTV LTR by glucocorticoid hormone. All protein components required for the transcriptional induction pre-exist and are merely functionally activated by the addition of hormone [12]. This observation is

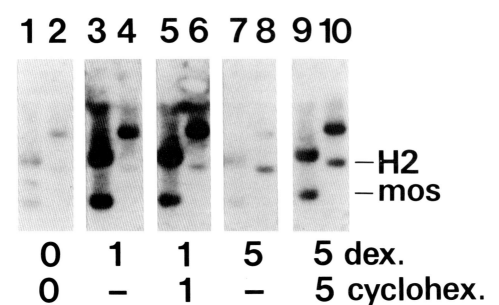

1 2 3 4 5 6 7 8 9 10

−H2
−mos

0   1   1   5   5 dex.
0   −   1   −   5 cyclohex.

Fig. 2.   Transcriptional rate measurements of the transfected LTR v-mos and endogenous H2 genes in NIH 3T3 cells. The transcriptional rates were measured in NIH 3T3 cells grown in the absence (lanes 1,2) or presence of 10^{-6} M dexamethasone (1 hr [lanes 3–6], 5 hr [lanes 7–10]). Cycloheximide was added to in inhibit protein synthesis to cells analyzed in lanes 5,6 and 9,10. ^{32}P-labeled, run-on RNA was synthesized in 10^6 isolated nuclei in vitro for 20 min at 26°C. RNA was extracted and hybridized to 1 μg of DNA restriction fragment separated by gel electorphoresis and immobilized on nitrocellulose filters. The DNA immobilized in lanes, 1,3,5,7,8 represents a v-mos containing plasmid. The position of a 1.3 kb restriction fragment is indicated as mos. The autoradiographic signal at this position is proportional to the LTR v-mos gene transcription rate. A H-2 L^d specific restriction fragment of 2 kb is immobilized in lanes 2,4,6,8,10 [25]. The hybridization signal is proportional to the transcription rate of the H-2 genes expressed in NIH 3T3 cells.

confirmed in Figure 2, lane 5, where the transcriptional rate of the LTR v-mos gene is measured 1 hr after hormone addition to the transfected cells. Protein synthesis was inhibited by cycloheximide simultaneously with the addition of hormone. The signal obtained is very similar to the signal produced in cells grown in the absence of the protein synthesis inhibitor (lane 3). A drastic effect of the protein synthesis inhibition, however, was observed 5 hr after hormone addition. Whereas p37 v-mos accumulated in cells grown in the absence of inhibitor and caused the transcriptional repression of the MMTV LTR (lane 7), inhibition of protein synthesis prevents p37 v-mos accumulation and a high level of MMTV LTR transcription is maintained (lane 9). The rates of RNA synthesis for major histocompatibility genes (H2) were measured simultaneously as controls and are shown in lanes 2,4,6,8, and 10. Similar rates are observed in the absence and presence of hormone (lanes 2,4, and 8). Cycloheximide seems to exert an induction of H2 transcription (lane 10).

These experiments show that the MMTV LTR transcription rate is specifically repressed in cells in which the oncogene product accumulates. Inhibition of oncogene product synthesis prevents the oncogene mediated repression.

P37 V-MOS ACTS VIA HORMONE RESPONSE ELEMENT; DOES NOT SUPPRESS EARLY INDUCTION

The interference of p37 v-mos with hormonally induced MMTV LTR transcription caused us to investigate possible mechanisms of action. The extensive studies on the sequence requirements for hormonal induction of MMTV LTR transcription were utilized to define the target of the signal originating at p37 v-mos. In vitro deletion analysis and recombination of MMTV LTR fragments with heterologous genes have yielded the definition of the hormone response element (HRE). This sequence is located at position -59 to -202 with respect to the viral RNA initiation site [9]. The HRE is necessary to confer hormonal induction to viral RNA transcription, but it also functions in an autonomous fashion when recombined with other genes. Hormonal responsiveness can be conferred ont the α-globin promoter when the HRE is combined either 5' or 3' in both possible orientations with the α-globin gene (HRE α-globin). Hormonal responsiveness is therefore dependent on the presence of the HRE in the vicinity of a promoter element, but relatively independent of the distance, orientation, and position with respect to the regulated gene [9,13]. This definition is similar to that of an enhancer element, i.e., the HRE can be described as conditional or inducible enhancer.

We investigated the effect of p37 v-mos on the constitutive transcription and hormonal induction of the HRE-α-globin gene construct. For this purpose HRE-α-globin transfected cells were infected with Moloney murine sarcoma virus (MoMSV) [8]. Cell clones expressing the p37 v-mos oncogene product were selected. The cells were induced with dexamethasone and the rate of transcription of the α-globin gene was determined. A basal level of transcription was observed in the absence of hormone. An increased rate was measured after 3 hr and a return to the basal level was observed after 5 to 16 hr (data not shown). This experiment shows that the oncogene effect is mediated via the HRE. The HRE enhancer function is repressed by a signal emanating from p37 v-mos, whereas the basal function of the α-globin gene promoter is not affected.

The inducibility of the HRE α-globin gene construct in MoMSV infected NIH 3T3 cells is not necessarily expected. The cells express p37 v-mos constitutively and thereby might interfere with the hormonal induction process even at early times after hormone addition. The observation that early inducibility is maintained in cells infected with MoMSV allows two conclusions: 1) the components that comprise the hormonal induction machinery (e.g., the glucocorticoid hormone receptor) are not affected in their expression by p37 v-mos; transcription, translation, and functional activation occurs in an apparently normal fashion in the presence of p37 v-mos, and 2) the formation of a functional complex involving the interaction of the HRE sequence with the glucocorticoid receptor and possibly other transcription factors like the NF-1 (= CTF) [14,15] precedes the interference by the p37 v-mos generated signal. It seems likely that the interaction of factors is disturbed and not their expression.

MODEL FOR P37 V-MOS INDUCED INTERFERENCE WITH MMTV LTR TRANSCRIPTION

An integration of the experiments and observations described here and elsewhere was attempted and a partially hypothetical model is shown in Figure 3. The model originates at the interaction of the glucocorticoid receptor (GR) with the cellular protein hsp 90 (1 in Fig. 3). This interaction is thought to mask the DNA binding ability of the GR. Experimental support for the postulation of such a complex comes from: 1) the molecular weight studies of unoccupied receptor [16], 2) the demonstration that partially purified cytoplasmic receptor can possibly be dissociated

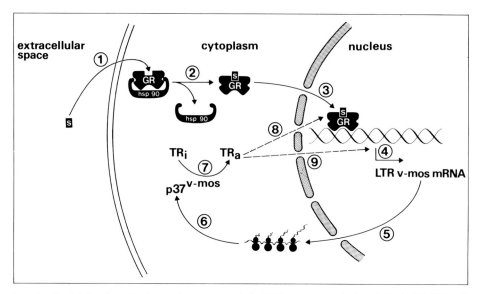

Fig. 3.   Model for the activation and repression of the LTR v-mos gene in transfected NIH 3T3 cells. (1) Glucocorticoid hormone (S) binds to the glucocorticoid receptor (GR). The formation of the GR-S complex is accompanied by the dissociation of the heat shock protein 90 (hsp 90) from the GR (2). The GR-S complex binds to the hormone response element (HRE) of the MMTV LTR (3) and possibly triggers the binding of additional transcription factors NF-1 and F-i [Ref. 15]. Transcription of the LTR v-mos RNA is initiated (4) and mRNA accumulates (5). The mRNA is translated (6) and p37 v-mos is synthesized. The p37 v-mos causes the transition of an inactive transcriptional regulator (TR$_i$) to an active one (TR$_a$). TR$_a$ interacts with either the GR (8) or the complex of transcription factors (9) and functionally interferes with the initiation of LTR v-mos RNA.

from hsp 90 and thereby gain specific DNA binding ability [17], and 3) the in vivo genomic footprinting experiments that show that unoccupied receptor is not bound to HRE sequences [18]. The association of steroid hormone with its receptor is thought to result in the release of the masking protein in vivo (2 in Fig. 3) and binding to specific HRE sequences located in the vicinity of steroid regulated genes (3 in Fig. 3). The binding of the GR to the HRE is thought to cause the enhancer activation and increased transcription from the MMTV LTR (4 in Fig. 3). This process, most likely, does not merely activate a pre-existing transcriptional complex [15]. The identification of additional factors involved in MMTV LTR transcription has shown that the nuclear factor-1 (NF-1) binds to sequences between position -58 and -81 in the MMTV LTR [19]. This factor is identical to the transcription factor CTF, which is responsible for the selective recognition of eukaryotic promoters with a CCAAT box element [14]. A second factor (F-i) was described that binds to sequences from -41 to $+1$ in vitro [15]. The binding of both factors in vivo seems to be dependent on GR binding to the HRE, i.e., cooperate interactions between the GR and at least two other factors are required to establish a transcription complex [15]. A cascade of binding events, led by the recognition of the HRE by GR, has been proposed. The GR binding might result in the subsequent NF-1 and F-1 binding [15]. In such a model all the transcription factors are present and potentially active [20,21]; they require, however, an initiating binding event by the GR for their functional activation [15].

The binding of GR and the other transcription factors to the HRE in the MMTV LTR promoter region results in an increased rate of LTR v-mos transcription (4 in Fig. 3); mRNA is accumulated (5 in Fig. 3) and translated (6 in Fig. 3). The p37 v-mos oncogene product then generates a signal (7 in Fig. 3) that results in the interference with LTR transcription (8 or 9 in Fig. 3). The subcellular location of p37 v-mos as a cytoplasmic, soluble protein [22] makes it unlikely that p37 v-mos interacts directly with the HRE or the HRE-GR complex. For this reason, we postulate an interaction with a hypothetical transcriptional regulator (TR). The influence on the functional activity of the TR could possibly be exerted by the protein kinase activity ascribed to the p37 v-mos oncogene product [23]. This change from an inactive TR (TR_i) to an active TR (TR_a) could be conceived as a reason for the influence of p37 v-mos on a variety of cellular genes. TR_a might be capable of up-regulation of a set of genes and down-regulation of a different set. Our data support the notion that TR_a does not change the expression or functionality of the transcription factors involved in MMTV LTR transcription. The maintenance of early induction in MoMSV infected cells suggest an interference of TR_a with the assembled components. Several possibilities can be envisaged. 1) A secondary modification of one of the interacting components might occur at a site that becomes accessible only after interaction with the other transcription factors (8 in Fig. 3). 2) The TR_a might recognize only complexes of transcription factors and not its individual components (9 in Fig. 3). 3) New DNA binding sites might become accessible for TR_a binding only after the transcription complex formation [24]. All of these possible interactions could interfere with the functionality of the complex. These involved models have to be taken into consideration to accommodate the present data. The experiments described here bring together the well-defined MMTV LTR HRE sequence and its binding proteins and oncogene interference with inducible enhancer action. This system promises insights into a molecular understanding of some aspects of oncogene regulation of cellular gene expression. This regulatory potential of oncogenes might in turn be the basis for the generation of the complex transformed phenotype.

REFERENCES

1. Bishop JM: Science 235:305–311, 1987.
2. Varmus HE: Ann Rev Genet 18:553–612, 1984.
3. Bishop JM: Cell 42:23–38, 1985.
4. Kingston RE, Baldwin AS, Sharp PA: Cell 41:3–5, 1985.
5. Jaggi R, Salmons B, Müllener D, Groner B: The EMBO J.5:2609–2616, 1986.
6. Weber M.J., Friis RR: Cell 16:25–32, 1979.
7. Hynes NE, van Ooyen A, Kennedy N, Herrlich P, Ponta H, Groner B: Proc Natl Acad Sci USA 80:3632–3641, 1983.
8. Van Beveren C, van Straten F, Galleshaw JA, Verma IM: Cell 27:97–108, 1981.
9. Ponta H, Kennedy N, Skroch P, Hynes NE, Groner B: Proc Natl Acad Sci USA 82:1020–1024, 1985.
10. Scheidereit C, Geisse S, Westphal HM, Beato M: Nature 304:749–752, 1983.
11. Groner B, Hynes NE, Rahmsdorf K, Ponta H: Nucleic Acids Res 11:4713–4725, 1983.
12. Ringold GM: Annu Rev Pharmacol Toxicol 25:529–566, 1985.
13. Yamamoto KR: Ann Rev Genet 19:209–252, 1985.
14. Jones KA, Kadonaga JT: Cell 48:79–89, 1987.
15. Cordingley MG, Tate Riegel A, Hager GL: Cell 48:261–270, 1987.
16. Joab I, Radanyi C, Renoir M, Buchon T, Catelli MG, Binart N, Mester J, Bauleiu EE: Nature 308:850–853, 1984.

17. Willmann T, Beato M: Nature 324:688–690, 1986.
18. Becker PB, Gloss B, Schmid W, Strähle K, Schütz G: Nature 324:686–688, 1986.
19. Nowock J, Borgmeyer K, Püschel AW, Rupp RAW, Sippel AE: Nucleic Acids Res 13:2045–2061, 1985.
20. Sen R, Baltimore D: Cell 47:921–928, 1986.
21. Lee W, Haslinger A, Karin M, Tjian R: Nature 325:368–372, 1987.
22. Papkoff J, Nigg EA, Hunter T: Cell 33:161–172, 1983.
23. Maxwell SA, Arlinghaus RB (1985) Virology 143:321–333.
24. Ptashne M: Nature 322:697–701, 1986.
25. Ponta H, Ball R, Steinmetz M, Groner B: EMBO J 4:3447–3453, 1985.

Growth Regulation of Cancer
221–237 (1988)

Molecular Genetic Analysis of Glucocorticoid Actions in Human Leukemic Cells

E.B. Thompson, Y.-S. Yuh, J. Ashraf, B. Gametchu, M. Linder, and J.M. Harmon

Department of Human Biological Chemistry and Genetics, The University of Texas Medical Branch, Galveston, Texas 77550 (E.B.T., Y.-S. Y., J.A., B.G., M.L.), and Department of Pharmacology, Uniformed Services University of the Health Sciences, Bethesda, Maryland 20814 (J.M.H.)

One of the most profound effects of glucocorticoids is lymphocytolysis. Thymic involution was observed as one of the striking results of administration of corticosteriods during the early period of their study, and it has remained a focal point of scientific interest. The mechanism by which corticosteroids kill lymphocytes is still not clear. It is known, if course, that the growth of normal lymphoid cells depends on various growth factors; the production of many of these growth factors is itself glucocorticoid sensitive. Thus for example, IL1, IL2, and gamma interferon are down-regulated by glucocorticoids [1–9]. To the extent that a given cell depends on these for its existence, this down-regulation will affect their growth. However, it seems that the down-regulation is not absolute. Basal production of the factors may remain even in the presence of glucocorticoids, and consequently not all cell growth may cease after administration of the hormones. Based on the early observation that there was loss of lymphoid tissue after corticosteroid administration, clinical scientists quickly applied these hormones to the treatment of many leukemias and lymphomas [10,11]. In those cases where it has been found empirically that they were of value, they remain an important part of treatment. Occasionally, leukemic cells may retain partial or even considerable dependence on growth factors for their proliferation. In such cases the above noted down-regulation of growth factor production by glucocorticoids undoubtedly plays a role in the effects of glucocorticoids in their behavior.

Received April 6, 1987.

For the most part, however, it seems that leukemic cells have lost dependence on exogenous growth factors—at least the well-known ones—and the effects of glucocorticoids seem to be direct on the leukemic cell. It still remains to be seen whether these effects are due to the switching off of some as yet undetected autonomous growth factor(s) or to the induction of a lethal substance. In any case it does seem that the glucocorticoid receptor plays a central role in mediating the effects of the hormones on the sensitive cells.

Lymphoid cells were used in some of the earliest demonstrations of glucocorticoid receptors [12], and receptors from this class of cells have been studied extensively in several species. In acutely dispersed rat thymocytes, corticosteroids have been shown to fill binding sites that fit the classic criteria defining glucocorticoid receptors: they are found in the cytosol in dilute extracts of the cells, they appear as one class by binding kinetics, and their occupancy correlates with the lethal effects of the steroids on the cells, as well as other biochemical effects [9]. These lethal effects have been studied extensively and numerous mechanisms for explaining the cell killing have been advanced, although none of them as yet have been generally accepted [reviewed in 13]. A more recent theory suggests that the effect of the steroid is to increase the activity of an endonuclease for DNA and that this leads somehow to cell killing [14,15]. This is an intriguing lead; however, the definitive proof that it is the critical step in the cell killing provoked by steroids remains to be seen.

To take advantage of the power of cell genetics, a number of groups have employed cultured cell lines to study the steps involved in glucocorticoid-provoked lymphocytolysis. Genetic methods were first applied to rodent systems and extensive studies have been carried out in both mouse and rat cell lines. A number of mutant phenotypes, as well as variant cells not clearly defined as mutants, have been identified that show resistance to steroids. Some of these are resistant due to lesions in the receptor, whereas others appear to have extrareceptor forms of resistance. The varieties and types of these have been reviewed recently [16,17] and therefore are not discussed here except in contrast to our studies on cultured human leukemic cells.

A MODEL FOR HUMAN LYMPHOID LEUKEMIA CELL RESPONSE TO GLUCOCORTICOIDS

In order to study a human leukemic cell for its sensitivity and acquisition of resistance to glucocorticoids, and thus to provide a model for direct application to at least one sort of human leukemia, we chose to develop the CEM line as a paradigm. CEM cells were cultured originally from the peripheral blood of a female child with acute lymphoblastic leukemia [18]. From this cell line, once we had determined that it was fundamentally glucocorticoid sensitive, we derived a number of subclones. These are described in Figure 1, which shows a "family tree" of several important types of glucocorticoid sensitive and resistant clones.

From the original uncloned CEM cells, a number of clones were obtained without steroid in the medium. Most of these were steroid sensitive, and clone C7 arbitrarily was chosen as the archetypical sensitive, wild type. One clone we found among the original unselected set displayed glucocorticoid resistance from the start. This clone, CEM C1, has been studied at the level of membrane resistance, steroid metabolism, glucocorticoid receptors, and enzyme induction. In all these properties the CEM C1 cells appear to be no different from the sensitive clone C7. Thus C1

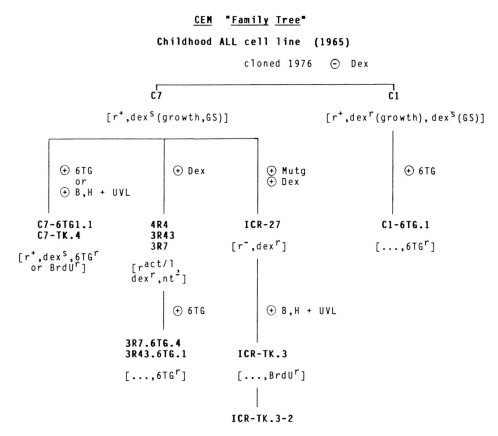

Fig. 1. A "family tree" of the CEM cell clones discussed in this paper. The original uncloned line was obtained and cloned in 1976, resulting in the glucocorticoid-sensitive clone C7 and the insensitive clone C1. Subclones from each were subsequently obtained by selection in the agents indicated to the right of the vertical lines. The phenotypes of the various clones are shown in brackets. Abbreviations used for the treatments: Dex, dexamethasone; B or BrdU, 5-bromo-2'-deoxyuridine; 6TG, 6-thioguanine; Mutg, mutagens 1CR-191 or N-methyl-N'-nitro-N-nitrosoguanidine; H, Hoechst dye 33258; UVL, ultraviolet light. Abbreviations for phenotypes: r^+, glucocorticoid receptor wild type; dex^s, sensitive to the effects of dexamethasone on (growth) or (GS, glutamine synthetase induction); dex^r, resistant to the same; $r^{act/l}$, glucocorticoid receptor mutant of the activation labile type; r^-, glucocorticoid receptor mutant of the low binding site type; nt^-, nuclear translocation defective; $6TG^r$, resistant to 6TG; $BrdU^r$, resistant to BrdU. Details of the origin, derivation, and properties of the various clones can be found in prior publications [19,21,22,53,54].

shows normal induction of the marker enzyme glutamine synthetase and normal physical properties for the glucocorticoid receptor, but does not lyse in the presence of high concentrations of glucocorticoids [19]. It has therefore been designated r^+ GS^+ but ly^- for lysis defective, following the nomenclature suggested by Bourgeois for mouse cells of a similar phenotype. The prototype sensitive clone C7 contains receptors equivalent in amount and in properties to those of C1. C7 shows induction of glutamine synthetase and also shows cessation of growth and cell lysis in the presence of concentrations of glucocorticoid that occupy receptors. Therefore the phenotype of the C7 clone is r^+ ly^+ GS^+. Some properties of C7 are listed in Table I. These cells grow with a doubling time of approximately 24 hr when in log phase, and virtually all the cells in culture are viable and cycling. Flow microfluorimetry

TABLE I. Glucocorticoid-Sensitive Human All Cells:
Proposed Genotype: r^+, ly^+, GS^+

1. Clonal, 47 chromosomes
2. Glucocorticoid responses
   a. early (6–24 hr)
      (1) decreased cell volume
      (2) glutamine synthetase induced

   b. late (24+ hr)
      (1) growth inhibited
      (2) lysed
      (3) endoDNAase ↑

3. Glucocorticoid receptors
   a. cytoplasmic in absence of steroid
   b. $M_r \sim 95,000$
   c. K_d for dexamethasone $1.9 \pm 0.2 \times 10^{-8} M$
   d. $14,000 \pm 6,000$ sites per cell

4. Do not make IL2, protective factors

studies have shown that the addition of glucocorticoids causes the cells to arrest in the G1 phase of the cell cycle where they die [20]. The glutamine synthetase induction, which occurs proportionately with receptor occupancy, precedes the cell killing by many hours [21]. Steroid must be present constantly for cell death to occur, and if the cells are washed free of steroid after as long as 24 hr, they will resume growth. After that interval in steroid, however, a growing proportion of the cells can no longer survive and will neither grow in mass culture nor form colonies. Microscopic examination then shows that they are indeed becoming pyknotic and lysing.

The effects of steroids on sensitive cells such as C7 can also be followed simply by counting cells. If one uses a device such as a Coulter counter to do so, however, the technicalities of machine "window" settings present difficulties in distinguishing all pyknotic dead cells from small live ones. Consequently, therefore, cloning is a more sensitive way of demonstrating viability of the cells. When several concentrations of dexamethasone were compared for their effect on cell growth as quantified by counting on a Coulter cell counter or by the ability of the cells to form colonies in soft agar, increasing concentrations of hormone had increasing effects on cell growth and cell kill. However, it was seen that at some times and some hormone concentrations the growth curves looked merely flat, although the "cells" being counted were not viable by the clonogenic assay [20].

Two major classes of glucocorticoid resistant cells have been isolated from C7. The first was obtained by simply growing out clonal survivors from C7 cells placed in $10^{-6} M$ dexamethasone (Fig. 1). The experiments were carried out by the method of Luria and Delbruck, so that a classic determination of the mechanism by which resistance occurred could be made. The results indicated that resistance occurred by spontaneous, independent, stable events, i.e., presumed mutations. These occurred at the rate of approximately 10^{-5} per cell per generation [22], consistent with a typical haploid rate in the human. It is not obvious why glucocorticoid resistance should occur at such a rate. Possibilities include: a large number of loci being hit, any of whose function is required for hormone sensitivity; dominant mutations at one of a pair of diploid alleles; a genetic "hot spot" with high probability of mutation; and functional or true haploidy at some critical site. CEM cells are nearly diploid, containing 47 chromosomes with one extra small chromosome and one abnormal chromosome 9. The abnormal 9 shows a pericentric inversion of the centromere plus partial loss from the q-arm [23]. These physical alterations do not define a haploid site for the glucocorticoid receptor, the gene for which has been mapped to chromosome 5 in the human [24,25]. Studies of the glucocorticoid receptor in the 50-odd independent clones of spontaneously resistant cells obtained through these experiments have shown that a persistant phenotype is seen. The cells contain measurable receptor sites, although in somewhat reduced amount compared to wild type, but these receptors do not associate with the nuclear fraction in broken cell extracts as do wild type receptors. Thus superficially the phenotype appears analagous to that described in mouse lymphoid cells as nt⁻ (nuclear translocation defective). More careful examination of the receptors shows them to be unique, clearly different from those described in the mouse system, in that they are capable of binding the glucocorticoid properly in the cold but lose the steroid when warmed to 20°. In the case of normal receptors, this will "activate" the receptor to a DNA binding form without loss of ligand. In other ways (size, affinity for steroids, inherent heat lability, etc.), the mutants seem to be quite similar to wild-type receptors. We have labeled this new class of glucocorticoid receptors, thus far seen only in the human cell system, as $r^{act/l}$, for activation labile [26,27]. The same mutant phenotype has been found in all three arbitrarily chosen clones from the 50 or so obtained; therefore it seems likely that it is the predominant mutation in these human cells. Properties of the activation labile class of mutants are shown in Table II. We describe their phenotype as $r^{act/l}$, GS⁻ ly⁻. Note that this is a phenotypic not a genotypic description; since the cells do not lyse in the presence of steroid, their phenotype is ly⁻. They may be capable of displaying the lysis function if they are supplied with normal receptors (see below). As yet no reports of steroid resistance in leukemic patients have been published on the basis of an activation labile receptor; however, a recent report from a Japanese group [28] has described a patient with primary glucocorticoid resistance and abnormal receptors whose properties, insofar as they have been examined, resemble those in our mutant clones of leukemic cells.

The other major class of resistant cells obtained from subclones of C7, was derived by treating the cells with chemical mutagens before selecting by growth in dexamethasone (Fig. 1). Again, a number of mutants were obtained and examined for their receptor properties. Nearly all of these mutants showed a severe lack of glucocorticoid binding sites, with only about 10% of the wild-type number of sites remaining [22]. They are therefore phenotypically receptor deficient, or r⁻, and of

TABLE II. Activation Labile Mutants of CEM C7 Cells: Proposed Genotype: $r^{act/I}$, ly⁺, GS⁺

1. Occur spontaneously
2. Rate ~ 10^{-5} per cell per generation
3. Receptors:
      high affinity
      binding sites ~50% r⁺
      nuclear transfer −
      "activation labile"
4. GS not induced

course, uninducible for glutamine synthetase and lysis deficient, or GS⁻ ly⁻. As the family tree in Figure 1 indicates, examples of all of these various clones of cells have been "marked" by a second selection, i.e., they have been selected either in 6-thioguanine or by a combination of bromodeoxyuridine followed by treatment with the intercalating dye Hoechst 33258 and then exposure to UV light. The former selects for mutants that are 6-thioguanine resistant and deficient in the enzyme hypoxanthine-guanine phosphoribosyl transferase. The second selection gives rise to mutants that lack thymidine kinase. These selective markers were placed in the cells to allow somatic cell hybridization studies to be carried out, as described below.

THE HUMAN GLUCOCORTICOID RECEPTOR AND ITS GENE

The human glucocorticoid receptor is a monomeric protein that migrates during electrophoresis on polyacrylamide gels under denaturing conditions with an M_r of approximately 95,000. It is phosphorylated at several sites, and in order to bind steroid must have a protector of thiol groups such as dithiothreitol present. The receptor specifically binds glucocorticoids (as opposed to other steriods) with high affinity. In the CEM cells this binding can be quantified by simple whole cell binding assays to give an apparent equilibrium dissociation constant of approximately 2×10^{-8} M. The receptor can be found in several states. If cells that previously have been free of glucocorticoids are exposed to hormone in the cold, the receptor-steroid complex can be shown in extracts to occur in a form much larger than that of the monomer. These oligomeric forms, which migrate on velocity sucrose gradients from 8–10 S, contain one or more receptors plus (quite probably) other proteins, such as the heat shock protein 90 which has been described in other glucocorticoid systems [29–31]. RNA may also be present in the complexes [32].

By treating in a number of different ways, the steroid receptor complex undergoes "activation" or "transformation," the result of which is to convert it to the monomeric holoreceptor-ligand form, which migrates at ~4 S on sucrose gradients. At the same time it becomes a protein with high affinity for DNA. This physical change can also be demonstrated by several types of ionic exchange columns. For example, during elution from DEAE cellulose by a salt gradient, the unactivated form elutes at approximately 0.22 M salt, whereas the activated form elutes at approximately 0.05 M [33,34]. This distinction has proved useful in studying both normal and mutant receptors. Limited proteolysis of the rat glucocorticoid receptor showed that it can be divided into steroid binding, DNA binding, and antigenic domains [35]. After trypsin digestion, the steroid binding domain comprised about one-third of the molecule. After chymotrypsin, the steroid binding region was found associated with a DNA binding domain in a peptide fragment of about 45,000, or roughly half the total size of the intact molecule. Eisen and coworkers [36] showed that the DNA binding domain could be obtained separately from the steroid binding domain, using a combination of immunologic and chromatographic techniques. Antibodies to the rat receptor indicated that the major antigenic sites of the molecule were located away from the steriod binding and DNA binding domains, although one particularly useful monoclonal antibody to the rat receptor remained close to the DNA binding region, allowing the study noted above to be done. It has been shown that the human glucocorticoid receptor has similar subregions, defined by limited proteolysis and antibody reactions [37,38].

Recently the rat, human, and mouse glucocorticoid receptors have been cloned [39,41]. The human receptor gene was found by selecting clones from an expression library, using polyclonal antiserum prepared against human leukemic cell receptor [42]. The sequencing of the complete cDNA for the human receptor gene has allowed its primary structure to be deduced, and this work shows it to be a peptide of 777 amino acids [43]. The molecular weight predicted by this sequence is below that which the protein demonstrates on gel electrophoresis; thus it appears to be one of those proteins that migrate anomalously. We find that slight variations in conditions can, without causing proteolysis, produce differences in migration corresponding to differences in apparent M_r of as much as $\pm$ 5,000 (E.B.T. et al., unpublished results). Analysis of the receptor gene and in vitro mutagenesis of it have confirmed and extended the above mentioned structural studies done at the protein level. Thus it has been shown that the steroid binding region is indeed subsumed by approximately one-third of the molecule at the carboxy terminal. The DNA binding region can be shown, as predicted by the proteolysis studies, to be in the center of the molecule, in a cysteine-rich area [44]. It is the amino terminal end of the molecule that is the strongest antigenic region. Figure 2 shows a simple diagram of these features.

We have carried out a computerized, theoretical analysis predicting the alpha helical and beta pleated sheet content of the receptor molecule. This analysis predicts that the cysteine-rich DNA binding region is likely to contain a helical structure between the several pairs of cysteines beginning at position 421 and ending at 481. The cysteines in the pairs are themselves separated by two or three amino acids, and are predicted to be in or near turns of the peptide chain. The DNA binding region of the glucocorticoid receptor, therefore, may fit the class of DNA binding proteins described in many procaryotes, in which a helix-turn-helix arrangement is essential to the DNA binding [45]. As pointed out by many others, the arrangement of cysteines and other amino acids in the DNA binding segment also resembles that found in the TFIII A peptide of *Xenopus* and in the *Krüppel* gene product of *Drosophila*, where "fingers" of amino acids are produced due to a complex between a pair of cysteines, a zinc molecule, and a pair of histidines, at the base of each finger. The complex holds the base firm, and the finger is formed by the 12 to 14 amino acids lying in the primary sequence between the pair of cysteines and the pair of histidines [46,47]. The spacing of the series of cysteines in the human glucocorticoid receptor DNA binding region suggests that they could serve a similar function. So far the analogy is based only on the visual evidence, but the predicted helical structure in the computer

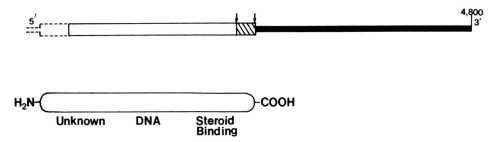

Fig. 2.   Diagram of the complete cDNA clone of the human glucocorticoid receptor (upper part) and of the receptor itself (lower part), with the general location of the steroid binding, DNA binding, and unknown function—but highly antigenic—regions indicated. Details of the topographical features of the cDNA clone can be found in ref. 25.

analysis adds to the idea that short helical fingers of peptide may indeed be the form used to give DNA binding. High helical content is seen in both the amino terminal and carboxy terminal ends of the protein.

The other remarkable structural feature of the receptor molecule has been its high homology with certain other proteins. As several other steroid hormone receptor genes have been cloned in the last two years, comparisons have been made between the structure of their predicted proteins. Regions of high homology exist in these proteins, including all the DNA binding regions and parts of the steroid binding regions. Furthermore, an unexpected homology was found with the *v-erb* A protein, a helper oncogene product [48]. Quite recently this homology was extended with a startling result, when it was found that the *c-erb* A protein, which also contains homologies in these DNA and hormone binding zones, is in fact a high affinity receptor for the thyroid hormone [49,50]. These results, obtained by others, have been presented in detail in the references cited and therefore are not described further here.

STRUCTURAL ANALYSIS OF THE GLUCOCORTICOID RECEPTOR, PROTEIN, AND GENE IN WILD-TYPE AND MUTANT CEM CELLS

Restriction endonuclease analysis of normal human DNA compared with that of CEM cells shows that CEM C7 cells contain no obvious rearrangements of the glucocorticoid receptor gene (M.L., and E.B.T., unpublished results). The receptor gene in CEM C7 cells, therefore, seems a good model to study for the behavior of the gene. Similarly, a limited set of restriction enzyme studies has been carried out comparing selected clones from the various types of resistant cells. None of them shows differences from the C7 wild type. Thus we can rule out the possibility that the receptor defective phenotype of the clone of r $^-$ resistant cell studied is due to a gross deletion or rearrangement of the receptor gene. Similarly, the chosen clones of activation labile mutants possess no great changes in the gene. Examples of these results are shown in Figure 3. Northern blot analysis of the RNA of C7 cells shows that the human receptor mRNA is expressed as a single, mature message of 7 kb. Comparing the quantity and size of message in the mutants with this, we found that the mutants all express message of normal size, although reduced in quantities from that of wild type. An example of the Northern blot showing this data is shown in Figure 4, and quantitative analysis of the data there is given in Table III. When the quantity of message in each cell type clone was normalized to α-tubulin mRNA (which was essentially equal in all lanes), the quantity of message found in the mutants can be seen to be about one-third of that in the wild type in this experiment. This does not fit exactly with the amount of binding sites for glucocorticoids seen in the mutants. As Table III shows, there are fewer binding sites in the r $^-$ mutant than the quantity of message would predict, and that is also true for one of the two activation labile mutants. At least three possibilities could explain such results. There could be a problem with translation of the mRNA, protein could be made with diminished half-life, or receptor of normal half-life but incapable of binding steroid could be produced. In order to explore this further, we took advantage of a new set of immunoreagents described below.

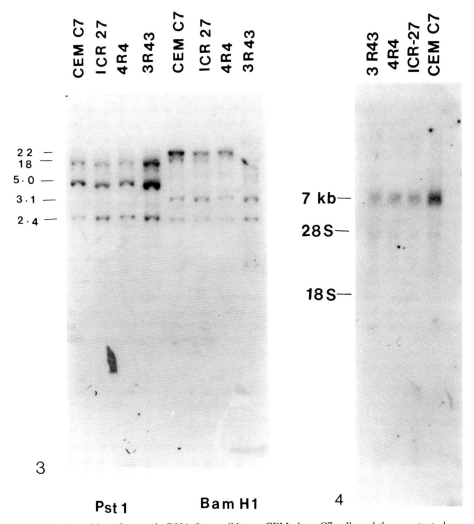

Fig. 3. Southern blot of genomic DNA from wild-type CEM clone C7 cells and three mutant clones, one r⁻ (ICR 27) and two r$^{act/l}$ (4R4 and 3R43) in phenotype. Each lane corrresponds to 10 μg of DNA. The DNA in the four left lanes was digested with Pst1, the four right lanes with Bam H1. The filter was probed with the full-length 4.8 kb cDNA shown in Figure 2, ^{32}P labeled by nick-translation. Numbers at the side refer to sizes of the fragments identified in kilobases.

Fig. 4. Northern blot of total RNA, 20 μg per lane, from the same four clones probed as in Figure 3. Indicated on the left are the size of the 7 kb mRNA identified by the probe and the location of the 28s and 18s rRNA bands seen after ethidium bromide stain of the original gel.

MONOCLONAL ANTIBODIES TO THE GLUCOCORTICOID RECEPTOR

We have recently prepared a set of monoclonal antibodies against human glucocorticoid receptor [51]. These react specifically with the receptor on the basis of shifting the monomeric 4S form of the receptor to a more rapidly sedimenting species on high salt velocity sedimentation sucrose gradients and also by standard immunoblot, in which receptor covalently labeled with treated radiated dexamethasone mesylate was electrophoresed, transferred to nitrocellulose paper, and then reacted with

TABLE III. hGR mRNA in CEM Cells and Mutants

Genotype	Clone	Ligand sites[a]	mRNA[b]
r[+]	C7	20,000/cell	100%
r[−]	ICR-27	1,000	33
r[act/l]	4R4	5,900	35
r[act/l]	3R43	3,500	30

[a]All from refs. 27 and 22.
[b]Normalized to α-Tubulin, and amount in C7 set at 100%; mRNA data from a single experiment.

antibody. The position of the radiolabeled receptor and that of the immunoreactive band exactly coincided. Examples of these results are shown in Figure 5. Using these monoclonals, we have examined cytoplasm from the mutants for the presence of immunoreactive receptor forms. The results show that both the activation labile and r[−] clones studied contained full-size immunoreactive receptor. In the r[−] clone particularly, the quantity of immunoreactive receptor exceeds that expected from the number of specific glucocorticoid binding sites measured in the cells (Fig. 6). Thus it seems that the mRNA that is present in these cells is being translated into receptor protein, which is in excess of what can bind steroid. This "silent receptor" phenomenon is similar to that described in rodent systems of cultured cells [44]. It is important to note that the residual 10% or so of glucocorticoid sites in the r[−] cells has an affinity for dexamethasone essentially unchanged from the wild type. Thus it does not appear that the mutant is producing a large quantity of receptor with poor binding properties, but rather two types of molecules, one that is immunoreactive but binds steroid not at all, and another that is both immunoreactive and a functional steroid binding molecule. It is interesting to note that although these cells are quite resistant to high concentrations of dexamethasone, they can be killed by an extremely potent, synthetic phenylpyrazolo glucocorticoid [52]. In binding studies, this molecule demonstrates a class of high affinity binding sites in the r[−] cells [53]. Thus the abnormal receptor in these cells may in fact be a truly functional glucocorticoid receptor but may exist in an amount too low to mediate cell killing when the cells are exposed to the usual glucocorticoids. When a higher affinity steroid is given them, it may be able to keep enough of the molecules saturated with steroid so that they can undergo the shift to their DNA binding form and carry out the lytic function.

SOMATIC CELL HYBRIDIZATION STUDIES

Somatic cell genetic analysis of the various classes of mutant cells has allowed further definitions of the lesions that they contain. Thus the "marked" subclones of the wild-type and mutant cells containing selective markers have all been hybridized with one another [54,55] in order to find answers to the following questions: Was any class of dexamethasone-resistant cells transdominant? Did mutant receptors show positive or negative complementation with one another? What was the ly[−] genotype in the r[−] and in the r[act/l] cells? In the CEM C1 clone (r[+] ly[−]), were the receptors present competent to mediate cell lysis when introduced into a potentially sensitive host?

The dominant/recessive test carried out between either the r[act/l] class or the r[−] class of mutant and the wild-type parent shows that in neither case does the mutant contain a dominant ly[−] function [54]. This result is consistent with the interpretation

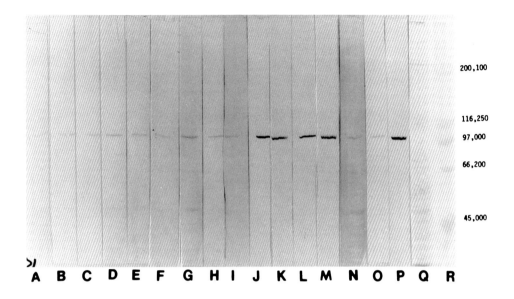

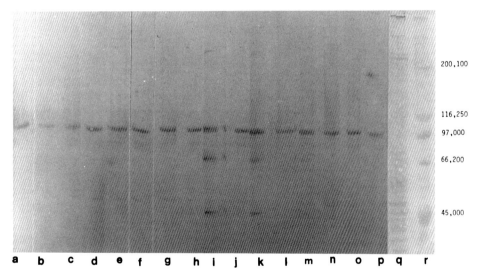

Fig. 5. Monoclonal antibodies to human glucocorticoid receptor. Crude cell cytosol was labeled with the covalent glucocorticoid ligand ^{3}H dexamethasone mesylate under conditions such that the majority of label attached to the glucocorticoid receptor. Aliquots of cytosol were then electrophoresed in a series of adjoining lanes in a slab gel under denaturing conditions. The proteins were transferred to a nitrocellulose filter that was immunoblotted with a set of independent monoclonal antibodies [50]. Antibody-receptor interactions were detected by a peroxidase reaction (upper panel, upper case letters). The filters were then exposed to X-ray film and a radioautograph allowed to develop (lower panel, lower case letters). Lanes A–P were blotted with one antibody each from 16 different clones. Lane Q, antibody-free medium. Lane R, protein size standards. Note that the dominant, radioligand labeled, holoreceptor bands in the lower panel exactly correspond to the immunoreactions in the upper panel.

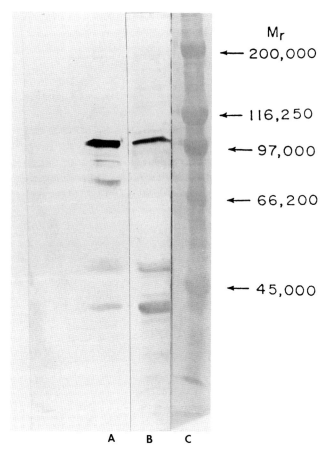

Fig. 6. Immunoidentification of receptor in CEM C7 (r$^+$) and ICR 27 (r$^-$) cell extracts. Receptor was prepared, electrophoresed, and immunoblotted from both cell types, using a pool of three monoclonal antibodies. Reactions were identified by the peroxidase technique. Lane A, 500 μg of total protein from CEM C7 (r$^+$) cells. Lane B, 500 μg total protein from 1CR 27 (r$^-$) cells. Lane C, protein standards.

that the mutants are affected only in the receptor molecule. A more complicated interpretation is that they are pleitropic, with mutant receptor and also some abnormal *cis* active element that prevents their lysis. We favor the simpler interpretation. Similarly, when the clone of the r$^+$ ly$^-$ resistant class was hybridized with the wild-type parent, no *trans*dominance of the ly$^-$ function was seen; therefore clone CEM C1 (r$^+$ ly$^-$) is not lysed by steroids due to some *cis* active property rather than a *trans*dominant antilysis function [55]. Hybrids between the r$^-$ and r$^{act/l}$ class of cells did not produce functional lysis; therefore these mutant clones do not give cross complementation. It has been suggested that glucocorticoid receptors act in dimers or oligomers at their specific DNA binding sites to enhance transcription. Since there was no dominance of either class of receptor mutant when crossed with the wild-type parent, if there is interaction of receptors at the genome to cause lysis or glutamine synthetase induction, these mutant receptors do not involve themselves in that inter-action. This seems unlikely, and therefore these results fit the view that the receptor-DNA interaction is a monomeric one. In terms of receptor binding sites, all the hybrids show quantities of sites representing close to the sum of the amounts contributed by each parent. Both glutamine synthetase induction and lysis are present in the hybrids between the sensitive and resistant clones.

Hybridizations between the r^+ ly^- clone C1 and a clone of r^- cells phenotypically ly^- allow one to test for the genotype of the r^- clone and the functionality of the receptor in C1 cells. Since the C1 ly^- phenotype is not *trans*dominant, one can by this hybrid see whether the genotype of the r^- clone is ly^+ or ly^-. The results of exposing such a hybrid to hormone are shown in Figure 7, and they clearly show that the hybrid is glucocorticoid sensitive. We can draw two important conclusions from this. First, the ly^- property of the C1 parent is not due to some subtle lesion in the receptor or a deficiency of a subclass of receptor that is specifically responsible for the lysis function, since this receptor can mediate lysis in the hybrid. Second, the genotype of the r^- clone can be defined as ly^+ since the cells lyse when supplied with appropriate receptor. The somatic hybrids also allow one to say that the genes supplied are in their correct location in the genome and in the correct proportion to the normal constituent complement of total DNA, as compared with transfection studies involving cloned segments of DNA in which it is difficult to control exactly the gene dosage and location.

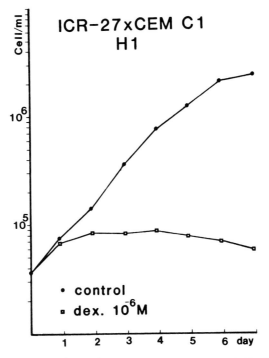

Fig. 7. Complementation of r^- ly^+ and r^+ ly^- cells in a somatic cell hybrid. C1-6TG.1 cells (r^+ ly^-) and ICR-TK.3-2 cells (r^- ly^+) were hybridized by facilitating cell fusion with polyethylene glycol and then selecting hybrids in medium containing hypoxanthine, aminopterin, and thymidine. The near tetraploidy of the hybrid clone shown was confirmed by flow cytometry. The hybrid clone was then tested for growth inhibition in 10^{-6} M dexamethasone, to which both parents were resistant. The hybrid (and all hybrids tested, as well as the uncloned mass cultures of hybrids) is clearly sensitive. Details can be found in ref. 54.

In sum, several conclusions may be drawn from the somatic cell hybridization studies. Dexamethasone resistance in the CEM clones examined, whether in receptor mutants or the ly$^-$ variant, is *not* dominant. The r$^-$ and r$^{act/l}$ mutations do not complement each other and are not dominant in a cross with r$^+$. When the r$^-$ clone tested was provided receptor, it showed its genotype to be ly$^+$. The r$^+$ ly$^-$ receptor can mediate cell lysis.

ORIGIN OF GLUCOCORTICOID-RESISTANT MUTANTS IN CEM CELLS: HYPOTHESIS

What is the basis for the observed genetics and biochemistry of the mutants we have thus far obtained from CEM cells? Key points to be explained are a spontaneous haploid rate of mutation leading to the r$^{act/l}$ state; and in the r$^-$ mutant, the discrepancy between the quantity of binding sites and the much larger amount of full-size immunologically reactive receptor. We propose that the CEM C7 sensitive clone is in fact haploid for the receptor gene. Thus the spontaneous mutation rate to resistance is entirely appropriate for a single gene. Such a condition was predicted, purely on the basis of genetic and biochemical evidence, for the mouse lymphoma line S49 [56]. Recent results from direct cloning and sequencing of the mRNAs from S49 cells have borne out the prediction [41]. We cannot explain the reason for the frequency of the r$^{act/l}$ phenotype, except to note that in vitro mutations of the hGR gene over a large portion of the molecule have affected steroid binding [44]. Thus r$^{act/l}$ may be the result of frequent mutations at a "hot spot" or of scattered mutations all resulting in a similar phenotype.

The r$^-$ clone studied could be the result of either of two alternatives. The first possibility is that the original haploid state consists of one normal allele and one mutant, down-regulated allele, making only about 10% of normal receptor amounts. Mutagenesis could have led to the normal gene producing a receptor quite incapable of binding steroid, with the residual expression seen coming from the original, mutated allele. The alternative model is that the original haploid state consisted of a silent mutant allele and a normal allele. Mutations causing enhancement of a cryptic splice site, as is seen in several β-globin gene mutations resulting in Thalassemia [57–59], could then explain the phenotype found. We are presently cloning and sequencing the mRNAs of these mutants to distinguish between these possibilities.

SUMMARY

The human glucocorticoid receptor is encoded in a sequence of nucleotides giving rise to a protein of 777 amino acids. Recent results from these clones and in vitro mutational analysis of them has allowed confirmation and extension of previous work defining the steroid binding, DNA binding, and antigenic regions of the protein. The DNA binding area of the molecule is striking in having a high content of cysteines that have an arrangement similar to that of the "zinc fingers" region of another DNA binding protein. Theoretical analysis of the helical content of the human glucocorticoid receptor by computer predicts that there is little helical structure in the DNA binding region but high helical content in both the amino terminus and carboxy terminus of the molecule.

The CEM cell line of human leukemic cells has been useful in studying the function of the receptor and its role in lysis of lymphoid cells by glucocorticoids. Lysis of wild-type cells requires constant occupancy of receptors by glucocorticoid in quantity sufficient to saturate them. Lysis is concomitant with capture of the cells in the G1 phase of the cell cycle, and it requires 24 hr or more to occur. These cells contain an inducible enzyme, glutamine synthetase, which is induced well before cell killing begins and which has been used as a marker for receptor function. Analysis of the genome by restriction endonucleases and Southern blots shows that CEM C7 wild-type cells contain the same arrangement of the gene as do normal human cells, and all the mutants fit this same pattern. Resistant variants and mutants have been cloned from the wild type, and these fall into three classes: a clone of pre-existing variant cells resistant to steroid, which show the phenotype r^+ ly^- (receptor normal but lysis defective), has been identified; and two classes of resistant clones selected from the wild-type parent by cloning in dexamethasone also have been defined. One is phenotypically nuclear translocation defective (nt^-), and biochemically it contains full-size receptors that bind steroid but cannot retain it when activated, i.e., are activation labile ($r^{act/l}$). The other class of mutant clones was found after mutagenesis and shows a paucity of receptor sites (r^-). The mRNA from these three classes shows that they all contain full-length 7 kb message, but the r^- and $r^{act/l}$ mutants contain less message than does the wild type. Immunological analysis has been possible by obtaining monoclonal antibodies to the human receptor. Immunoblots of mutant cytosols using these antibodies show that the $r^{act/l}$ and r^- clones examined contain full-size immunoreactive receptor, often in excess over that predicted from the number of binding sites in the cells.

Somatic cell hybridization analysis of the mutant clones shows that in no case is the resistant phenotype dominant over the sensitive. The $r^{act/l}$ and r^- mutants do not complement each other; however, the r^+ ly^- mutant variant complements the r^- mutant. Thus one can conclude that the mutant that is r^- is genetically ly^+.

ACKNOWLEDGMENTS

Supported in part by grant 1-RO1-CA41407 from the National Cancer Institute, National Institutes of Health, Bethesda, MD 20205. J.A. is a Fellow of Leukemia Society of America.

REFERENCES

1. Gillis S, Crabtree GR, Smith KA: J Immunol 123:1624, 1979.
2. Larsson E-L: J Immunol 124:2828, 1980.
3. Arya SK, Wong-Staal F, Gallo RC: J Immunol 133:273, 1984.
4. Adolf GR, Swetly P: Nature 282:736, 1979.
5. Zor U, Ben-Sori R, Maoz I, Wallach D, Gurari-Rotman D: J Gen Virol 63:359, 1982.
6. Adolf GR, Swetly P: J Interferon Res 2:261, 1982.
7. Kasahara T, Hooks JJ, Dougherty SF, Oppenheim JJ: J Immunol 130:1784, 1983.
8. Palacios R, Sugarawa I: Scand J Immunol 15:25, 1982.
9. Munck A, Guyre PM, Holbrook NJ: Endo Reviews 5:25–44, 1984.
10. Wolff J, Brubaker C, Murphy M, Pierce M, Severo N: J Pediatr 70:626, 1967.
11. Pearson O, Eliel L: JAMA 144:1349, 1950.
12. Munck A, Wira C: In Raspe G (ed): "Advances in the Biosciences 7." Pergamon Press, New York: 1971, pp 301–330.

13. Schmidt TJ, Thompson EB: In Sharma RK, Criss WE (ed): "Endocrine Control in Neoplasia." Raven Press, New York: 1978, pp 263–290.

14. Compton MM, Cidiowski JA: J Cell Biochem 11A:115, 1987.

15. Bourgeois S, Crepin M, Dean DC: J Cell Biochem 11A:100, 1987.

16. Pfahl M, Kelleher RJ, Bourgeois S: Mol Cell Endocrinol 10:193–207, 1978.

17. Gehring U: Mol Cell Endocrinol 48:89–96, 1986.

18. Foley G, Lazarus H, Farber S, Geren Uzman B, Boone B, McCarthy R: Cancer 18:522–529, 1965.

19. Zawydiwski R, Harmon JM, Thompson EB: Cancer Res 43:3865–3873, 1983.

20. Harmon JM, Norman MR, Fowlkes BJ, Thompson EB: J Cellular Physiology 98:267–278, 1979.

21. Harmon JM, Thompson EB: J Cell Physiology 110:155–160, 1982.

22. Harmon JM, Thompson EB: Mol Cell Biol 1:512–521, 1981.

23. Moore DE, Weise K, Zawydiwski R, Thompson EB: Cancer Genetics and Cytogenetics 14:89–94, 1985.

24. Gehring U, Segnitz B, Foellmer B, Francke U: Proc Natl Acad Sci USA 82:3751–3755, 1985.

25. Hollenberg SM, Weinberger C, Ong ES, Cerelli G, Oro A, Lebo R, Thompson EB, Rosenfeld MG, Evans RM: Nature 318:635–641, 1985.

26. Schmidt TJ, Harmon JM, Thompson EB: Nature 286:507–510, 1980.

27. Harmon JM, Schmidt TJ, Thompson EB: J Steroid Biochem 21:227–236, 1984.

28. Nawata H, Sekiya K, Higuchi K, Kato K-I, Ibayashi H: J Clin Endocrinol Metab (in press).

29. Housley PR, Sanchez ER, Westphal HM, Beato M, Pratt WB: J Biol Chem 260:13810–13817, 1985.

30. Sanchez ER, Toft DO, Schlesinger MJ, Pratt WB: J Biol Chem 260:12398–12401, 1985.

31. Mendel DB, Bodwell JE, Gametchu B, Harrison RW, Munck A: J Biol Chem 261:3758–3763, 1986.

32. Webb ML, Litwack G: In Litwack G (ed): "Biochemical Actions of Hormones," XIII. Academic Press, New York: 1986, pp 379–402.

33. Sakaue Y, Thompson EB: Biochem Biophys Res Commun 77:533–541, 1977.

34. Thompson EB, Sakaue Y, Harmon JM: In Sakamoto Y, Ishohashi J (ed): "Glucocorticoid Hormone: Mechanisms of Action." Verlag, Tokyo/Berlin:1986, pp 119–135.

35. Carlstedt-Duke J. Okret S, Wrange O, Gustafsson J-Å: Proc Natl Acad Sci USA 79:4260–4269, 1982.

36. Eisen LP, Reichman ME, Thompson EB, Gametchu B, Harrison RW, Eisen HJ: J Biol Chem 260:11805–11810, 1985.

37. Thompson EB, Zawydiwski R, Brower ST, Eisen HJ, Simons SS, Schmidt TJ, Schlechte JA, Moore DE, Norman MR, Harmon JM: In Eriksson H, Gustafsson J-Å (ed): "Steroid Hormones Receptors: Structure and Function." Elsevier, Amsterdam: 1983, pp 171–194.

38. Smith AC, Harmon JM: Biochem 26:646–652, 1987.

39. Miesfeld R, Okret S, Wikström A-C, Wrange O, Gustafsson J-Å, Yamamoto KR: Nature 312:779–781, 1984.

40. Weinberger C, Hollenberg SM, Ong ES, Harmon JM, Brower ST, Cidlowski J, Thompson EB, Rosenfeld MG, Evans RM: Science 228:740–742, 1985.

41. Danielsen M, Northrop JP, Ringold GM: EMBO J 5:2513–2522, 1986.

42. Harmon JM, Eisen HJ, Brower ST, Simons SS, Langley CL, Thompson EB: Cancer Res 44:4540–4547, 1984.

43. Hollenberg SM, Weinberger C, Ong ES, Cerelli G, Oro A, Lebo R, Thompson EB, Rosenfeld MG, Evans RM: Nature 318:635–641, 1985.

44. Giguère V, Hollenberg SM, Rosenfeld MG, Evans RM: Cell 46:645–652, 1986.

45. Pabo CO, Sauer RT: Ann Rev Biochem 53:293–321, 1984.

46. Miller J, McLachlan AD, Klug A: EMBO J 4:1609–1614, 1985.

47. Rosenberg UB, Schröder, Preiss A, Lienlin A, Côté S, Riede I, Jäckle H: Nature 319:336–339, 1986.

48. Weinberger C, Hollenberg SM, Rosenfeld MG, Evans RM: Nature 318:670–672, 1985.

49. Weinberger C, Thompson CC, Ong ES, Lebo R, Gruol DJ, Evans RM: Nature 324:641–646, 1986.

50. Sap J, Muñoz A, Damm K, Goldberg Y, Ghysdael J, Leutz A, Beug H, Vennström B: Nature 324:635–640, 1986.

51. Gametchu B, Thompson EB: In Puett D (ed): "Advances in Gene Technology: Molecular Biology of the Endocrine System." Cambridge Press, Cambridge: 1986, pp 282–283.

52. Harmon JM, Schmidt TJ, Thompson EB: Cancer Res 42:2110–2114, 1982.

53. Schlechte JA, Simons SS, Lewis DA, Thompson EB: Endocrinology 117:1355–1362, 1985.
54. Harmon JM, Thompson EB, Baione KA: Cancer Res 45:1587–1593, 1985.
55. Yuh Y-S, Thompson EB: Som Cell Mol Genet 13:33–45, 1987.
56. Bourgeois S, Newby RF, Huet M: Cancer Res 38:4279–4284, 1978.
57. Kazazian HH: Hospital Prac 20:55–69, 1985.
58. Steinberg MH, Adams JG: Am J Pathol 113:396–409, 1983.
59. Orkin SH, Kazazian HH: Ann Rev Genet 13:131–171, 1984.

Index